Dynamics of Oncology Nursing

Pamela K. Burkhalter, M.A., M.N., R.N.

Psychologist and Nurse Consultant
Honolulu, Hawaii

Diana L. Donley, B.S.N., R.N.

Oncology Nurse Consultant
Honolulu, Hawaii

McGRAW-HILL BOOK COMPANY

A Blakiston Publication

New York   St. Louis   San Francisco   Auckland   Bogotá   Düsseldorf
Johannesburg   London   Madrid   Mexico   Montreal   New Delhi
Panama   Paris   São Paulo   Singapore   Sidney   Tokyo   Toronto

No kā māua mau mea ma'i—i ka wā i hala, i keia manawa, a me ka wā mahope.

To our patients—past, present, and future.

Dynamics of Oncology Nursing

Copyright © 1978 by McGraw-Hill, Inc. All rights reserved. Printed in the United States of America. No part of this publication may be reproduced, stored in a retrieval system, or transmitted, in any form or by any means, electronic, mechanical, photocopying, recording, or otherwise, without the prior written permission of the publisher.

1 2 3 4 5 6 7 8 9 0 DODO 7 8 3 2 1 0 9 8 7

This book was set in Times Roman by Creative Book Services, subsidiary of McGregor & Werner, Inc. The editor was Orville W. Haberman, Jr.; the cover was designed by John Hite; the production supervisor was Jeanne Selzam.
R. R. Donnelley & Sons Company was printer and binder.

Library of Congress Cataloging in Publication Data
Main entry under title:

Dynamics of oncology nursing.

    "A Blakiston publication."
    Includes index.
    1. Cancer—Nursing. I. Burkhalter, Pamela K. II. Donley, Diana L. [DNLM: 1. Neoplasms—Nursing. WY156 B959d]
RC266.D96   610.73'6   77-22965
ISBN 0-07-009052-1

Contents

List of Contributors

Doris Y. Ahana, R.N., M.S.
Clinical Specialist in Oncology
St. Francis Hospital
Honolulu, Hawaii

Linda Alexander, Ph.D.
Clinical Associate Professor
  of Medicine
John A. Burns School of Medicine
University of Hawaii
Honolulu, Hawaii

Jeanie Barry, R.N., M.S.
Critical Care Nursing Instructor
Emergency Medical Services
  of Hawaii
Honolulu, Hawaii

LoRaine Carlson, R.N., M.S.N.
Assistant Professor of Nursing
School of Nursing
University of Hawaii
Honolulu, Hawaii

Graceann Ehlke, R.N., M.N.
Instructor of Nursing
School of Nursing
University of Hawaii
Honolulu, Hawaii

Rev. Dr. David Y. Hirano
Nuuanu Congregational Church
Honolulu, Hawaii

Sharon S. Ogi, R.N., M.S.
Former Project Director
Community Oncology Nursing Project
Queen's Medical Center
Honolulu, Hawaii

Patricia K. Sato, R.N.
Head Nurse, Oncology Service
Kuakini Medical Center
Honolulu, Hawaii

Judi K. Shabert, R.D.
Honolulu, Hawaii

Amy K. Takeuchi, R.N., B.S.N.
Oncology Nurse
CARES at Home
St. Francis Hospital
Honolulu, Hawaii

Luana L. Venard, R.N., B.S.N.
Project Director
Comprehensive Cancer Care Project
Queen's Medical Center
Honolulu, Hawaii

Melvin S. Y. Whang
Former Professional Education
  Coordinator
Hawaii Division
American Cancer Society
Honolulu, Hawaii

Preface

Nurses in every area of practice have numerous opportunities to care for people who have or are recovering from cancer—oncology patients. Cancer is one of the most threatening and widespread of the illnesses known to humanity. It strikes people of all ages, often in a seemingly indiscriminate manner. Twenty years ago oncology nursing as a specialty did not exist. Today the oncology nurse is making dramatic and significant contributions to the care, treatment, and recovery of thousands of cancer patients each year.

Because cancer is such a pervasive health problem in our society (being the second leading cause of death in the United States) and because it has a tremendous impact on people's biological, psychological, emotional, and social stability, it becomes imperative that nurses learn not only about the nature of cancer but also about their role in facilitating the patient's treatment and recovery. Thus, the purpose of *Dynamics of Oncology Nursing* is to provide in-depth information on the status of cancer as a major health problem, the treatment methods used to intervene when cancer strikes, and the ever-expanding role of the nurse in the care of oncology patients.

The title of the book, *Dynamics of Oncology Nursing*, clearly represents the underlying philosophy of its contents. Oncology nursing is characterized by change: changes in treatment modalities, changes in knowledge and skill required of nurses caring for the oncology patient, and changes in the nature of nursing interventions applied to this patient population. Even the nursing specialty name has changed from "cancer nursing" to "oncology nursing."

The practice of oncology nurisng, therefore, is not static or inflexible; it is dynamic, ever-changing, and continuously developing. Within this philosophy lies a second basic philosophical belief that emphasizes the hopeful side of oncology nursing. As the oncology patient utilizes various treatment modalities, the nurse must seek to retain a constant focus on the qualitative aspects of the experience. Although a cure for each patient's cancer is not always possible, maintenance of quality of living is not only possible but should represent a major goal of nursing intervention.

The book is divided into five parts. Part One presents extensive background information on the nature of cancer from both the physiological and the sociocultural viewpoint. In Part Two, the role of the nurse is explored in terms of present contexts of practice as well as evolving and extended role development. Significant nursing implications of treatment methods are emphasized throughout and are based on a comprehensive model of assessment. Part Three focuses on supportive aspects of the nurse's role in a variety of settings, hospital and community. Major issues the nurse faces while caring for the oncology patient e.g., counseling and care of the dying person, are emphasized.

In Part Four, unique roles in oncology nursing are considered. Within this context information is presented on the development and establishment of the oncology nursing unit. Educational aspects of oncology nursing are presented in Part Five which includes an emphasis on community and continuing education components of nursing practice.

Ideally this book can be used as a professional reference in the nurse's daily practice. While content clearly focuses on the adult oncology patient, information contained in these chapters in many instances is applicable to the pediatric oncology patient as well.

Contributors to the book are current practitioners in the field of oncology nursing. Each believes that while oncology nursing can be extremely demanding of one's personal resources, at the same time it is perhaps the most beautiful, challenging, and fulfilling area of nursing practice. Nowhere are the skills and abilities of the nurse more tested or needed than with the oncology patient. With this book, it is hoped that the enthusiasm and commitment shared by these nurses will be communicated to each reader.

Pamela K. Burkhalter
Diana L. Donley

Part One

The Nature of Cancer

Chapter 1

From the Inside Looking Out . . . A Personal Experience with Cancer

Grace Ann Ehlke

What is it like to have cancer? Being a nurse, I was familiar with the word "cancer" and had seen patients who had the disease. Seeing cancer patients had left me with very negative feelings about the illness. In fact, I remember thinking that if I was ever diagnosed as having cancer, I would commit suicide. And then it happened.

SEPTEMBER 1966

I was a registered nurse, a graduate of an associate degree nursing program. I was back in school to obtain my baccalaureate degree in nursing. At the time I started back to school, in September of 1966, I was tired of working. I had worked for the better part of two years and felt like I wanted to know more than I did; thus I was in school. I was excited about being in school again, although it was also a very serious time for me.

Because of my prior academic performance, it was mandatory that I maintain a certain grade point average over the first two quarters of my program. Although I performed satisfactorily, the pressure to achieve higher grades began to mount prior to Christmas 1966. I became anxious and a little panicked as I realized that my academic performance *had* to be higher if I was to remain in school.

FEBRUARY 1967

It was a cold, wet, dreary day. The date was Friday, February 3, 1967. It had started out as all Fridays did for me in those days—busy. I had attended classes all morning, and now I was on my way to work. I was driving a bit fast. I was in a hurry. After parking, I rushed to nursing office to pick up my paycheck. As I remember, I needed the money badly—I must have written some checks the night before that needed to be covered by money in the bank.

When I got to nursing office, Pat, the secretary, told me that because I had not gotten my annual chest x-ray I could not be paid. "But Pat, I had a chest x-ray taken in September when I started to school, and I really don't need another as this is only February." Pat said, "You are right; however, I still cannot give you the check until I have a carbon copy of that September x-ray report. Since all of the employee reports are kept in emergency room, just run down and get the copy and bring it back to me."

Time was ticking away. I had to be at work in 10 minutes, but I still had time. I had to get that x-ray report because I absolutely needed that money today.

As I hurried toward the emergency room to get my x-ray report, I heard Code 500 Emergency Room blare over the loudspeaker system. When I got to the emergency room there was no one there to help me. With very few choices left and the minutes ticking away, I decided it would be faster to go and get another chest x-ray, which I did.

I look back on this situation with awe. Fate is a funny thing.

It was busy that evening at work. There were numerous patients who had just had surgery that day and who needed a great deal of care. It was hectic. In the middle of the confusion and busy work schedule, I received a call from one of the physicians in the radiology department.

I picked up the telephone, "This is Miss Ehlke."

"Hi, this is Dr. Morse. How are you feeling?"

"I am fine. Why do you ask?"

"You aren't having any difficulty swallowing or any trouble breathing?"

"No, of course not. What is this all about?"

"You just had a chest x-ray taken, didn't you?"

"Yes, and I feel fine and there isn't anything the matter with me. You must have mixed my x-ray up with someone else."

"Who is your doctor, Grace Ann?"

"Dr. Walsh."

"I am going to call him right now, and I want you to go in to see him tomorrow morning."

"But tomorrow is Saturday, and that is the only day I have to sleep in. What is the matter?"

"Well, I don't know but your x-ray is abnormal and I want you to get checked by Dr. Walsh tomorrow."

"Well, what might it be?"

"Well, it could be any number of things: tuberculosis, a tumor, or sarcoidosis."

"Okay, I promise I will go in to see Dr. Walsh tomorrow."

The telephone conversation ended and I said to my charge nurse, "Guess what, I have an abnormal x-ray but I know they mixed mine up with someone else's because I feel fine."

IMMEDIATE REACTIONS

About that time the supervisor came on the floor, and I told her. We discussed the situation, and she promised to go down to the x-ray department and find my x-ray so that I could look at it. Then I would be able to show the doctors that they had made a mistake.

I wasn't too upset because I was sure an error had been made, and the supervisor was going to get the film so that I could prove that the doctors had made a mistake. I wasn't angry—I just wanted to get them going on the right track, and that track was not me.

Although I do not remember being angry, I obviously was concerned and upset. I didn't know what sarcoidosis was, and I asked a physician on the floor what the worst thing was that could happen to you with sarcoidosis. His response was "blindness."

I can't remember what I said after that. I was very shaken. I realized that I was single, I had to support myself, and I thought that might be difficult if I was blind. The rest of the night was a blur. I was really upset about being blind, but my spirits lifted as I went to coffee about 8:30 P.M. because I knew that the supervisor probably had found my x-ray by that time and I would be able to see that all of this worry was for nothing.

When I got to coffee and asked the supervisor about the x-ray, she told me that she had been unable to find it, that probably they had already sent it to Dr. Walsh's office so that it would be there when I got there in the morning.

I wasn't particularly upset by this as it just delayed my proving my point by one day. It just irritated me that I had to get up early the next day when all of this was unnecessary.

As I thought back over the day, I was satisfied. It was Friday. I had gotten my paycheck and during dinner had gone to the bank and gotten the check taken care of. Things were back on schedule and the weekend was going to be a good one. I had a number of papers to complete for school, and maybe it was good that I was being forced to get up and get an early start; after all, I would be home from the doctor's office long before I usually arose on Saturday.

On Saturday I saw Dr. Walsh along with another physician who was a medical chest specialist. Interestingly enough, I did not ask to see my x-ray nor did I tell the doctors that I thought they were all mixed up. I did ask what was wrong with me, and the physicians told me that they would have to do some tests because they really did not know what was wrong with me at this point. While in the doctor's office, I really do not remember feeling anything. I was in a crisis state, and all I wanted at that particular time was to be given direction—and the physicians were giving me direction by telling me that I had to be at the clinic at certain times for more testing. I was numb, nonreactive, and nonfeeling at this particular time.

After talking to Dr. Gorden, the medical chest specialist, and scheduling some of the tests I was to take, I went home and attempted to tackle some of my homework. My roommate was gone for the weekend, and suddenly Saturday evening I began to fall apart. I felt rather sorry for myself. This whole trip just wasn't fair.

I was beginning to feel things close in upon me and decided to call my parents who lived in Honolulu, Hawaii. I needed some support, and I was sure they would give it to me. As it turned out, I was a poor judge of character. When I told my parents that I had an abnormal x-ray, my mother's immediate response was, "If you had quit smoking like we had told you to do, this would never have happened." In their shock and frustration they were not able to give me the support that I needed.

I was scared. I flared, got very angry, and told my parents that I would never talk to them again. With my outburst of anger and my mounting frustration, I hung up and felt worse than prior to the telephone call. I felt very alone and abandoned and of course very angry that this was happening to me.

Sunday I worked. It was a day that I remember little of. It probably had little significance. At least by working I was with people and not left with the feelings of isolation and depression that encompassed me Saturday evening.

Thus between February 4, 1967, and February 16, 1967, I went through every test in the book. I had skin testing done for tuberculosis; I had all kinds of blood work done; I had all of the thyroid studies; I had more chest x-rays taken. All of this work was done at a large medical center in Seattle.

DIAGNOSTIC TESTING PERIOD

Monday and Tuesday I spent essentially in the clinic getting tests done. This was a particularly traumatic time as I was having to miss classes—which I knew I could not afford to do.

Although at this time I did not have any formed opinions of what was the matter with me, my thoughts most often drifted to having tuberculosis. The world began to spin and became more and more frustrating. I had difficulty making decisions. I could not decide whether to buy groceries for one day or for one week. I could not decide whether to get a dollar's worth of gas or five dollars worth of gas. I did not know whether to give the landlord notice that I would be leaving my apartment or to pay the next month's rent. My indecision was based on lack of knowledge about my condition. I did not know whether I should study at night or not. Where would I be in a week or a month? Would I be in Hawaii or would I be in a tuberculosis sanitorium? Would I be recuperating from surgery or would I be lying in a hospital bed dying? These were the thoughts cascading through my mind.

By Thursday, February 9, 1967, I was a wreck. At that time I didn't care what they told me, just so I would know what I was doing besides existing in suspended animation.

FINDING OUT

Thursday afternoon I had another appointment with Dr. Gorden. I loved Dr. Gorden dearly. I had complete faith in him. When I went into his office, I had great anticipation that I would finally find out what was wrong with me.

Dr. Gorden sat me down and said, "Well, the best thing I can say to you, Grace Ann, is that you look great and you haven't lost a single pound, because you have a massive tumor." I have to add an editorial note to say that I really was not grossly overweight as I weighed about 150 lb and am 5 ft 5 in tall. I was shocked and stunned but I did feel that Dr. Gorden was telling me the truth. I very much appreciated that and am very grateful to him. The frustration of the unknown was finally over.

Dr. Gorden then said to me, "Come, let me show you the x-rays." I was numb, but I managed to go with him to the x-ray department, where he had me put on the special glasses and showed me the oblique x-rays that had been taken of my chest. The tumor was easy to see. It was centrally located in the middle of my chest. It was long, extending from the top of my sternum to the end of it. It was about 3 in in width. I will always be grateful to Dr. Gorden for showing me my x-ray. The interesting thing about being in a crisis is that anything someone does for you that you interpret positively is like getting a million dollars. When a person is not in a crisis situation, many times these actions do not seem very significant. However, in a crisis situation they are very significant. Perhaps that is because the individual in crisis is so shattered that the smallest positive gesture becomes very magnificent.

SURGICAL BIOPSY WAS NEXT

As we left, I remember Dr. Gorden saying "Great teaching film," and marking the films "teaching." I was happy because I felt that at least I would be remembered in some way.

We then went back to Dr. Gorden's office and he said, "Now who do you want as your surgeon?"

"I guess Dr. Hugh."

"Dr. Hugh is going to be out of town for 10 days, and you can't wait that long."

"Well, then, I guess Dr. Hall."

"Fine." With that Dr. Gorden called Dr. Hall's office and told him about my situation and that I would be right down.

Everything was happening so fast. I really did not have a chance to think. But I was grateful to finally know what was wrong. As I went to Dr. Hall's office I remember wishing he would say that we could walk right over to surgery and get this over with. Now that I knew that I had a tumor, I just wanted to get it removed—the sooner the better.

In talking with Dr. Hall I found out that there were a few more tests to be done, but the main point of the visit was to schedule me for a biopsy—a mediastinoscopy. I asked Dr. Hall if I couldn't wait a little while as there were only 3 more weeks of school before finals. He said no. Surgery was scheduled for the following Friday, February 16, 1967. It is interesting to note that Dr. Gorden had told me I could not wait 10 days and yet I had not really absorbed the seriousness of the situation, which was indicated by my asking Dr. Hall if I couldn't wait.

I returned home from Dr. Hall's office and had many mixed feelings. I was glad to finally know what was the matter, but visions of the patients I had taken care of kept flashing through my mind. The most frequent flash was of a beautiful, beautiful lady that I had taken care of from the beginning of her illness. By the time she died, she wasn't beautiful. She was old and haggard as well as emaciated and weak.

The telephone rang and interrupted my thoughts. It was Dr. Baily. He just wanted to know how I was doing. He told me that the type of tumor that I had—a thymoma—was a good tumor to have if you had to have a tumor. He told me that it did not metastasize readily. I was grateful that he had called and felt much relieved.

I had felt well in control of things when I left Dr. Gorden's office for Dr. Hall's office. Other people, as I learned later, thought I looked shaken. Thus one of the nurses who had seen me leave had asked Dr. Baily to call me.

The next day I went up to the university and withdrew from classes. I was able to obtain passing withdrawals. I had mixed feelings about this experience. I was relieved that I would not be flunking out of the university, and at the same time I was angry that my tuition for the quarter would not be refunded. Again I found myself saying that it wasn't fair. I hadn't asked for this to happen. Why couldn't I have my money back?

Somehow I managed to get through the rest of the week. I had had no further communication with my family. They had written, but I refused to write back.

I had many friends and a good support system. They all seemed very cheery and not in the least worried about my surgery. This helped me not to worry.

On Wednesday I was at two friends' apartment. Our discussions got around to my folks, and they convinced me to call them. The intent of the call was to notify my parents of the surgery, which was less than 48 hours away. It turned into a long conversation with many tears on my part. As it turned out, my father was to come to a meeting in California. He would call me from the airport when he arrived in Seattle to change planes.

This may seem rather hard and cruel, but my parents are German and have a tendency to believe that no one ever gets sick. I did not feel that it was hard and cruel. I am sure my parents were rather stunned at this point. I thought it was great that my father was going to call to see how I was.

Wednesday evening was spent with other nurse friends. I told them that I was worried. When they asked what I was worried about, I said "pain." One of them asked what I thought the pain would feel like. I was unable to tell her. All I was able to say was that I didn't want to scream like some of those patients I had seen in intensive care.

In looking back at this situation I think it is most interesting that the one thing I was afraid of I could not describe. Never do I remember being afraid of dying, but the pain I was concerned about. It is obvious to me now that my concern was with loss of control, but I was totally unable to identify that at the time.

Thursday arrived, and I was admitted to the hospital. Prior to going to my room, I had the routine laboratory work done. I was in great spirits as I was going to spend the evening visiting.

It is interesting to look back and note that I did not really consider myself a full-fledged patient as I did not change into patient attire. Perhaps that was my way of attempting to maintain my individuality and not lose my identity.

The nursing staff on the floor that I was admitted to had decorated my room. They had all brought food, and we were going to have a party later.

The hospital house staff was a bit irritated with me as I was never in my room, and finally they paged me so that they could get the history and physical done as well as discuss my preoperative preparation with me. I did comply, but grudgingly, as I really did not see the necessity for it.

The evening was fun. Many friends visited from school and elsewhere. I do not remember being apprehensive about anything other than the possible pain. I was very high. Perhaps all of the fuss and attention allowed me time to deny the seriousness of the situation.

Friday morning arrived. I had had my preoperative medication but was not really sleepy. In the induction room I gave the staff some trouble as I did not want to take off my patient gown. When they wheeled me into the operating room I didn't want to move onto the operating table as I did not have any clothes on. I wanted to see Dr. Hall before they started the anesthesia, and when I knew that the Pentothal had been started, I sat up on the operating table and thanked everyone in the room. At the time I did not think any of my responses to be strange.

I remember very little after my initial performance. When I awoke, I was in the recovery room. The stuffed dog that I had been given and that I insisted on taking to surgery was with me. I vaguely remember being nauseated, vomiting, and having the sheets changed. I remember very little else from this experience.

I was back in my hospital room. It was dinner time, and I was famished. I was brought a regular dinner tray that I attempted to eat. I got nauseated and was unable to eat very much.

I remember little else. I was anxious for the next morning. It would be Saturday, and my dad would be calling. I would find out the results of the mediastinoscopy and what they were going to do with me. To my knowledge, I experienced nothing that I thought was pain. My biggest problem that evening was my sore throat. It was very sore, and I was glad I had Life Savers to relieve the soreness.

Saturday arrived. My dad called. He was anxious to know the results of the biopsy. At the time, I did not know the results. He said that he would call again on Friday after his meeting in California.

The physicians came in and told me that they did not know the results of the biopsy yet but they would send me home that day. I remember again feeling very frustrated. I didn't understand why no one could ever tell me anything. They should never have said they would give me the results if they couldn't produce. I was very disappointed.

I left the hospital with friends. I had lots of time on my hands. I wasn't working or going to school. I played bridge, read, and visited with lots of friends. Underlying the experience was again frustration very similar to that experienced prior to the biopsy.

THEN MAJOR SURGERY

A week following the surgery I was visiting with friends. I showed them my incision and the terrific swelling around the incision. One of them felt the area, and I remember she looked rather startled; however, at the time I didn't think much of her reaction. It was not until later that I thought back on the experience. She said, "I think you'd better call Dr. Hall in the morning and go in and show this to him."

In the morning I did see Dr. Hall. He entered the examination room and put on sterile gloves. He picked up a large syringe and came over to me. He felt the swelling and said, "I don't think there is enough fluid in your neck to take out." I was so relieved that I sat up and heard little else of what he said. However, I do remember him telling me that they would do surgery on Wednesday and for me to come into the hospital Tuesday afternoon. I was relieved. Finally they were going to get this thing out of my body. I do not remember anyone ever referring to the "thing" as anything other than a tumor. The words "cancer" and "malignancy" were never mentioned. In fact, it was not until I got my bill that I knew I definitely had cancer. The diagnosis on the bill was "malignant thymoma."

My father called that afternoon after his meeting, and I was shocked when he said he was coming back to Seattle after I told him that I would be having the surgery on Wednesday. I couldn't imagine him taking time off from work to be in Seattle while I was having surgery; however, I will have to admit I was glad he was coming.

The days flew by, and it was soon Tuesday. Again I entered the hospital. Again I refused to enter the patient role, dressing in my own clothes rather than hospital clothes. Again the interns and residents were annoyed with me. The house staff services had changed that day as it was the first of March. I thought it was ridiculous that I had to have another history and physical, and I told them so. Finally they told me to just sit down and be quiet. I did.

Again I was concerned about the pain I might experience, and I was troubled by a new thought. I kept looking at myself in the mirror, finding it difficult to imagine that by tomorrow at that time I would never look the same. It was a very difficult idea to absorb. I was to have a sternal split done. I was rather big busted, and I knew I would never look the same again.

My dad was there. A family friend took him for dinner that night, and I was pleased that his time was occupied, although he did not seem particularly upset.

I was amazed at all of the kindnesses people were showing me. I acquired a number of nightgowns and robes along with bedroom slippers, cards, and flowers. I knew that I was to be in intensive care and that one of the gals I had worked with a lot was coming in on her day off to take care of me. This was a kindness I could not express my appreciation for. Sally had five small children, and I wondered why she was doing this for me. I was very grateful. It helped me feel peaceful and secure.

I was fine until 11:00 P.M., when all my friends left. I knew the gals that worked nights, but because I had primarily worked evenings, I was much closer to the people who worked that schedule. I was pretty lonely after they left and felt rather abandoned. Although I received sleeping pills, I was unable to sleep.

I was glad when morning arrived and I would soon be on my way. About 9:00 A.M. I was given my preoperative medication. I knew that it was going to be stronger than the preoperative medication given to me prior to the biopsy because the anesthesiologist had said so the night before. I have never known what I received for medication because I never asked. It is interesting that I did not question what was said to me.—I believed everything that was said.

My mouth became very dry and I felt parched. Numerous friends were there, and finally the operating room supervisor—my friend—came and took me to surgery. I remember thinking what an awful experience this must be for children. I had no control, and all I could see was bars (the side rails), a person's face upside down, and the walls and ceilings. Whether I liked it or not, I was on my way to surgery and there was no way to stop the procedure. I no longer had control over what was happening to me. My dad was there, and I knew he would be present when I got out of surgery. That was comforting. I thought about how lucky I was that I knew everyone and how frightening it must be for someone who did not know the staff.

I woke up with lots of people looking at me. I was groggy. My friends were teasing me. A friend showed me her engagement ring that she had gotten the night before.

The next thing I remember is waking up with a start. I expressed my concerns about voiding and getting out of bed. People listened to me and assisted me. I was able to drift back into sleep.

I next remember waking up and begging for something to drink. I was so thirsty. I apparently was not supposed to have anything, but Nancy brought me a sip of 7-Up. I vomited the 7-Up and asked for more. I knew at this point that it was night. Nancy was there, and she worked nights. I remember thinking that it must be awful for other patients. If I had not known the nurses, I would have had no concept of what time it was. In intensive care the lights were on all of the time and it was always busy, although I do not remember a thing that was going on around me. There were no windows in the intensive care unit, which made things worse for patients as they had no idea what was happening outside—whether it was day or night.

I then noticed that I had a rose on my bedside table, and I felt special. I knew that flowers were not allowed in the intensive care unit. It was nice. It gave me a feeling of something other than machinery. It was real.

Nancy then came over and gave me a bath. It felt wonderful. She didn't ask if I wanted a bath, she just gave it. If she had asked me if I wanted a bath I would have probably refused, thinking that I was being a bother. Nancy also put powder on me. It smelled so good, and I felt that it put the personal touch on my bath.

My assumption that first night was that they had gotten all of the tumor. I did not ask anyone. It was never anything I even thought about.

I experienced nothing that I thought was pain. My chest muscles felt very sore—as though I had been jogging for 2 weeks straight—but that was the only discomfort I felt.

I do remember trying to cough and finding the experience very difficult. I would never have thought that it would be difficult for a patient with a sternal split to cough, but it was. It wasn't sore, there just was not enough pressure to do an effective job of coughing.

The first significant things that happened to me that first postoperative day were the visits by my numerous physicians. For example, Dr. Hall came to see me. He had a big smile on his face as he came toward me. He told me that they had gotten 99 percent of the tumor. That was my first realization that things were not okay. I knew that the tumor had grown from less than 1 percent so I wondered what he was saying to me. I asked no questions. I remember feeling confused. I also remember feeling sure that there was tumor still inside of me. I did not think of dying. I just assumed they would take care of the situation.

I enjoyed the many visits from people that day. My father was there although I remember nothing of his visits other than the fact that I was glad he was there.

I received intravenous solutions for several days. The pain from the infiltrated intravenous solutions was greater than the incisional pain.

One day in intensive care faded into the next. I had difficulty sleeping. No position was comfortable. I usually slept on my stomach, but with two chest tubes and a sternal split incision that was impossible. Even sleeping on my side was impossible.

One of the residents came in to talk with me. He informed me that my phrenic nerves had been cut and I might experience some difficulty breathing. I was sitting straight up in bed at the time. I lay back down and immediately had difficulty breathing. It is amazing what the power of suggestion will do. Apparently I had had difficulty breathing since surgery but I had not been aware of it.

A resident told me that I could have Librium anytime I wanted it so to be sure to ask for it. I wondered why he was telling me this. I didn't think I was upset or agitated, but I began to wonder if I should be.

The intravenous infusions were stopped on about the third day postoperatively. I breathed a sigh of relief. I was especially grateful that the physicians decided to continue the antibiotics orally rather than intramuscularly.

Harriet was able to sneak into intensive care to see me. She was one of my best friends and worked at the hospital. I remember having a good visit with her. I later found out that she had to be taken out of the unit because she was crying, she thought I looked so awful. I do not remember that nor do I remember feeling bad or thinking that my condition was anything but great.

I have nothing but good feelings about the experience of hospitalization. I knew everyone at the hospital, so I was constantly among friends. I did wonder what kind of an experience it might be for individuals who did not know the staff.

The entire intensive care experience was one of fading in and out. The unit was always busy, and it was rather difficult to sleep.

I never experienced anything I thought was pain. I do not remember asking for any pain medication nor do I remember receiving any pain medication while in the intensive care unit. I have since learned that I did receive pain medication.

On Sunday, my fifth day in intensive care, one chest tube was removed, and the following day the second was removed. I was never bothered by the chest tubes—again, they did not cause me any pain except when I would catch one and it would pull. The chest tubes did cramp my style. I could not go very far with them. While the chest tube was being removed, there was a split second when I felt like my breath had been taken away, but it in no way caused me any difficulty breathing or any pain.

I was then moved out of the intensive care unit. My father was with me the entire time. When I was safely housed in my room, my father left for home—Hawaii. I was so glad he had been there. Mother was to arrive in a few days, so I in no way felt abandoned.

One of the first significant things that happened to me when I left intensive care was that my telephone began to ring. One of the first calls I received was from my friend Joan. Her son Michael wanted to talk to me. He told me that he was going to come to visit me. I didn't think this was possible as he was 4 years old. However, he arrived later that day with his mother. Joan came up to get me. She put me in a wheelchair and took me to the lobby. Michael came running toward me with his blanket, which he gave to me. He said he know that I needed it and I could have it for 1 day. I was overwhelmed. I took the blanket as if it were a treasured gift that could only be so from a 4-year-old boy.

COBALT TREATMENTS WERE BEGUN

It was on that first day out of intensive care (Monday) that the doctors told me that I was to receive cobalt treatments and that they were to begin the next day. I don't remember feeling anything at all except that I hoped I would not be nauseated. I don't remember wondering if I would die, nor do I remember feeling sure that the cobalt would cure me.

Tuesday arrived, and I went down to the x-ray department for my cobalt treatment. I was not in the least apprehensive. I was put on the table on my back, and suddenly I couldn't breathe. The treatment was not done. I returned to my room. I was a little disturbed by this, but the inhalation therapist came to see me. He had rigged up a portable Bennett machine and would have it for me the next day when I went down to cobalt. He was sure that the problem would be solved. Because he was positive about the situation, I, too, was positive about it.

Monday evening Joan came to see me. She brought with her a pretty mint green nightgown and dry shampoo. Again I was overwhelmed. Here was a person who had a family with two relatively young children, and yet she came to see me and do things for me without my having to ask. I wondered why I was so important to people. I began to realize that hundreds of things had happened to me that I would never be able to repay people for in money. The things that were done for me and the companionship of people were worth more than money could ever buy. If I had not before, I knew at this point that I *must* live to pay all of these good deeds back to all of these people.

One of the most important experiences centered around the individuals and families who sent me so many Get Well cards. The feeling I was left with was not that it was just a socially acceptable thing to do, but that these people had not forgotten me—they had not abandoned me.

It was at this time that I remembered Dr. Hall had come to see me the day of surgery prior to going to the operating room. He had come between cases to see how I was doing. I found that remarkable, and again I found that there were not enough words or deeds to show my gratitude.

A number of anonymous gifts arrived. One was a stuffed dog with a radio. It was from a patient in the hospital who had heard about me. I was never able to find out who the patient was, but I did relay messages regarding my gratitude to the patient.

The next day I was able to begin my cobalt experience. What a trip. I became intimate friends with Maxine, Peggy, and Dr. John. They were my constant companions during these fleeting moments of therapy.

I was able to breathe using my portable Bennett machine. Peggy and Maxine left the room. I suddenly felt very alone. I could not move. The room was an awful green, and the walls were bare. Through the intercom Peggy and Maxine kept me informed of what they were doing, but the experience was very frightening nevertheless. As the weeks passed with my cobalt therapy, I wondered why there wasn't something to look at while a patient was having treatment. There were no mobiles or pictures of any kind in the treatment room. I decided I would have to do something about that when I was able to get around a little better. I constantly wondered if there was any chance of the cobalt machine falling on me. Cobalt therapy is a strange experience and one that health professionals should not take lightly.

I had continued to receive many cards while I was in the hospital. I wanted to see all of them all the time. I asked one of the nurses to make a string clothesline for me, which she did. On this line I put all my cards. I could see them all. This made me feel as though my family and friends were always there. It was comforting.

On the eleventh day of hospitalization I was discharged. I was to stay with the Lewises. I was staying in their bedroom in the basement. There was no bathroom in the basement. Joan was afraid that if I needed something she might not hear me, so Bob fixed up a call bell next to my bed. I was connected to the doorbell. Again I was overcome with appreciation.

The next day my mother arrived. It was good to see her. She was glad to see me. She was to stay for 3 weeks. By then I would be almost through with my cobalt treatments.

Friends of my brother Tommy were leaving for California for vacation and asked if we wouldn't like to stay in their home while they were gone. So after staying with Joan for a few days, we moved into the Anderson home—a lovely house with a lovely view. My brother, who was attending school in Portland, Oregon, spent Easter vacation with us. During this time I had my twenty-fifth birthday.

I remember that one of those days we were at the Andersons, the linen needed to be changed on the bed. I went upstairs to the bedroom to help my mother with the linen. I was so incredibly tired after walking up one flight of stairs that I had to sit down for 10 minutes before I could do a thing. I was shocked at how tired I was.

I began to get discouraged. I never really felt good. I was nauseated, and I resorted to carrying around a box of crackers all the time. My best period of the day was the evening. It was a blessing to have my mother there as I did not have to cook or drive. I wondered what people did who did not have all the help I had.

I became depressed during this time and asked Peggy and Maxine what would happen to me if the cobalt therapy did not work. I was surprised at their response. They told me I shouldn't talk like that, and they called Dr. John. He arrived and asked what this was all about. I repeated the question, and he told me I need not think about that. I became frustrated and a little irritated. It was my life. How did he know that everything was going to be okay? It was false reassurance. I had just asked a simple question to which I had not been able to get an answer from anyone.

I overhead my mother talking to one of her friends in California. She said that I was still able to swallow and didn't seem to be having trouble with hot or cold foods at the present time. I was surprised. I didn't know they had anticipated any trouble—and I wondered why everyone but me knew about this.

Everyone was cheery, and I never doubted that I had been cured—at least most of the time I didn't. My mother had to leave all too soon. I assured her that I would be fine. I had about 2½ weeks of cobalt left.

At that point I began driving myself to cobalt every morning. One day towards the end of therapy, I had to stop the car because of the nausea. I did finally make it to the hospital but had to remain there for several hours because of the nausea. My biggest problem with the nausea continued to be in the morning. I was grateful to friends who would stop by after work in the evening and fix soup for me which they placed at the side of my bed. I set the alarm clock for 3:00 A.M. I would wake up then and drink the soup in an effort to avert the dry heaves I was experiencing on arising.

GOING HOME

At the completion of the cobalt therapy I returned to Hawaii for 6 weeks of rest. I was happy to be home. I was not in the least concerned about dying. I was sure I was cured. The physicians in Seattle had given me orders concerning things to be cautious of, such as getting sunburned, prescriptions to be filled if necessary, and signs and symptoms to watch for. I did not equate any of these directions with anything other than the physicians' being overly concerned.

Within about 10 days after I arrived home, I felt much better. I was no longer nauseated, tired, or depressed. I enjoyed being with my parents, and they very much seemed to enjoy being with me. It was a very pleasant ''R and R.''

STARTING OVER

I returned to Seattle in June of 1967. I again began taking classes at the University of Washington and working evenings. I continued to have frequent checkups with my doctors. I was feeling fine, and no additional treatment was planned.

The major changes in my life concerning this experience occurred in several areas. The first area was and continues to be checkups. Whenever a doctor's appointment is scheduled, a great deal of psychological preparation is done by me for me. I always have to say to myself that I can handle anything that is said to me. I also remind myself that if I went through a cancer experience at the age of 24 I can go through anything. I do this very conscientiously. I do remember one month during the last few years when I didn't make a doctor's appointment because I felt I couldn't handle any bad news that particular month.

The second area of major change has been body image. During the first 6 years following the surgery, I did not realize that I was adjusting to an altered body image. About 4 years ago I bought a dress that had a neckline that did not hide my scar. I suddenly realized that this dress was the first garment I had bought since the surgery which showed my scar. I suddenly wondered how many things or concepts one does not realize one is working through. Now I often wonder whether I am still working through many aspects of the surgery. It is 10 years since the surgery, and I do not have the answer to that question. I do know that it takes a very long time, meaning many years, to work through some aspects of a catastrophic experience.

The third area that has had major changes for me is life focus. I used to be primarily a future-oriented person. At the present time I am a person who focuses primarily on the here and now. Interestingly enough, life is much more exciting from this viewpoint. I feel like I am the lucky one because I believe I see and experience much more of the life that is going on around me daily. But I am not totally a here-and-now person: Since having the surgery I have completed a baccalaureate and a masters degree in nursing and am now thinking about pursuing additional education. I am teaching student nurses and am very active in a number of organizations that have future orientations.

The experience of having cancer can be a very meaningful and good experience. I feel that having a positive experience with a disease such as cancer necessitates much support from collegues, friends, and family. I am grateful that I received such support. The challenge for the health-related professions is to recognize that cancer is not equated with a death sentence. It is only through this recognition that health professionals can give the cancer patient support, which is perhaps the key to a positive experience with the disease.

Chapter 2

Sociocultural Aspects of Cancer

Pamela K. Burkhalter

Persons who have cancer tend to have a unique status within society. They are frequently showered with compassion, concern, and caring by family and friends, but their status as employees and productive members of society is jeopardized. The intellectual acknowledgment by family, friends, and coworkers that cancer is a tragic illness and is often fatal can become clouded by the emotionally based fears of cancer that reside in each person. This ambiguous approach of society to cancer and cancer patients is reflected in the attitudes and myths about cancer that seem to be perpetuated.

ATTITUDES TOWARD CANCER

Throughout each person's growth and development, attitudes toward self and others are shaped by life experiences, parental and societal value systems, and culturally prescribed behavior codes.

Fear

The prevailing attitudes toward cancer and the person afflicted with the disease center around the emotion of *fear*. The word "cancer" engenders feelings of dread, anxiety, and fear in many people because of the chronicity and debilitation often associated with its treatment and eventual outcome. In spite of the fact that certain forms of cancer have a high probability for remission, eradication, or cure, these feelings of dread can be aroused in most people when a diagnosis of cancer is a possibility.

The fear of cancer has contributed to the development of positive, adaptive societal attitudes toward the disease. For instance, there is an increased public awareness that early screening and detection of cancer *is* possible and, if done in a comprehensive manner, can result in successful early intervention. In terms of a general modification of attitude, this acknowledgment of the hopeful side of cancer care is truly a change from the denial of cancer's reality which was present many years ago. The fact remains, however, that most people do possess an attitude of fear toward cancer. Although the fear is justified, it *can* act as a motivating simulus for preventive health care measures and for effort to seek early intervention when the disease's presence is suspected.

Challenge

A second societal attitude toward cancer is represented by the word "challenge." Work directed at identifying the cause(s) of cancer and designing new treatment approaches is often referred to as "the war on cancer," the "fight against cancer," or the "conquest of cancer." Each of these phrases and others implies the acceptance of a challenge: the taking up of the gauntlet and the embarkation on a crusade that will result in victory for the forces opposed to cancer. The American ethic of "can do" is readily reflected in this attitude of challenge. The statement "If we can put a man on the moon and land on Mars, surely we can find a cure for cancer" represents this belief that cancer *can* be cured by hard work, sincerity of purpose, and a hopeful attitude. Without a doubt, this attitude has done more to advance scientific understanding of cancer, its possible causes, and the development of spectacular treatment modalities than has any other attitude toward the disease. When the challenge is accepted, defeat is negated and hope and promise are fostered. It is this kind of attitude, supported by society's resources, that will make the eventual cancer cure breakthrough possible.

Attitudes toward cancer are reflected not only in overt ways such as expression of fear or attempts to overcome the disease. Each facet of the cancer care problem owes its existence, continuation, or demise to attitudes. These belief systems either propel or impede human behavior. Thus, the remaining sections of this chapter will discuss the impact of attitudes on the sociocultural aspects of cancer. As each topic is presented, the delineated attitudes and the role they play will be presented.

MYTHS OF CANCER

Many attitudes toward cancer and the cancer patient are reflected in the cancer myths that have arisen over the years. These unfounded beliefs have contributed to negative or ambivalent feelings toward the cancer patient. Dispelling myths that perpetuate incorrect information is a vital responsibility for all health professionals and public information agencies.

The "Contagious" Myth

Perhaps the most common myth about cancer is that it is a contagious disease; i.e., another person can "get" it from a cancer patient. Clearly cancer is *not* a communicable disease: it is not transmitted by contact with the cancer patient or the patient's belongings. Although few health professionals would harbor such a misconception (we hope), the author has had the occasion to observe the following incident. Prior to giving complete nursing care to a bedridden cancer patient, the nurse's aide assigned to the patient put on a gown, mask, and gloves. She then prepared to enter the patient's room to care for him. Before she saw the patient, she was asked, "Why are you dressed for isolation?" The aide replied, "I just don't want to *get it!* Get cancer." This person was expressing her fear of cancer in an obvious, protective manner.

The impact of such behavior on the recipient of care, the cancer patient, probably is immense. Not only does the individual face learning how to cope with the disease and its treatment, but he or she may also face rejection by care givers who have not dealt with their own feelings toward cancer.

The example cited above probably is not representative of the many overt ways rejection is experienced by some cancer patients. It does, however, illustrate an important point: health professionals *may* express such attitudes and subscribe to such cancer myths without realizing the impact of this behavior on their care-giving actions. *Awareness* of such attitudes on the part of the nurse, physician, or other care giver is the crucial first step in the process of eventual attitude change.

The "Pain" Myth

The fear of cancer has led to the development and prepetuation of a second major myth. Many people believe that once an individual is diagnosed as having cancer, that person's course of illness will follow a trajectory of pain: pain that will be unremitting; pain that cannot be controlled. Such inevitable suffering *is* frightening, but in many cases the fear can be reduced or alleviated.

While some cancer patients do experience pain as the disease progresses, others do not. Some cancer patients with widespread metastatic disease never express or appear to be experiencing pain. They require little to no medication or other pain relief measures. The inconsistency among patients, the differences in tolerance and expression of pain, and the variance in response to pain intervention measures contribute to the pain myth's continuation. What is uncertain, unquantifiable, or unpredictable often can lead one to formulate parameters within which the feared idea or concept can be proscribed. With pain and cancer, an assumption of cancer equals pain can be made as an attempt to structure an unknown, feared experience.

The public, health professionals, and, most of all, cancer patients need to be counseled regarding the nonfactual basis of the pain myth. Discussion and literature should emphasize the fact that pain may be associated with the illness or treatment process but that an inevitable progression in severity of pain does not occur with *every* person who has the disease. By no means does this position imply a Pollyanna attitude toward pain and cancer. It does, however, imply that the myth and the fear it generates can be abbreviated with correct information and clarification of misconceptions about the relationship between cancer and pain.

The "Hidden Cures" Myth

Tremendous effort has been expended to find a cure for cancer, and the work continues throughout the United States. Yet, in spite of this concerted effort on the part of scientists, a cure for cancer has not been found. Unfortunately, many people harbor a belief that such a cure, or cures, has been found but that for various unethical, cold-hearted reasons, it is not made available to the public. Thus, the "hidden cures" myth has evolved over the years, getting most of its support from the purveyors of quack cancer cures (see Chapter 21). Tragically, a cancer patient unable to benefit from available, reputable treatment modalities for the disease may seek one of these hidden cures. Perpetuation of the myth occurs, then, as cancer patients or people who fear they may have the disease seek the "miracle" that will free them from it.

The arguments offered as support for the existence of a hidden cure focus on a conspiracy theory. This theory maintains that the entire medical establishment, the pharmaceutical industry, the federal and state governments, and health professionals in general do not want the "truth" to be revealed. If this truth were made available, the cancer care business would flounder. Clearly the argument is easily refuted. Is it reasonable to believe that physicians, nurses, or government officials would allow themselves or family members to suffer with cancer if a cure was available? The answer is obviously no!

The hidden cure myth is clearly unfounded. Cures for cancer are not being hidden from those who could benefit from them. When treatments that possess curative potential are discovered, tested, and thoroughly evaluated, they *are* made available to the cancer patient.

The "Treatment" Myth

A certain number of persons with cancer will hesitate to have their suspicions confirmed and to embark on a course of treatment because of a belief that such treatment will always be long and torturous. This treatment myth is difficult to dispel. Cancer treatment *is* often long, expensive, and taxing. However, treatment measures are coordinated with the type of cancer present. As a consequence, some forms of cancer *do* require long courses of treatment. On the other hand, other types of cancer may be treated in the physician's office and require little or no hospitalization.

It is truly imperative that health professionals work to clarify the treatment misconceptions they become aware of. The delay in seeking treatment which can occur with belief in the myth can be extremely costly to the patient.

The "Mutilation" Myth

In some people's minds, cancer is equated with disfigurement and mutilation in an inevitable sequence of occurrence. For the person who suspects a diagnosis of cancer, this fear of what *may* occur can impede the acceptance of early intervention. Some forms of cancer treatment do involve radical surgery, radiation therapy, or temporary or permanent loss of function. With comprehensive rehabilitation, however, the changes in appearance or functioning can be compensated for in many cases (see Chapter 10).

The mutilation myth remains unfounded. It cannot be accurately applied to each cancer patient. A more logical approach would involve consideration of each type of cancer and the treatment that it may entail. For the cancer patient, belief in a positive outcome is crucial. Dispelling the idea of mutilation, with its inevitably negative connotation, therefore becomes a vital responsibility of public education agencies and health care givers in general.

The myths of cancer act to perpetuate negative attitudes toward the disease and those afflicted with it. Reducing the impact of unfounded beliefs involves a commitment on the part of society to reject illogical, fear-based attitudes.

EMPLOYMENT AND THE CANCER PATIENT

Society's attitudes toward the recovered cancer patient are clearly reflected in employment policies. Many rehabilitated cancer patients are denied employment despite the fact that capability to perform the required duties is present. Some employers and employees do not wish to associate with someone who has had cancer. Perhaps they fear contagion when in close proximity with the person or they become anxious when faced with the reality of the disease. Whatever the reason, employment problems are very real for the person who wishes to reestablish competence, productivity, and a feeling of self-worth. Opportunities for meaningful employment are reduced to a greater extent, however, for those persons with functional impairment due to cancer treatment or the disease process.

The employer may believe that the person who has had cancer is a risk in terms of continued employment. Apprehension regarding reduced productivity and absenteeism may arise if the patient is in remission but has not entered the "recovered" category of cancer treatment.

Attitudes toward the recovered employee seem to be changing in certain areas. Some large businesses are following a policy of reinstating valued, trained employees after recovery from cancer. These companies are finding that absences for cancer treatment are of a low frequency when compared with absences due to other diseases or illnesses. The fear of the economic impact of cancer from the employer's viewpoint may have no basis in fact.

Of equal importance is the trend toward employee advocacy by certain labor unions. When a union member is denied relicensure or return to employment, the union may initiate appropriate action to ensure the individual's right to fair and impartial consideration. The result, of course, is of benefit not only to the recovered cancer patient but to the employer as well.

Changes in societal attitudes toward the person who has recovered from cancer *are* occurring. Each individual who reestablishes the ability to make a contribution to society after recovery from cancer enhances the trend toward change of attitudes.

INSURANCE COVERAGE

The recovered cancer patient may be considered a potentially expensive health risk by insurance companies that provide coverage for private business or government sectors. The inability to obtain insurance coverage can directly relate to the individual's difficulty in finding suitable employment; i.e., companies may be unwilling or unable to hire the person who is not eligible for insurance coverage. A vicious cycle can develop in which employment is withheld when insurance coverage is not allowable, while insurance coverage is not extended to the unemployed recovered cancer patient.

Individuals seeking to obtain personal health insurance after a bout with cancer may also have difficulty in finding an insurance carrier willing to cover them. Generally, a detailed health history is required. Disclosure of a history of cancer may result in refusal to insure. In addition, patients who have recovered from cancer or have had the disease process arrested may be able to obtain personal insurance coverage only after delays as long as 10 years. Many insurance policies contain a rider that excludes treatment for cancer while covering all other medical problems.

Insurance coverage, whether health or personal, is frequently difficult to obtain when an individual has had cancer. This inequity fosters fear and anxiety in the recovered cancer patient, who often has considerable apprehension about recurrence of the disease. Again, societal attitudes toward the disease and the economic burden it can create for the individual, the insurance carrier, or the society have frequently made it difficult for the individual to obtain insurance coverage.

FINANCIAL CONSIDERATIONS

Cancer is considered both an acute and a chronic illness with direct and indirect financial costs. Direct costs result from diagnositc, treatment, and rehabilitation efforts for the patient. Hospital costs, outpatient charges, home care nursing services, and nursing home costs also contribute to the direct financial impact. Indirect costs consist of loss of income, decreased or halted productivity, or costs for supportive services not directly related to treatment. Additional indirect costs, which greatly increase the economic burden of cancer for the patient and family, include items such as wigs, special clothing, labor-saving devices for performance of household duties, or home structural modifications. To enhance the patient's comfort when cared for in the home, family members may add an extra telephone, television set, or air conditioner. Each of these items is costly for a family with great financial burdens. These financial considerations and many others result in an annual economic expenditure for cancer that exceeds tens of billions of dollars.

While the overall costs of cancer are astounding, the impact on the individual cancer patient and the patient's family can have an equally devastating impact. One study found that total costs related to the illness ranged from $5,000 to $50,000.[1] While most patients have some form of medical insurance, charges for treatment and care may exceed the coverage. When this occurs, the patient's financial resources can be drained. The costs incurred in treating cancer are, of course, subject to variation in relation to the type of cancer, time of diagnosis, response to treatment, and presence or absence of complications. Nevertheless, the financial burden of cancer represents a most tangible concern to the individual, family, and society.

THE POLITICS OF CANCER

Considerable controversy exists with reference to the political aspects of the war on cancer. Hundres of millions of dollars are expended on this war annually via the National Cancer Act of 1971. Therein lies the source of the controversy. On the one hand, it is clearly acknowledged that the search for a cure for cancer is of paramount importance. At the same time, some critics of these expenditures point out that many other health problems receive a disproportionately small amount of government research support and attention.

The support for research aimed at identifying the causes and cures for cancer originates with each person. The fear of cancer and its ever-present threat of appearance is a powerful force for expanding financial backing for cancer research. In one sense, the large annual governmental expenditures reflect society's concern about the disease of cancer and the strong drive to eradicate its continued threat.

CARE TRENDS

Sociocultural values are often reflected in the way health services are delivered. Attitudes of fear and anxiety about cancer have an influence on *how* and *where* care is received. For example, the chronically ill cancer patient may be cared for in a general hospital, nursing home, or private home. Availability of financial resources will influence where care can best be given or most economically administered. The willingness and capability of the family to care for the patient directly influence where care is received. Some terminally ill cancer patients are returning to their homes for the chronic care they need. Family or home health nursing services provide the necessary treatments and continuous care necessary to ensure optimal comfort and well-being. The large majority of cancer patients, however, continue to receive acute and chronic care in the general hospital or the skilled nursing facility.

A promising trend in offering comprehensive, highly sensitive care to the terminally ill cancer patient is in the evolutionary stage of development. The "hospice" (half home, half hospital) approach to terminal care seeks to promote comfort, peacefulness, dignity, and pain-controlled life until the time of death. The emergence of the hospice concept in the United States reflects a change in societal attitude toward the cancer patient with a concomitant recognition that terminal care can be humanely and lovingly administered.

SUMMARY

The values and attitudes of a society or culture are reflected in the way in which a devastating illness is handled. Cancer evokes a primary emotion of fear, which may translate into rejecting or isolating behaviors exhibited toward the cancer patient.

Some attitudes are negative, while other, very positive attitudes are demonstrated via the extensive research being conducted and supported by governmental and private agencies. The ambivalence toward cancer will not be eliminated until its causes and cures are found. Until that time, cancer will continue to foster feelings of fear, ambivalence, and hope.

REFERENCE

1 *The Impact, Costs and Consequences of Catastrophic Illness on Patients and Families.* New York: Cancer Care, Inc., 1973, p. 20.

BIBLIOGRAPHY

Byrd, B. F. and Johnson, W. V. (co-chairmen). *Human Values and Cancer,* New York: American Cancer Society, 1972.

Eisenberg, Lucy. "The Politics of Cancer," *Harper's Magazine,* **243**: 100–102+, November 1971.

"For Cancer Survivors, Life Still Presents a Plethora of Problems," *Medical World News,* **15**: 18–19, February 8, 1974.

The Impact, Costs and Consequences of Catastrophic Illness on Patients and Families. New York: Cancer Care, Inc., 1973.

Knox, Gerald M. "Ten Common Misconceptions about Cancer," *Better Homes and Gardens,* **52**: 22–28, 1974.

Levin, D. L., Devesa, S. S., Godwin, J. D., and Silverman, D. T. *Cancer Rates and Risks, 2nd Edition,* 1974, U. S. Government Printing Office, 1974.

Pekar, Peter P. "Cost Analysis and Consequences of the National Cancer Plan," *Federation Proceedings,* **33**(11): 2225–2230, November 1974.

Pilgrim, Ira. *The Topic of Cancer.* New York: Thomas Y. Crowell, 1974.

"The Politics of Cancer," *Time,* **94**: 40–41, July 5, 1971.

Rosenbaum, Ernest H. *Living with Cancer*. New York: Praeger Publishers, 1975.

Rother, Russell. "What Have We got to Show for the 'War on Cancer'?" *Modern Medicine,* **43**: 46–49, January 1, 1975.

Schottenfeld, David. *Cancer Epidemiology and Prevention*. Springfield, Ill.: Charles C Thomas, 1975.

Ward, Audrey W. M. "Terminal Care in Malignant Disese," *Social Science and Medicine,* **8**: 413–420, 1974.

Chapter 3

Theories of Causation

Pamela K. Burkhalter

Evidence of the presence of cancer in human ancestors as early as 2500 B.C. in ancient Egypt has been reported. Hippocrates (ca. 400 B.C.) attributed the cause of cancer to an imbalance of black bile, one of the body's four humors responsible for health and homeostais. Although current theories of causation have evolved to a higher level of sophistication over the ensuing centuries, clear evidence for the disease's cause remains a mystery to a large extent. The purpose of the present chapter, then, is twofold. First, an overview of the complexities involved in the "etiology" (or study of causes) of cancer will be explored. Second, the major theories of causation will be presented as a means of preparing the nurse for content to be included in subsequent chapters.

CONSIDERATIONS IN THE ETIOLOGY OF CANCER

In seeking to identify the cause(s) of cancer, scientists derive information from and base decisions on three kinds of data:

1 Epidemiological studies of the incidence and distribution of cancer according to age, sex, socioeconomic status, ethnocultural background, etc. This information is analyzed to identify factors common to each patient group.

Usually correlations are drawn between descriptive characteristics of the cancer patient (age, sex, etc.) and these common factors. The correlational approach is valid in identifying agents or possible cancer-causing factors that require in-depth study to determine their potential for cancer initiation. However, considerable concern is aroused in the public and professional sectors when correlational data between a particular type of cancer and an agent found to coincide with the cancer are discussed in cause-and-effect terms.

Correlations represent a statistical occurrence of two or more factors, agents, or situations. To attribute a cause-and-effect relationship to such findings is misleading. A correlation does not clarify the *link* between a supposed causative agent and the appearance of a cancer. It *does* suggest and arouse suspicions about the possible role the agent may have. With these concerns in mind, the correlational method of identifying agents that *may* have a connection with cancer causation can be an invaluable tool in narrowing the number of possible factors to receive in-depth study.

2   Controlled experimental research with laboratory animals serves as the major avenue to identify cancer-causing environmental agents as well as internal initiators of cancer. For obvious ethical and practical reasons, experimental research into possible links between human cancers and potential causative factors cannot be conducted. To circumvent these problems, animals (e.g., rats, hamsters) are used in studies designed to determine (a) the potency of certain agents to start cancerous growth and (b) the sequence of events responsible for cancer initiation, growth, and ultimate outcome.

While the animal research model is the accepted scientific approach to identifying cancer-causative agents or factors, it has a definite limitation. Data revealing clear evidence of cancer causation in experimental animals cannot be accepted as conclusive confirmation of similar causative hypotheses for humans. In spite of this limitation, however, an overriding implication for humans arises from animal research: factors or agents found to cause cancer in animals *must* be considered as *potential* causative factors in humans. As a result, bans on certain consumer products found to be harmful to laboratory animals reduce exposure of humans to potential cancer-causing agents. In terms of preventing cancer, it truly is more beneficial to take the necessary precautions with suspected harmful agents than to hesitate until conclusive links of causation are established.

3   Factors found to be associated with cancer are studied from two points of view. The first focuses on the nature of the agent—its biochemical or molecular structure—and how and under what conditions it functions. The second attempts to identify and isolate the agent in its natural habitat, whether external or internal to the body. The data gathered from this work have resulted for example, in the compilation of lists of potential cancer-causing substances, such as nitrogen mustard and its derivatives.

These three types of data form the foundation upon which effort to determine the cause(s) of cancer is based. Once a cause is known, scientists seek to use this information to delineate preventive and treatment measures specific to the particular form of cancer. Thus, while the search for the cause(s) of cancer may at times appear to be frustrated, it is a crucial step in the ultimate conquest of the disease. The time, effort, and financial resources expended in the search are revalidated with each instance of research that clearly identifies a link in the chain of cancer causation.

THEORIES OF CANCER CAUSATION

Any discussion of the causation of cancer tends to result in one conclusion: there is no single theory that accounts for the causation of cancer in its many forms. The trend in the etiology of cancer is toward a *multiplicity* theory in which a number of factors converge and result in the appearance of cancer.

In the study of the cause(s) of cancer, carcinogens play a dominant role. "Carcinogens" may be defined as physical, chemical, or biological factors or agents that increase the probability of cancer appearance in humans or animals. Many of the factors that converge with an incident of cancer are carcinogenic agents. Carcinogens may act at the initial contact site, at the site of a specific organ where they are localized or accumulated, at the site of metabolism, or at the site of excretion. Certain carcinogens are site-specific, while others affect numerous sites. A carcinogenic process consists of the action of such an agent(s) on a susceptible organism. The organism may become susceptible as a result of the associated external (originating outside the body) and/or internal factors (within the body), as depicted in Figure 3-1. Any cell that divides may be subject to a carcinogenic process. Given an association of potential causative events, however, the appearance of a cancer is *not* guaranteed. For many unknown reasons, the convergence of carcinogenic agents with a susceptible organism does not result in cancer in some people, while it does in others. This incongruence continues to be studied in an attempt to identify the discriminative element(s) that prevents or impedes cancer development in such a selective manner.

Because of the intimate interaction that takes place between external and internal carcinogenic factors, it is not possible to label each of the carcinogenic agents as solely originating or acting in one sphere or the other. As a consequence, the major theories of causation will be discussed with reference to the external and internal carcinogenic characteristics each possesses.

Chemical Carcinogens

Occupational Carcinogens Human cancers brought about by exposure to external chemical agents tend to be associated with industrial or occupational situations. Workers coming in direct contact with certain chemicals and chemical by-products have an increased incidence of certain types of cancer. Table 3-1

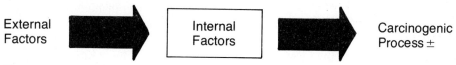

Figure 3-1 The carcinogenic process: External factors influence internal factors, leading to carcinogenesis.

Table 3-1 Occupational Human Carcinogens

Carcinogen	Site and type of cancer

Polycyclic aromatic hydrocarbons
  Examples: soot, pitch, coal tar and
  products, antracine
	Skin: epitheliomas and other skin cancers

Aromatic amines
  Examples: benzidine, beta-naphthylamine,
  4-aminobiphenyl
	Bladder: papillomas and other bladder cancers

Metals	
Asbestos	Lung: mesotheliomas; gastrointestinal tract: carcinomas
Chromium compounds and uranium	Lung: bronchogenic carcinomas
Nickel	Upper respiratory tract: various carcinomas
Cadmium	Prostate gland: various carcinomas
Miscellaneous	
Vinyl chloride	Liver: angiosarcoma
Chloromethyl methyl ether	Lung cancer

contains a brief summary of the more common industry-related carcinogens and resulting types of cancer. These cancers appear infrequently, but they appear among certain industrial workers at a rate significantly greater than that found in the general population. Many of the companies requiring use of such chemical compounds have initiated safeguards to protect the employee. Recent research indicates that aniline dyes, one of the polycyclic hydrocarbons used in hair dyes, may have carcinogenic potential when used for the purpose of hair bleaching and color dyeing over long periods of time.

Dietary Carcinogens Carcinogens associated with food intake have received considerable attention over the past several years. A large number of these agents are harmful to animals, but as yet clear evidence is lacking for the role of these carcinogens in human cancer development. One animal carcinogen, DDT, has been largely banned as a pesticide based on the appearance of cancers in certain animals who ingested the material. It is not possible at this time to state unequivocally that DDT residues in human tissues, acquired through the food chain, will cause cancer to develop at a later date. Suffice to say that a potential danger has been identified and steps have been taken to preclude the development of such a cause-and-effect relationship.

Food-related carcinogens with potential for development of certain human cancers include the nitrosamines. When nitrates, used as food additives or preservatives (found in most canned or smoked meat and fish), combine with naturally occurring or dietary amines (from certain drugs or nicotine) to form nitrosamines, certain types of human cancers may develop. Foodstuffs (e.g., coffee) containing phenolic materials may enter into this combining process by acting as catalysts in the formation of the nitrosamines. The naturally available sources of nitroso compounds, however, are quite limited in distribution and availability.

Where large quantities of peanuts, corn, rice, peas, soybeans, barley, fruit, milk, certain meats, and cheddar cheese are accumulated or stored, a lactone-produced fungus, aflatoxin B_1, which is a highly potent carcinogen to the liver in humans, may form. Contamination with this fungus seems to be prevented by refining processes. In addition, protein intake stimulates abundant gastric juice secretion, dilutes the toxin, and promotes its elimination, thereby reducing the danger of cancer formation.

The artificial sweetener sodium cyclamate, *may* have a carcinogenic potential for humans, although this cause-and-effect relationship has not been conclusively demonstrated. Other suggested foodstuffs or food-related substances considered to have carcinogenic potential include benzpyrene (found in bread, smoked foods, and roasted coffee beans); cycad nuts; excessive sugar intake; excessive alcohol intake; and diets containing large amounts of refined carbohydrates, animal protein, and fat.

Drug Carcinogens   Certain drugs have been associated with increased risk in humans. Chlornaphazine has been associated with the appearance of bladder cancer, while Thorotract, a contrast medium, has been found to produce cancer in both laboratory animals and humans. Thorotract has been discontinued as a contrast medium because of its cancer-inducing potential.

Potential chemical carcinogens are innumerable. The number of these agents definitely linked to human cancer causation, however, is relatively small.

Radiation Carcinogens

Cause-and-effect relationships have been clearly established between certain forms of human cancer and both ionizing and nonionizing radiations.

Ionizing Radiations   Exposure to x-rays and radioactive atoms, as ionizing radiations, have been found to cause certain forms of human cancer. Significantly higher rates of leukemia are found in radiologists and in individuals treated by irradiation for several years for the treatment of ankylosing arthritis. When the pregnant female is exposed to abdominal x-rays, the risk of radiation carcinogenesis for the child is significantly increased. Survivors of the Hiroshima and Nagasaki atomic blasts, experienced a peak incidence of acute and chronic myeloid leukemia 6 to 8 years after the explosions.

Diagnostic or therapeutic irradiation may be responsible for the appearance of certain cancers in later life when the exposure (1) takes place during fetal life or (2) is for treatment of such conditions as hyperplasia of the thymus or lymphadenitis during the first 2 years of life.

Appearance of cancer in later life may also be related to long-term low-level exposure to radiation, which promotes premature aging. Aging tends to bring about progressive deterioration of nucleic acid molecules. This deterioration fosters the accumulation of noncorrectable errors in the synthesis of protein. Over time, normal cells may lose their ability to repair such errors, as a result, normal cell function or division may fail—a situation potentially conducive to cancer development.

Ultraviolet Radiations   Nonionizing radiations responsible for skin cancers are primarily ultraviolet radiations from sunlight. Excessive exposure to sunlight over a long period of time has been repeatedly associated with skin cancer attributed to the absorption of the rays by the epidermis.

Viral Carcinogens

The most enticing current theory of cancer causation focuses on the possibility that certain viruses may be carcinogenic to humans. Research suggests that viral agents *may* play a role in the initiation of leukemia and lymphatic tissue tumors, although definitive causative relationships for humans have not been established. Animal studies with chickens, rabbits, and mice have identified viruses as animal carcinogenic agents. But in spite of the fact that certain human viruses may stimulate tumor growth in laboratory animals, animal-originated viruses have not been identified as human viral carcinogens.

Periodic clustering of cases of Hodgkin's disease and leukemia have revitalized the viral hypothesis of cancer causation. To date, Burkitt's lymphoma appears to have a link with viral carcinogenesis. The Epstein-Barr virus (EBV) has been identified as the probable cause of infectious mononucleosis in humans and has been found in some types of leukemia as well as in Burkitt's lymphoma, a cancer endemic in the tropical and subtropical regions of New Guinea and Africa.

Viruses and chemicals may interact in certain carcinogenic processes. For example, laboratory research with animals indicates that chemical carcinogens may stimulate viral carcinogenesis by altering cellular susceptibility to viral agents or by impairing immunologic surveillance mechanisms. Viruses in turn may stimulate chemical carcinogenesis by interfering with cellular detoxification of chemicals or by altering cellular permeability to chemical affects.

The viral hypothesis continues to receive considerable research attention but as yet has not been established as a definite cause of human cancers.

Genetic Factors

Genetic Inheritance   In seeking to identify the relationship between genetic inheritance and the incidence of cancer, it is necessary to emphasize that characteristics or traits are not inherited. Only *genetic material* is inherited, establishing an individual's range of potential reactions. Rarely is cancer inherited in the genetic sense, i.e., direct transmission of a "cancer" gene to offspring. There are, however, several hereditary syndromes that are associated with the appearance of certain cancers (see Table 3-2). These cancers may be related to an autosomal dominant or recessive pattern of inheritance.

Heritable human cancers may occur in response to an overall genetic constitution of an individual which increases susceptibility to the disease. In addition, evidence indicates an increased tendency for the development of certain forms of cancer within families. For example, female breast cancer among close relatives appears with greater frequency when the patient is premenopausal and the cancer is bilateral.

Table 3-2 Summary of Some Heritable Forms of Cancer in Humans

Site of cancer	Disorder	Autosomal status
Colon and rectum	Familial polyposis coli	Dominant
	Gardner's syndrome	Dominant
	Turcot's syndrome	Recessive
Bone and connective tissue	Multiple exostosis, chondrosarcoma	Dominant
Skin	Xeroderma pigmentosum	Recessive
	Multiple nevoid basal cell carcinoma	Dominant
	Cutaneous melanoma	Dominant
Eye	Multiple trichoepithelioma	Dominant
	Retinoblastoma, intraocular melanoma	Dominant
Brain and central nervous system	Turcot's syndrome, glioblastoma multiforme, medulloblastoma	Recessive
	Neurofibromatosis, sarcoma, pheochromocytoma	Dominant
	Von Hippel-Lindaus syndrome, hemangioblastoma of cerebellum, pheochromocytoma	Dominant
Esophagus	Esophageal cancer	Dominant
	Celiac disease, esophageal carcinoma, lymphoma	Dominant

Somatic Mutation and Oncogenesis Clear relationships between the on-cogene theory of cancer causation and somatic mutations have not been established. The "oncogene" hypothesis suggests that each cell contains structural genes that normally are repressed. Malignancy can be produced either spontaneously or via the effect of carcinogens when the cells undergo derepression. Derepression may result from germ cell mutation or somatic mutation (including chromosome deletion), which alters all cells arising from the mutant cell. This mutation is then transmitted to offspring. The gene carrier may develop none, one, or multiple cancers according to this theory.

The oncogene theory, then, maintains that all cells contain the potential for cancer development. When this potential is activated or a malfunction of the genetic mechanism occurs, cancer appears.

The role of genetic factors in human cancer causation has partially been identified. Determination of conclusive links between heredity and cancer is difficult when family medical histories and pedigrees are incomplete or absent. In addition, persons who may carry an inherited cancer tendency may die from other causes prior to the cancer's appearance. Further complication of the process of confirming cause-and-effect relationships occurs when chromosomal aberration is identified in family members *after* a cancer has developed. For example, in one family in which the mother had carcinoma of the breast, four out of five children had chomosomal aberrations. Three of the children developed cancer—chronic myelogenous leukemia, myelofibrosis and carcinoma of the breast, and squamous cell carcinoma of the lip, respectively. Of considerable interest is the fact that the mother and two of the affected children had been exposed to possible occupational carcinogens. In this instance, then, the issue became clouded with the identification of the external carcinogen.

Conclusions made regarding genetics and cancer therefore remain tentative. Statistically only three statements can be made:

1 Identified heritable cancers are characterized by comparatively early onset; e.g., a hereditary form of basal cell carcinoma may appear at the average age of 15 while the nonhereditary form appears at an average age of 50.
2 Heritable cancers are characterized by multiplicity of primary tumors, as depicted in Figure 3-2.
3 Virtually every type of human cancer occurs in both a heritable and a nonheritable form.

Failure of Immunologic Mechanisms

The immune system acts as a primary internal protective mechanisms. When intact, the system rejects foreign substances, proteins, or any substance or cell not recognized as "self". This process of immunological defense is referred to as "immunological surveillance."

Impaired Immunological Surveillance Cancer may result when the normally functioning immunological surveillance mechanism is impaired. Malnutrition, age, and chronic disease are examples of conditions that may be factors in

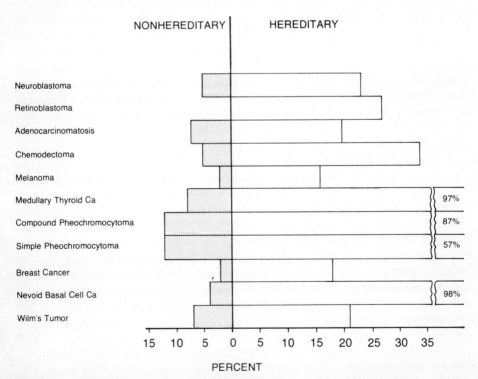

Figure 3-2 The percent frequency of multiple primaries in hereditary and nonhereditary forms of neoplasms. (*Reprinted with permission from David E. Anderson, "The Role of Genetics in Human Cancer," Ca—A Cancer Journal for Clinicians, 24:130–136, May/June 1974, p. 134.*)

the breakdown of the immune mechanism. Weakening of the surveillance system is not, however, considered to be the sole instigator of cancer. Research has indicated that suppression of immunity may facilitate cancer development in patients receiving large quantities of immunosuppressive agents. Kidney transplant patients who receive large quantities of immunosuppressive drugs to prevent rejection of the grafted organ have a higher rate of reticular cell sarcoma, lympholeukosarcoma, or gastrointestinal leiomyosarcoma than does the general population. In addition to suppression of immunity by such preparations, the kidney transplant patient usually tends to suffer from end-stage glomerulonephritis—a chornic autoimmune disease consisting in part of malfunctioning of the immune system.

An impaired immunosurveillance system may also contribute to cancer development by "setting the stage" for other carcinogens to act on an unprotected body. When protection is lowered, chemical or viral carcinogens may have easier access in order to directly foster cancer growth or to activate an inherited tendency for cancer development.

Evolutionary Reversion   Revival of the evolutionary reversion theory of cancer causation has occurred within recent years in conjunction with research being conducted on immunological theories of carcinogenesis. The evolutionary reversion theory maintains that inherent ancestral types of cells are prevented from gaining cellular dominance by a competent immune system. These regressive ancestral cells may overwhelm the rejection ability of the immune defenses when cellular reproduction processes accelerate for all body cells. Cell division may increase as a result of biochemical, radiation, or traumatic irritation or by the action of chemical, thermal, or mechanical agents. The primitive cells theoretically become dominant over the host cells because there is a greater metabolic demand for nutrients. A weakened immune mechanism then may facilitate the establishment of the neoplasm.

According to the evolutionary reversion theory, single as well as multiple tumors may appear when these primitive cells become entrenched in tissue. For example, neonates born with agammaglobulinemia (which includes a defective immune system) have an unusually high incidence of neoplasms such as leukemia and lymphoma. It is hypothesized that the incompetent immune system allows the inherent regressive cells to become established, resulting in cancer growth.

Research into the immunologic theory of cancer causation indicates that defects in the protective system alone or in combination with various carcinogenic agents may play a definitive role in the appearance of certain human cancers.

Hormonal Imbalances

Whether hormonal imbalances brought about by (1) ingestion of hormone preparations or (2) internal changes in the levels of these substances directly cause cancers or establish an environment in which other carcinogens may act has not been determined. Animal research has demonstrated definite relationships between steroid ingestion and the appearance of cancers such as breast carcinoma in male mice. In humans, carcinoma of the liver has been associated with anabolic steroid treatment in a limited number of cases. In addition, correlations have been found between breast cancer in menopausal and postmenopausal women and intake of estrogen supplements. Long-term use (15+ years) of the estrogens correlates with a breast cancer risk twice that found in women not taking such hormonal preparations. Recent evidence suggests that a rare form of vaginal cancer may be linked to maternal intake of diethylstilbestrol prescribed for the prevention of spontaneous abortion. This seemingly very unusual long-term potential effect of a hormonal preparation on offspring indicates a need for careful follow-up of patients receiving such preparations.

Interest in hormones primarily the estrogens and progesterones (the hormones most frequently used by the general public), as potential carcinogens, should continue to receive considerable research attention as the long-term effects of birth control pill ingestion by millions of women become evident.

Chronic Wounds, Trauma, and Precancerous Lesions

The appearance of cancer at the site of chronic wound injury, trauma, or preexisting lesion has been reported in cause-and-effect terms. The exact carcinogenic mechanism is unclear. It has been hypothesized that with the existence of damaged tissue, a "co-carcinogen" may act to initiate a malignant change. In each case, the proportion of persons developing cancer is extremely small, ranging from 0.25 to 2 percent.

Chronic Wounds   Degeneration of a chronic wound to a cancerous state may occur 20 to 40 years after the original injury, depending on the wound. A small percentage of chronic burn wounds may be subject to development of squamous or basal cell carcinoma usually located in lower extremities, on the face, or on the upper extremities. Acute burn scars may give rise to malignant degeneration when the area has exhibited premalignant change prior to the burn. Patients with chronic draining osteomyelitis may develop squamous cell carcinoma in the skin surrounding the sinus or within the drainage tract.

Chronic lower-extremity ulcers may develop squamous cell carcinoma, which tends to occur more often in elderly individuals than in younger persons. Both squamous cell carcinoma and adenocarcinoma have been found in perianal sinuses. Chronic rectal or urinary fistulas and pilonidal sinuses have occasionally degenerated to squamous cell carcinoma.

Several factors have been identified which help to explain the relationship between chronic wound degeneration and malignancy. These factors consist of the following:

1 Burns resulting from certain carcinogenic substances may enhance eventual cancer development.

2   Infection or delayed healing may lower the effectiveness of the immune system.

3   The depth of the wound may be related to the development of cancer; e.g., basal cell carcinoma is more likely to develop following a superficial burn in which sweat glands and their follicles are uninjured.

4   Chronic irritation of chronic wounds may predispose to cancer growth.

5   Trauma to the scar may foster a cancerous degeneration process.

Trauma   The difficulty in attributing causation of cancer to trauma centers on two factors: (1) The cancer may have been present but unnoticed until the time of injury; e.g., a breast mass is identified following chest injury. (2) The cancer development interval between injury and appearance may not coincide with substantiated evidence for the usual developmental time period reported for the particular type of cancer. Nevertheless, cases continue to be reported in which traumatic injury is thought to be the initiator of the disease. To date no experimental evidence exists to support this position.

Coincidental appearance of certain cancers with traumatic injury has occurred. Malignancies commonly reported as having a potential causal relationship with trauma include malignant melanoma, testicular cancer, and bone and soft-tissue sarcomas. It seems clear that the evidence for a trauma theory of cancer causation is at this time largely circumstantial.

Precancerous Lesions   Certain preexisting conditions may precede the appearance of cancers. The progression from a precancerous state to a malignant one is not predetermined by the lesion itself, for not all such lesions inevitably become cancerous. Precancerous lesions that have been associated with progression to malignancy include leukoplakia, and arsenic and senile keratosis. Compound and junctional nevi subject to irritation may be precursors of melanoma. Based on clinical observations, adenomatous polyps of the stomach and gallbladder may also be considered precancerous. Correlation between the appearance of hepatic carcinoma and development of cirrhotic liver changes has been reported but has not been conclusively supported by experimental research. Villous polyps found in the large intestine are considered to be precancerous, and their early removal is usually encouraged if they are easily accessible.

It appears, then, that while various cancers may be correlated with chronic wound degeneration, traumatic injury, or precancerous lesions, definitive cause-and-effect relationships between such conditions and inevitable progression to a malignant state have not been established.

Demographic Variables

The incidence of various cancers is influenced by a number of variables that can be characterized as descriptive in nature. Human characteristics predetermined or subject to individual control may operate to enhance susceptibility to particular cancers. Conclusive statements, however, cannot be made based on present epidemiological evidence.

Age   Cancer can appear at any age. In general, the risk seems to increase with age. The incidence of certain cancers, however, is higher during the first 5 years of life than in the succeeding two 5-year periods. Several cancers are often congenital in nature: Wilm's tumors of the kidney, neuroblastomas, chondromas, and hemangiomas. Leukemia occurs more frequently in the adult years, while Hodgkin's disease appears most commonly during young adulthood.

It is clear that certain types of human cancer occur with greater frequency in certain age groups. These correlations do not support specific cause-and-effect relationships.

Sex   In general, the female cancer rate is slightly higher than that of males. This fact may be attributed to the increase of female lung cancer. Males under 10 years of age have a higher incidence of cancer than do females in the same age group. The incidence of cancer for females between 20 and 60 is higher than for males in the same age group and may partially be attributed to the appearance of uterine and breast cancer during the 35- to 50-year age period. Site-specific cancers for each group differ; e.g., prostate cancer exists in males and uterine cancer in females. Breast cancer is the most common malignancy for females, but has a low incidence among males. For as yet undetermined reasons, the appearance of some cancers seems linked to the sex of the individual.

Behavior Patterns   Smoking is perhaps the most common cancer-related behavior pattern. The causal relationship has repeatedly been demonstrated but continues to be questioned by some researchers. Links between long-term smoking habits and cancer of the esophagus (due to swallowing of the inhaled gases) have tentatively been made. Smoking *does* have a relationship with cancer in that life expectancy is shortened for those who smoke; e.g., smoking 10 cigarettes or less each day may shorten life expectancy by from 2.8 to 4.6 years. As a result of these projections and established risks to human health, cigarette manufacturers have decreased tar content by as much as 60 percent over the past 20 years because tar is considered to have human carcinogenic potential.

Alcoholism and the incidence of certain cancers may be related in a causal fashion. With addition of a correction factor for persons who smoked, research has revealed that some patients with cancer of the esophagus, mouth, hypopharynx, or larynx regularly consumed larger quantities of alcoholic beverages than did control subjects. The incidence of digestive system cancers has been found to be five times more frequent among alcoholics than among the general populations of certain areas. In addition, liver cell cancer frequently arises in cirrhotic livers, a condition found in many alcoholic patients. While a causal link may exist between cancer and alcoholism, it must be remembered that alcoholics may suffer from malnutrition and/or anemia, which may also predispose them to cancer (see Chapter 17).

Alcohol *may* exert a carcinogenic effect in a number of ways:

1 Prolonged tissue contact with alcoholic substances may directly engender carcinogenesis.
2 Alcohol may act in concert with tobacco to initiate cancer development.
3 Drinking of alcohol may establish an environment in which other carcinogens, e.g., viruses, can be effective.
4 The physiological consequences of prolonged drinking, such as malnutrition and poor hygiene, may predispose the body to the growth of cancer.

Culturally defined eating behaviors have been associated with cancer development. For example, oral cavity cancers found in Asiatic populations have been causally linked to the chewing of tobacco and betel nuts. Gastric cancer in Iceland, Chile, and Japan has been associated with high dietary intake of fish, which may contain nitrates. Contamination of food and alcoholic beverages with nitrosamines has been hypothesized to be responsible for the high incidence of esophageal cancer in certain areas of France and Zambia.

Geographic Location Where people live may determine in part the exposure to known or suspected carcinogenic agents. Lung cancer mortality appears to be related to geographic location with an emphasis on the presence or absence of air pollution. Increased levels of organic air pollutants may act as a carcinogenic factor in the higher rates of lung cancer found in urban populations. With occupation and smoking pattern taken into consideration, evidence continues to implicate air pollution as a carcinogen.

Demographic variables undoubtedly play a role in cancer causation. The extent of influence of these descriptive factors, however, can only be hypothesized. Age, sex, behavior patterns, and geographic location probably act in conjunction with one or more suspected carcinogens and a decreased immunosurveillance system in the facilitation of carcinogenesis in susceptible humans.

Psychological Correlates of Cancer Causation

Over the past several years, a number of studies have been conducted which have attempted to identify the role of psychological factors in cancer causation. Results from the studies indicate that the personalities of cancer patients differ significantly from those of persons in the general population. Extreme caution is necessary in evaluating the data obtained. First, the data collection is carried out with cancer patients. The dilemma of "Which comes first, the personality pattern or the cancer?" precludes drawing cause-and-effect conclusions from the information. Second, it continues to be extremely difficult to specify exactly *when* a cancer develops. The disease process may be undetectable for several years. As a result, the cancer may be present as the person's personality characteristics are evolving.

Malignancies reported to correlate with psychological characteristics range from leukemias and lymphomas to uterine and lung cancer. The cancer patient is characterized as being a tense, rigid, inner-directed, and authoritarian person who uses excessive repression of affect as a primary coping style. Patients with rapidly progressing disease tend to be significantly more apologetic, acquiescent, and polite and to be unable to decrease anxiety. Cancer patients who respond well to therapy, who go into remission or who are cured, generally tend to be more expressive.

Events preceding the development of cancer may contribute in some way to development of susceptibility to the disease. These prior life events or personality patterns include the following:

1   Loss of an important relationship or a history of bereavement
2   Unresolved tension or conflict with regard to parental relationships or childhood experiences
3   Inability to express emotions, especially hostile feelings, resulting in a repressive personality pattern
4   Tendency to respond to loss of a significant person or life event (retirement, job loss) with despair, hopelessness, and/or helplessness

These events or personality patterns may influence the ability of the immune system to ward off carcinogens, which in turn are able to initiate carcinogenesis. Evidence indicates that stress and emotional distress may influence the immune system's functioning. The personality characteristics discussed are associated with emotional stress and varying levels of anxiety. Therefore, it is theoretically possible that with a defective immunologic defense system, the presence of stress or emotional upheaval, and a certain personality pattern and coping style, certain persons *may* be more likely to develop cancers than may persons lacking these elements. Controlled prediction studies are needed before confirmation of this hypothesis can take place.

SUMMARY COMMENT

The cause of cancer remains a mystery enshrouded in "possibles," "probables," and "potentials." It seems clear that there is no *single* theory of cancer causation. It is equally clear that the solution to the causation question will be answered only as science seeks to identify the mechanism determining the interaction of a multiplicity of carcinogenic factors both internal and external to the body.

As depicted in Figure 3-3, the possible and partially confirmed carcinogenic factors are numerous. The interaction of factors, and in some cases the *origin* of factors, is unclear. Unraveling this complex puzzle is necessary to truly gain an understanding of the cause of cancer—perhaps humanity's most fearsome disease.

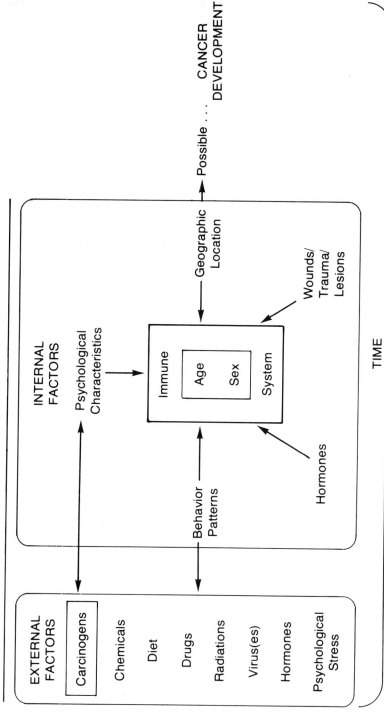

Figure 3-3 Suggested interaction of factors in cancer causation. Partially confirmed and unconfirmed carcinogens influence the internal factors. Age and sex are predetermined, while the immune system is influenced by a number of factors, as indicated by arrows. Psychological characteristics and behavior patterns, in turn, both influence the body while being influenced by external factors. Genetic inheritance overlays all factors. Time for the entire process act as the governing element.

41

BIBLIOGRAPHY

Anfinsen, C. B., Potter, Michael, and Alan N. Schechter (eds.): *Current Research in Oncology 1972,* Academic Press, New York, 1973.

Bahnson, Claus B.: "Psychophysiological Complimentarity in Malignancies: Past Work and Future Vistas," *Annals New York Academy of Sciences,* **164**:319–334, 1969.

Becker, F. F. (ed.): *Cancer 2: A Comprehensive Treatise.* Plenum Press, New York, 1975.

Beland, Irene L., and Joyce Y. Passos: *Clinical Nursing: Pathophysiological & Psychosocial Approaches,* Macmillan, New York, 1975.

Castro, Bruce, and Joseph A. DiPaolo: *Progress in Medical Virology,* **16**:1–47, 1973.

Challis, B. C., and C. D. Bartlett: "Possible Carcinogenic Effects of Coffee Constituents," *Nature,* **254**:532–533, April 10, 1975.

Comings, David E.: "A General Theory of Carcinogenesis," *Proceedings of the National Academy of Sciences USA,* **70**:3324–3328, December 1973.

Epstein, Samuel S.: "Environmental Determinants of Human Cancer," *Cancer Research,* **34**:2425–2435, October 1974.

Fialkow, Philip J.: "The Origin and Development of Human Tumors Studied with Cell Markers," *New England Journal of Medicine,* **291**:26–35, July 4, 1974.

Fortner, J. G., and A. I. Holleb: "Transplantation and Cancer," *CA—A Cancer Journal for Clinicians,* **22**:148–150, May–June 1972.

Graham, William P.: "Malignant Degeneration in Chronic Wounds," *Pennsylvania Medicine,* **76**:65, July 1973.

"Hair Dyes and Cancer," *Lancet,* **2**(7927):218, August 2, 1975.

Hickling, Lee: "Studies Find Cancer Related to Personality," *Honolulu Star-Bulletin & Advertiser,* C-5, December 28, 1975.

Holland, James F., and Emil Frei: *Cancer Medicine,* Lea & Febiger, Philadelphia, 1973.

Hoover, Robert; Gray, Laman A.; Cole, Philip; and Brian MacMahon: "Menopausal Estrogens and Breast Cancer," *New England Journal of Medicine,* **295**(8):401–405, August 19, 1976.

"Immunosuppression and Malignancy," *British Medical Journal,* **3**:713–714, September 23, 1972.

Keller, Mark (ed.): *Alcohol & Health: New Knowledge* (preprint edition), U. S. Government Printing Office, Washington, D.C., June 1974.

King, Brian B.: "Eating Habits Linked to Cancer Development," *Honolulu Star-Bulletin,* 2, July 29, 1975.

Knudson, Jr., Alfred G., Strong, Louise C., and David E. Anderson: "Heredity and Cancer in Man," *Progress in Medical Genetics,* **9**:113–158, 1973.

Leibowitz, Stewart, and Robert S. Schwartz: "Malignancy as a Complication of Immunosuppressive Therapy," *Advances in Internal Medicine,* **17**:95–125, 1971.

Lewinsky, B. S., and D. G. Baker: "The Genetic Control of Immunity and Its Relationship to Carcinogenesis," *Oncology,* **26**:481–494, 1972.

Low, Hans: "Nitroso Compounds," *Archives of Environmental Health,* **29**:256–260, November 1974.

Lynch, Henry T.: "Cancer Genetics, Part I: Historical Background and Animal Studies," *Nebraska Medical Journal,* **58**:360–365, October 1973.

———: "Cancer Genetics, Part II: Studies in Humans," *Nebraska Medical Journal,* **58**:401–407, November 1973.

Magee, P. N.: "Carcinogens in the Environment," *Proceedings of the Royal Society of Medicine,* **67**(8): 741–743, August 1974.

Marcus, Mary G.: "The Shaky Link between Cancer and Character," *Psychology Today,* 52–54, 59 and 85, June 1976.

McAllister, Robert M.: "Viruses in Human Carcinogenesis," *Progress in Medical Virology,* **16**:48–85, 1973.

Meek, Edward S.: "Viruses as Possible Factors in Human Cancer," *Journal of Iowa Medical Society,* **62**:535–538, October 1972.

Monkman, George R., Orwall, Gregg, and John C. Ivins: "Trauma and Oncogenesis," *Mayo Clinic Proceedings,* **49**:157–163, March 1974.

Moore, Condict: *Synopsis of Clinical Cancer,* C. V. Mosby, St. Louis, 1970.

Nizze, Horst: "Exposure to Asbestos and the Genesis of Pleural Plaques and Neoplasia," *Archives of Pathology,* **95**:213–214, March 1973.

Parkes, H. G.: "Occupational Bladder Cancer," *Practitioner, 214*(1279):80–86, January 1975.

Prescott, David M.: *Cancer: The Misguided Cell,* Bobbs-Merrill, Indianapolis, Ind., 1973.

Rapp, Fred: "Herpesviruses and Cancer," *Advances in Cancer Research,* **19**:265–302, 1974.

Richards, Victor: *Cancer: The Wayward Cell,* University of California Press, Berkeley, 1972.

Ryser, Hugues J.: "Special Report: Chemical Carcinogens," *CA—A Cancer Journal for Clinicians,* **24**(6):351–360, November–December 1974.

Scholefield, P. G. (ed.): *Proceedings of the Ninth Canadian Cancer Research Conference,* University of Toronto Press, Toronto, 1972.

Schwind, Justin V.: "Cancer: Regressive Evolution?" *Oncology,* **29**:172–180, 1974.

Shafer, N., and R. W. Shafer: "Potential Carcinogenic Effects of Hair Dyes," *New York State Journal of Medicine,* **76**(3):394–396, March 1976.

Solomon, George F.: "Emotions, Stress, the Central Nervous System, and Immunity," *Annals New York Academy of Sciences,* **164**:335–343, 1969.

Spratt, John S.: "Your Behavior and Cancer," *Missouri Medicine,* **71**:22A–24, January 1974.

Wein, A. J., Graham, W. P., and H. P. Royster: "The Malignant Change in Chronic Wounds," *Industrial Medicine,* **41**(1):12–14, January 1972.

Wurster-Hill, Doris H., Cornwell, Gibbons, G., and O. Ross McIntyre: "Chromosomal Aberrations and Neoplasm—A Family Study," *Cancer,* **33**:72–81, January 1974.

Chapter 4

Pathophysiology of Cancer

LoRaine Carlson and Diana L. Donley

Cancer represents one of the most fundamental and challenging areas for study in the basic biological sciences. It is an area in which the knowledge and skills acquired in many different disciplines will have to be applied if an understanding of the problem is to be achieved.

Cancer is often thought of as a modern disease caused by pollution, chemicals, radiation, or the by-products of industrialization, but it may in fact be one of the most ancient of diseases. Its occurrence has been recorded in the earliest writings of humanity. Hippocrates first used the Greek world *kapklvoo,* which means "crab," to describe the malignancy that spread its pincers throughout the body to choke off life. The word "cancer" is the Latin word for "crab."

Cancer is one of the most widely varying forms of cellular derangement. Cancer, like a crab, ignores straightforward progression in its movement. Instead it progresses sideways in its refusal to behave in a purposeful manner, its need to invade neighboring tissues and to send some of its cells far from its point of origin, that is, to metastasize.

Cancer seems to be a fundamental derangement of the normal mechanisms controlling the rate of growth, division, and migration of cells. The basic nature and origins of cancer are complex and not completely understood. Research has so far shown that more than 100 viruses and over 1000 chemicals are capable of producing cancer in animals when the concentration of these substances is high. The vagaries, manifestations, and courses of the disease and its prognosis are many. In the past 25 years, revolutionary advances in genetics, virology, biochemical studies of protein synthesis, membrane function, and immunology have brought about a set of organizing principles that explain, at least partially, normal and abnormal cell growth and the transfer of hereditable information. Therefore, an explanation of the fundamental biology of the cell is necessary to an understanding of the pathophysiology of cancer.

THE BIOLOGY OF THE NORMAL CELL

To gain an appreciation of cellular biology, one must understand the evolution of life. While explaining the evolution of life would require too extensive an exploration back into time, there are a few principles regarding these origins which seem essential for anyone who desires an understanding of the cancer cell.

"Life" can be defined as the ability of a substance or organism to take in or ingest matter, to utilize energy, to reproduce itself, and to mutate and pass these mutations on to progeny. In nature, such an ability has existed for billions of years. It existed long before the appearance of animal and human species and is thought to have originated with the evolution of large molecules known as "nucleic acids." Nucleic acids form deoxyribonucleic acid (DNA), which is the material genes and chromosomes are composed of, riboxynucleic acid (RNA), and ribosomes. All living cells and organisms must do two things. First, they must transform and transfer energy. Second, they must communicate and transfer information so that reproduction and replication can occur.

Studies of single-celled organisms and of cells growing in tissue cultures yield much information regarding the structure and composition of cells. The cell (see Figure 4-1) is surrounded by a membrane, and the internal constituent of the cell is given the general term "cytoplasm." Many of the structures of the cell are contained in the cytoplasm, and much of the work of the cell occurs here. In the cytoplasm of all dividing cells is the nucleus, which is separated from the cytoplasm by its own membrane, called the "nuclear membrane." Many of the proteins in the cell serve as enzymes that stimulate cellular functions or act as catalysts that speed up and facilitate chemical reactions within the cell. DNA is found only in the nucleus, while RNA is found in both the nucleus and the cytoplasm. Ribosomes are found only in the cytoplasm.

DNA, RNA, and the Formation of Protein

DNA is composed of two strands of protein twisted around each other to form a double helix (see Figure 4-2), while RNA is a single strand of protein. Although there is only one type of DNA, there are three distinct forms of RNA. These are messenger RNA (mRNA), transfer RNA (tRNA), and the ribosome, or ribosomal RNA. Both DNA and RNA are composed of a sugar, four different bases or amino acids, and phosphoric acid. In DNA the sugar is deoxyribose,

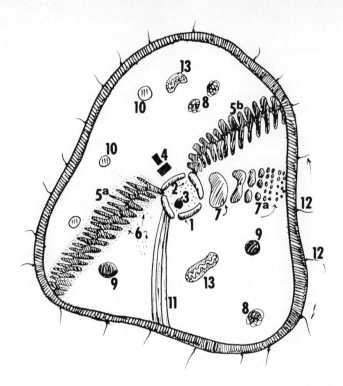

Figure 4-1   The normal cell.
   1   The nucleus is present in all cells that divide. The nuclear membrane folds back upon itself and forms perinuclear cisterns through which various substances move in and out of the nucleus.
   2   Chromatids are loosely coiled strands of DNA plus supporting structures. Genes are present as part of the DNA. When the cell prepares for division, the strands tighten into a coil and are then called "chromosomes."
   3   The nucleolus is a site of RNA storage and may be the site where RNA is transformed into one of the three basic types: tRNA, mRNA, or ribosomal RNA.
   4   The centrioles are located outside the nucleus and are at right angles to each other. These structures move apart and form the mitotic spindle when the cell prepares to divide.
   5   The endoplasmic reticulum (ER) is a complex series of tubules in the cytoplasm and may be either rough (5a) or smooth (5b). A rough ER has ribosomes attached to the membrane and is found in cells that secrete protein. A smooth ER may form protein, but for the cell's own use rather than for secretion, and may be involved in lipid synthesis.
   6   Ribosomes are found on the ER or are free in the cytoplasm and are the sites of protein synthesis.
   7   Golgi complexes are collections of tubules and vesicles. Their functions are (a) to encase the protein in a membrane; this is then called a "zymogen granule" 7(a), which migrates to the cell wall and extrudes its contents; (b) to produce some lysosomes; and (c) to help produce glycoproteins.
   8   Glycogen appears as a dark mass without a coating.
   9   Lipids are larger than zymogen granules and are a solid dark mass.
   10   Lysosomes are the digestive system of the cell; they contain many digestive enzymes surrounded by a protective membrane.
   11   Microtubules have the function of intracellular transport and are involved in cellular division.
   12   Microfilaments are found only in the white blood cells and are used for movement of the cells. They are composed of contractile proteins.
   13   Mitochondria are the powerhouses of the cell and assemble adenosine triphosphate (ATP) for the rest of the cell's needs. It is thought that mitochondria once were viruses that invaded the cell and now aid in cellular life.

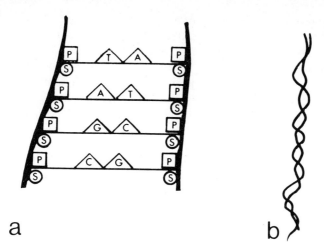

Figure 4-2 Structure of DNA. (*a*) DNA is composed of a sugar (S), a phosphoric acid (P), and a base, or amino acid, represented by the triangles in the center of the chain. (*b*) Each chain of DNA consists of two strands of protein–sugar–phosphoric acid twisted around each other to form a double helix.

while in RNA the sugar is ribose. The amino acids differ in that uracil (U) appears only in RNA and thymine (T) appears only in DNA. The three remaining amino acids, adenine (A), guanine (G), and cytosine (C), are found in both DNA and RNA. Adenine pairs only with thymine to form DNA, but with uracil to form RNA. Cytosine and guanine are always found paired in both RNA and DNA (see Figure 4-3).

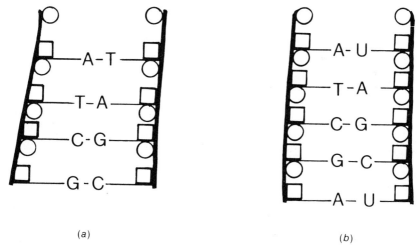

(*a*) (*b*)

Figure 4-3 Structure of DNA and RNA. (*a*) Composition of DNA. (*b*) A strand of mRNA (on the right) is being formed on the DNA template. Note the presence of U in place of T when RNA is formed.

Replication of DNA is accomplished by the separation or unwinding of the two strands. New amino acids migrate in to fill the now vacant spaces, and two new chains of DNA are formed. DNA also serves as a template for the formation of new protein. When a new protein is needed by the body or the cell, the DNA receives a signal to begin its unraveling at a specific point along the chain, so that only a specific number of sites in a specific sequence are exposed. These sites are then paired with the amino acids that compose RNA, and messenger RNA is formed. mRNA is then transported to the cytoplasm through small holes in the nuclear membrane called "perinuclear cisterns." In the cytoplasm, transfer RNA is joined to the mRNA. One function of tRNA will be to help the ribosome release the amino acids to the newly formed chains of protein. The strand of mRNA plus tRNA moves to the ribosome, which "reads" the message on the strand (see Figure 4-4). Each set of three amino acids on the mRNA is called a "codon." Each codon has a significance to the ribosome. Some codons serve to notify the ribosome that a specific amino acid is needed to form the required protein, while others notify the ribosome that the chain of newly constructed protein is completed and may be released. The reason for the existence of the remaining codons has not yet been discovered. These codons are currently referred to as "nonsense syllables."

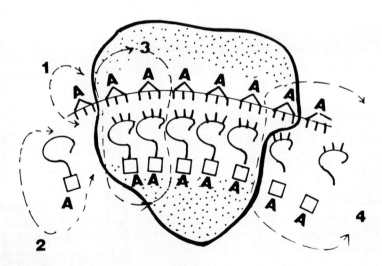

Figure 4-4 Protein formation.
1 Each three amino acids on the mRNA is one codon.
2 Each codon refers to a specific amino acid (A_1, A_2, A_3, A_4, etc.) to be used to construct the new protein.
3 The ribosome "reads" the codon's message and brings in another amino acid on a carrier to fill the space as directed.
4 The carrier protein is released, and the carried amino acid is retained, being added onto the chain to form the new protein.
The dotted area indicates that the entire process occurs *inside* the ribosome.

Genetic Mutations

There are two basic kinds of genetic mutations or errors. Genes are composed of four proteins. A type I genetic mutation occurs when one gene is omitted completely. A type II error is seen when one amino acid is omitted and the new gene or protein is therefore not constructed according to the specifications of the DNA template. The errors may occur at the site of formation of the mRNA, during DNA replication, or in the ribosome. These mutations may be beneficial or harmful or may not be influential at all. The mutation may be retained by the cell or may be destroyed by the cell itself or by the immune system, which usually recognizes such aberrant proteins as foreign to the normal structure of the proteins of that particular individual.

Another type of error has recently been discovered. The type III error occurs when a compound *adds* an additional codon to the mRNA or an additional protein or amino acid to the newly constructed protein. This error occurs in the presence of certain acridine dyes and may be the mechanism of action when viruses cause transformation of a normally innocous bacteria into a virulent bacteria. It is postulated that this third type of error may be the operant factor in the viral induction of cancerous states.

These mutations are of great interest to the cancer researcher, for the cancer cell is a changed cell and does not behave normally. These changes may be the result of a mutation. Cancer may be the direct result of a mutation within the "genome" (or the entire genetic information) of the cellular DNA. But the cell may also be influenced by carcinogenic agents from outside the cell. The origin of cancer may one day be found to be linked to these genomal and extragenomal changes in the normal cell. All the information about cell functions and about life itself is contained in the DNA. But each cell utilizes only the particular information which is necessary for its specific function.

Differentiation

"Differentiation" is the increasing complexity of structure and organization of cells and tissues during development. Thus, several cells may all begin in identical surroundings from identical parent tissues, but as they continue to divide, they become altered so that they no longer closely resemble one another in their mature forms. An example is the blood cells, which all develop from one common stem or parent cell yet vary widely in both appearance and function in their adult or mature state. For some cells and tissues, differentiation is a one-way process, allowing only for increasing differences between these cells of common origin. Yet some cells, such as the immunocytes, may reverse this process and again become immature when additional cells of a specific type are needed. This process of de-differentiation may also be seen in certain types of cancer cells. The de-differentiated cancer cells may be so different from the parent tissues and cells that it is impossible for the pathologist to determine where the site of origin has been. This type of cancer cell may be referred to as an "anaplastic cell" and differs from the parent tissues and cells in both its function and the shape of the cells and tissues.

The essence of differentiation is the choice to activate certain portions of the DNA along the chromosomes and to repress others. The etiology of the "choice" may be chemical, as in chemical carcinogenesis; viral, as in viral carcinogenesis; or unknown. The concept of differentiation has received experimental verification in studies at the Institut Pasteur by François Jacob and Jacques Monod, who won the Nobel prize in medicine in 1965 for their work in differentiation. Jacob and Monod were able to show that cells contain DNA that affects structure and other types of DNA that control function. DNA that controls function has the power to start and stop the activity of the structural DNA and, ultimately, to initiate or prevent the formation of enzymes.

The common theme underlying cellular growth and differentiation is DNA control. Variations on this theme are demonstrated by the presence of specific cellular enzymes; the organization of cells into tissues and tissues into organs; the control of mitosis, aging and death; and the balance between cellular regeneration and destruction. Since the coding of the cell is in its DNA, one gains an understanding of the importance of DNA.

DNA is activiated or destroyed by the chemical messengers voyaging within and around the cell. Extracellular or environmental factors also control the hereditary information, as is seen in the adoption of the chemicals and bacterial products that can cause mutations of the cell. Thus differentiation is the result of complex intracellular and extracellular interactions of DNA and its products, the body proteins and enzymes. Tissues and organs are sensitive targets of chemical messengers, or hormones, and therefore are susceptible to a variety of alterations from these combined effects.

Each cell and each tissue has the potential for specific self-replacement and for differentiation. In humans and animals there are potentials for breakdowns in the DNA control mechanism. If control DNA does not properly direct the structural genes, it is possible that ultimate deterioration of cell function and differentiation will occur and result in cancer. When there is a breakdown in tissue homeostasis, (i.e., in its essential stability), a wayward cell appears. If the wayward cell is not eliminated by the immune surveillance system, the process becomes carcinogenesis, with its single most important characteristic being abnormal cell growth. Since cancer is a disease of the cell, it is equally capable of expression in all higher organisms.

THE BIOLOGICAL NATURE OF THE CANCER CELL

Cancer can arise from a normal useful cell anywhere in the organism. Whereas normal cells divide and stop dividing after a certain size has been reached, cancer cells do not. Their proliferation occurs in an anarchistic fashion. What seems to complicate the matter is that there is limited knowledge of how a normal mammalian cell is notified to stop dividing. Bacterial cells and viruses continue growth until their sources of food and energy are exhausted or until they are destroyed by their own toxic products, but normal mammalian cells must live in balance. While the balancing factors are not known, researchers postulate they may be immunologic in nature or may be the result of the functioning of the regulator, or control, DNA, or may result from contact inhibition.

Researchers have established that there is communication between normal cells by inserting a microelectrode into one cell and another microelectrode into an adjacent cell and observing the passage of an electric current. This electric current is an ion flux, or the movement of electrically charged atoms, and is essential for normal intercellular communication. When the same procedure is repeated with cancer cells, one discovers that a high resistance to the ion flux is present. Thus, the cancer cells do not communicate normally.[1]

If normal cells are placed on a glass surface, they stop moving and growing only when they are in direct contact. It is presumed that this contact is a type of communication that inhibits further growth, and it is called "contact inhibition." If cancer cells are placed on a glass surface, however, they do not stop moving and dividing when they touch another cell. While normal cells grow in vitro on solid surfaces in single layers, cancer cells show less affinity for the solid surface and grow in irregular masses several layers deep. This type of growth indicates that there must be some disturbance in the normal communication between cancer cells. The cancer cell, then, does not act as part of a system, but rather operates independently of the laws that govern normal cellular growth. This tendency to operate independently is called "autonomy" and is considered to be the most important single characteristic of cancer, since without it there could be no cancer growth.

The inability of the cancer cell to control itself in relation to its neighbors is also manifested in the ability of cancer cells to disseminate. Normal cells adhere to one another and have a "home" of their own. A kidney cells stays in the kidney and a lung cell in the lung unless tissue integrity is disrupted by surgery or trauma. Even then, should these cells gain access to the bloodstream and be disseminated, they are incapable of growth in other than their own particular tissues, while the cancer cell may grow anywhere. Cancer cells may be said to belong nowhere and to have no proper residence. This characteristic is extremely puzzling to the scientist, for in comparing the chemical composition of normal cells to that of cancer cells, one sees the same components, although in slightly different amounts and relationships. For example, the DNA content of a cancer cell is greater than that found in a normal cell. At present, cancer cannot be explained on the basis of chemical differences alone. Perhaps when more is known about the bases, or amino acids, and their exact sequence, more light may be shed on the functioning of the normal cell, and the significance of the differences between normal and abnormal cells may be seen more clearly and understood.

Cancer, once induced experimentally in animals by carcinogens, undergoes the transformation from normal to malignant, and the succeeding generations are malignant also. This is true only at the cellular level, for a mother cannot transmit cancerous cells or cancer, except in very unusual circumstances, to her unborn child. In general, cancer cells remain cancerous. They do not revert back to a normal state, and when a person is "cured" of cancer, the cancerous cells have died rather than returned to normal. Theoretically, it is possible that the transformation could be reversed, but the secrets involved in the reversal of the cancerous state are not yet known.

Invasiveness and Malignancy

Two clinically important characteristics that distinguish malignant from benign tumors are the abilities of the former to (1) invade underlying tissues and (2) detach small groups of cells from the tumor mass which then move through the blood and/or lymph channels to distant sites where the cells may grow and new tumors may arise. It is this capacity of malignant cells to become widely disseminated in a host that makes cancer such a dangerous and often incurable disease.

Certain tumors of the endocrine glands (e.g., islet cell tumors and adrenal and extra-adrenal chromaffin tissue tumors) may be highly toxic or even lethal when only microscopic in size, because of an excessive secretion of their specific hormones. Such tumors may show limited cell division and may not invade or metastasize during the early period of their development. These tumors are malignant not in the sense of invasion or metastasis, but in the sense that they may kill their hosts by secreting of lethal amounts of their products, the hormones, while still localized. When examined by a pathologist, these cells do show reversion to the de-differentiated state associated with cancer. Other types of tumors, while benign both in the cellular appearance microscopically and in their inability to metastasize, may be malignant by virture of their location. If the tumor presses against essential nerves, arteries, veins, or other vital structures, its pressure is injurious to the body and therefore may be termed malignant.

Certain cancers invade local tissues but rarely metastasize, while others metastasize widely despite a minimum of local invasion at the original site. Other cancers can be transplanted but do not commonly invade or metastasize. Instead, they continue to grow autonomously, reach a huge size, and ultimately cause death by simply overwhelming their hosts (see Figure 4-5).

Oncogenesis is now known to be, in many instances, a multistep process that progresses in a series of continuous or gradual changes from the benign to the malignant state. It may also progress in a series of discontinuous or abrupt changes. Foulds[2] has proposed a set of six general principles underlying this phenomenon, which he calls "tumor progression." (Tumor progression may also be the term used to refer to the natural course of a specific cancer.) Foulds's principles may be explained by using the following example. First, a chemical carcinogen may convert normal cells into tumor cells that do not immediately proliferate into a cancerous growth. These tumor cells can then be stimulated by a promoter, or co-carcinogen, such as croton oil or other chemicals, to develop into a cancerous growth. Each stage in the multistep process may be facilitated by specific chemicals that may not be active as promoters at other stages in the process. This is an example of the gradual changes that may occur. In other instances, the transformation of the normal cell into a fully autonomous, rapidly growing cancer cell appears to occur as a single step, as is represented by the discontinuous, or abrupt, theory of cancer progression.

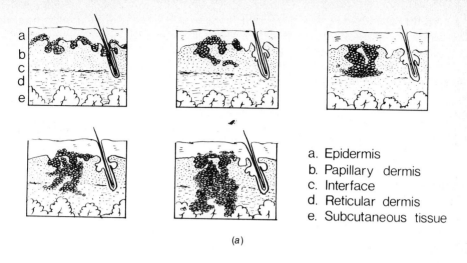

a. Epidermis
b. Papillary dermis
c. Interface
d. Reticular dermis
e. Subcutaneous tissue

(a)

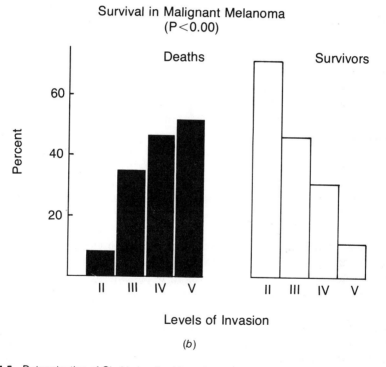

(b)

Figure 4-5 Determination of Clark's levels of invasion requires recognition of the interface of the papillary and reticular dermis, a histologic landmark that is sometimes difficult to identify in skin from the elbow, knee, palm, sole, subungual area, or vulva. The difficulty most frequently encountered when using Clark's levels is in distinguishing a deep level II from a level III lesion. (a) Clark's levels of invasion in cutaneous malignant melanoma. (b) Comparison of levels of invasion and survival for 208 cases of cutaneous malignant melanoma. (*Reprinted with permission from W. H. Clark, L. From, E. A. Bernardino, and M. C. Mihm, Jr., "The Histogenesis and Biologic Behavior of Primary Human Malignant Melanomas of the Skin," Cancer Research, 29:705–726, 1969.*)

Learning about properties of cancer cells may offer new ways to control cell growth. For example, invasion may occur because the extracellular matrix, which cements normal cells together, is destroyed by cancer cell enzymes. The surface of the cancer cell is altered from that of a normal cell, and so cell-cell interactions are altered as well. One result of this alteration, as alluded to previously, is that cell motility continues after the cells contact each other, instead of being inhibited. Researchers are now trying to determine the biochemical nature of the cell-surface structural alterations that are involved in implantation. This discovery may lead to ways of blocking implantation of circulating malignant cells and preventing their colonization of previously uninvolved areas.

MECHANISMS OF METASTASIS

Cancer can be spread by the circulation of the blood or of the lymph.

Entry of the Malignant Cell into the Blood

The malignant cell may enter the blood circulation in one of four ways:

1 Intravasation of free malignant cells through a blood vessel wall can occur, particularly through the capillary plexus of the organ(s) in which the cancer is growing.
2 Cells may become detached from a cancer that invades a vein in which circulation is still present.
3 Cancer cells may pass from the lymphatic system draining the cancerous area or from lymph nodes that contain metastases.
4 Free malignant cells may pass from the peritoneal cavity to the blood if there is an intra-abdominal tumor.

A combination of more than one means of bloodstream entry could occur in the same person.

Venous Invasion   The phenomenon of venous invasion by cancer occurs frequently and is responsible for the majority of blood-borne metastases. The clusters of cancer cells occasionally found in peripheral blood and circulating, large, malignant emboli are almost certainly a consequence of venous invasion. Surgeons and pathologists first noted the invasion of veins by cancers over a century ago, and so it is not a recent finding. Venous invasion bears a definite relationship to the type of cancer, its method of and potential for spread, and the prognosis. Most evaluative data on this type of relationship are found in the histories of carcinoma of the colon and rectum, possibly because the venous drainage of such cancers may be followed more easily and so may be compared with other statistics.

The actual detachment of malignant cells from a mass of neoplastic tissue invading a vein depends on the size of the vein and the rate of blood flow. A large vein with a rapid flow is more likely to be the site of detachment than is a small vein with a sluggish flow. The degree of intercellular adhesiveness of the cancer cells plays an important part also.

Intravasation "Intravasation" is defined as the passage of malignant cells from extravascular tissues into the bloodstream through defects in the vessel wall. It usually occurs when the extravascular pressure is greater than the intravascular pressure. There need be no actual invasion of the vein wall by the cancer. The tissue pressure in cancer is considerably greater than that of normal tissue and may well exceed the pressure in the veins. Under certain conditions, then, malignant cells may pass through the wall of a vein by direct intravasation. These conditions could include pressure on the tumor mass arising from such occurrences as manipulation during surgery, pathological fractures, or movement that puts pressure on the tumor mass. The raised extravascular pressure may collapse the walls of the blood vessels in the vicinity of the cancer by mechanical pressure, thereby diminishing the blood supply to and from the tumor.

Deposition of Cancer Cells into the Bloodstream through the Lymphatics Lymph channels communicate directly with veins in many locations. When lymphatic spread occurs as far as the thoracic duct, a source of blood-borne dissemination is produced. In cases of gross invasion of the thoracic duct, pulmonary metastases are almost invariably present.

Intra-abdominal Cancers and Bloodstream Invasion Although there is no direct evidence that malignant cells in the peritoneal cavity can pass directly into the bloodstream, Baum[3] has shown that some abdominal lymphatic channels communicate directly with veins. Therefore, this mode of metastasis is not proven but is highly probable.

Routes of Dissemination

The usual routes of dissemination of detached tumor cells are through the lymphatic vessels or blood vessels as emboli, through serous cavities, and occasionally by transport in the spinal fluid or through hollow structures such as the bronchi or ureters. The lymphatic vessels are the most common route of dissemination for carcinomas, while sarcomas favor the venous route. Once cancer cells invade lymphatic vessels, they detach to become emboli, or they may form a continuous growth in the vessel itself. The latter mechanism is known as "lymphatic permeation" and usually accounts only for the local spread of the disease. The more common process is for detached cancer cells to be carried as emboli to the peripheral sinus of a regional lymph node, where the cancer cells multiply and invade the lymphoid pulp and supporting stroma. Thus, the entire lymph node gradually becomes completely replaced and considerably enlarged by the metastatic cancer. With a knowledge of the primary site, the most likely sites and distribution of lymph metastases can be surmised. Cancer of the breast, for example, metastasizes to the axillary lymph nodes, and cancer of the scrotum to the inguinal lymph nodes. Because of the vagaries of lymphatic flow or obstruction, metastasis in a distant or unusual site may occur.

Metastasis through blood vessels is the common route for sarcoma dissemination, but carcinomas frequently metastasize that way as well. Certain carcinomas, such as those of the lung, breast, kidney, prostate, and thyroid, are particularly likely to show blood-borne metastasis. Once the cancer cells from the main cancer mass have invaded blood vessels, they may detach as tumor emboli, either as single cells or, if a thrombus forms around them, as cellular aggregates of various sizes.

Cell Embolism

Cancer cells embolize as all emboli do in that they are transported through their respective vascular systems. Cancers of organs that normally drain into the portal vein system tend to metastasize to the liver. Cancers of organs draining into systemic veins tend to metastasize to the lungs. Since it is easier for cancer cells to invade veins and venules than to invade arteries or arterioles, metastasis by the arterial route is of less significance than that by the venous route except in the case of cancer of the lungs or in secondary brain tumors. Just as with lymphatic metastasis, blood-borne metastases may at times appear at unusual sites because of retrograde metastasis following venous obstruction or aberrant vascular anastomoses.

The metastasis represents a colony from the primary tumor; therefore it usually resembles the primary mass in color, consistency, and microscopic appearance. Although the metastasis may be less differentiated than the parent tumor, the histologic resemblance is usually such that it is possible to estimate the nature and growth of the primary cancer from a microscopic study of the metastasis.

How Many Cells Are Needed for Metastasis?

What is the number of circulating cells necessary for metastases to be established? Although the transmission of leukemia in animals has been accomplished by injection of a single malignant cell, there is no evidence that a solid tumor can be transplanted by intravenous injection of one cell. All available information suggests that a considerable number of circulating cells must be present before the cells can grow in previously unaffected tissues. The higher the number, the greater the likelihood of growth. In experimental animals, the percentage of "takes" increases in proportion to the number of injected cells, and there must be a high number of cancer cells circulating for metastasis to occur. The question of whether individual cells or small clusters of cells are more effective in the establishment of metastases has not yet been resolved. Factors enhancing the establishment of metastatic growth are trauma, physical agents, chemical agents, metabolic stress, and decreased host immune resistance to the establishment of blood-borne metastases.

The fate of cancer cells circulating in the bloodstream has yet to be completely explained. The presence of circulating cells at the time of a mastectomy, for example, does not correlate with recurrence of disease, metastases, or the length of life after surgery. In the majority of patients, the malignant cell does not give rise to secondary cancer sites simply because it is circulating. It should be noted, however, that cancers take many years to make their presence known, and such may also be the case with metastases. The disease-free interval that is considered to indicate a curative effect of breast cancer surgery was formerly 5 years; now it is 10 years.

CLASSIFICATION OF CANCER

While the word "cancer" is used to describe the invasive or malignant properties of this pathologic process, each type of cancer may be seen as a different disease because of the variations in causation, multiplication and spread of cells, treatment, and prognosis. Thus, classification of cancer is no easy task. Many classifications have been proposed. Although some fragments of them persist, most are of limited or no practical use. Classification of cancers on a basis of site of origin or of the substances they produce has seldom been satisfactory. When the classification is based on etiology, the problems are that (1) the etiology of most cancers is poorly understood; (2) the same agent may produce cancers of several different types; (3) cancers that are exactly alike morphologically and clinically may be induced by completely different agents; and (4) once a cancer has developed, the agent is usually no longer necessary for its continued growth. The classification is therefore usually a combination of two approaches. One is based on the histogenesis, or the presumed tissue of origin, and the second on the anticipated behavior of the cancer.

The histologic, or cytologic, classification is made after microscopic examination of the cancer has been done and the tissues or cells from which the neoplasm seems to arise or of which it consists are recognized. This method is particularly useful for cancers arising from tissues that are themselves distinct, but minor difficulties arise because some normal tissues are difficult to classify according to this method. Problems also arise when only a metastatic lesion is present for the diagnosis and the cells are so de-differentiated that the site of origin cannot be distinguished.

The second method of classifying cancers considers the known or anticipated biologic behavior. Tumors are classified as neoplasms, which are then designated as benign or as malignant. The latter are rapidly growing and destructive tumors. This type of classification is illustrated in Table 4-I.

GRADING AND STAGING OF CANCER

Grading

An estimate of the degree or grade of malignancy of a cancer may be useful for prognosis and for determining the type of treatment, as in Hodgkin's disease. Cancers in some locations may be graded roughly by their appearance. More

Table 4-1   Benign/Malignant Classification of Cancers

Tissue	Benign tumor	Malignant tumor
Connective tissue		
Adult fibrous tissue	Fibroma	Fibrosarcoma
Embryonic fibrous tissue	Myxoma	Myxosarcoma
Cartilage	Chondroma	Chondrosarcoma
Bone	Osteoma	Osteosarcoma
Fat	Lipoma	Liposarcoma
Muscle		
Smooth muscle	Leiomyoma	Leiomyosarcoma
Striated muscle	Rhabdomyoma	Rhabdomyosarcoma
Endothelium		
Lymph vessels	Lymphangioma	Lymphangiosarcoma
Blood vessels	Hemangioma	Hemangiosarcoma
Lymphoid tissue	Nonrecognized	Lymphosarcoma
Bone marrow	Nonrecognized	Leukemia
Neural tissue		
Nerve sheath	Neurilemmoma	Neurogenic sarcoma
Glial tissue	Glioma (rare)	Glioma
Primitive nerve cells	Nonrecognized	Neuroblastoma
Epithelium		
Squamous epithelium	Papilloma	Squamous cell carcinoma (epidermoid carcinoma)
Transitional epithelium	Papilloma	Transitional cell carcinoma
Glandular epithelium	Adenoma	Adenocarcinoma
Liver cells	Benign hepatoma	Malignant hepatoma
Sweat glands	Hidradenoma	Hidradenoid carcinoma
Islets of Langerhans	Islet cell adenoma	Islet cell carcinoma
Miscellaneous		
Placental trophoblasts	Hydatid mole	Choriocarcinoma
Totipotential cells	Benign teratoma	Malignant teratoma

*Since there are almost limitless varieties of tumors, a complete table of classification would require many pages. Any shortened version is not only necessarily incomplete, but also likely to be confusing. This classification is meant only to show some examples and to be a general guide to nomenclature. Extensive classifications of tumors of respective organs and tissues, including synonyms, and related terms, are presented particularly well in the various fascicles of the *Atlas of Tumor Pathology* published by the Armed Forces Institute of Pathology.

    Source: William A. Meissner and Shields Warren, "Neoplasma," in W. A. D. Anderson (ed.), *Pathology*, 6th ed., vol. I, C. V. Mosby, St. Louis, 1966, p. 403.

frequently they are graded microscopically, with two factors being considered: first, the degree of anaplasia or of de-differentiation of the cancer cells, and second, an estimate of the rate of growth. Customarily, cancers are graded into three or four grades, with the lower grades implying a lesser degree of malignancy. Evidences of differentiation are based on the resemblance of the cancer cell to the normal cell prototype. For example, a well-differentiated cancer arising from squamous epithelium would be expected to form considerable amounts of keratin and intracellular bridges. One method of estimation of rapidity of growth is based on the number of mitoses per unit of tissue and on the presence of nuclear chromatin.

Although grading of cancers is a fairly common practice, it has limited clinical usefulness because of several difficulties. While generally cancers are uniform throughout the mass in histologic appearance, others may vary considerably from portion to portion. The edges of a large tumor are frequently better nourished than the core, and the core may become necrotic because of poor circulation. Thus, a biopsy from one region could give a false impression of the degree of malignancy in another area. The estimation of degree of malignancy must also take into consideration the primary site of the cancer. The grading standards that prove satisfactory for epidermoid carcinoma of the lip would be unsatisfactory for the grading of epidermoid carcinoma of the bladder.

Staging

Staging is the evaluation of the extent of a cancer, usually based on gross and clinical findings. It is independent of the grade of the cancer. Staging is a useful method of describing the extent of an individual cancer at a given time.

A new approach toward a classification system for malignant tumors is evolving from the work of the International Union Against Cancer and the American Joint Committee for Cancer Staging and End Stage Reporting. The designations T for primary tumor, N for regional lymph nodes, and M for metastasis are used in this system. Subscripts are used to describe the progression of the disease and the presence or absence of metastasis. TIS denotes tumor in situ. T_1, T_2, T_3, and T_4 describe the increase in tumor size. N_0, N_1, N_2, and N_3 describe the advancing modal involvement. M_0, M_1, M_2, and M_3 describe the advancing mestastases. Clinical staging is determined by evaluation of the cancer at accessible sites such as the cervix, skin, or tongue. Surgical procedures and biopsies allow for surgical staging (see Table 4-2.)

Table 4-2   TNM Staging System

Tumor	
TO	No evidence of primary tumor
TIS	Carcinoma in situ
T1 T2 T3 T4	Progressive increase in tumor size and involvement
T	Tumor cannot be assessed
Nodes	
NO	Regional lymph nodes not demonstrably abnormal
N1 N2 N3	Increasing degrees of demonstrable abnormality of regional lymph nodes. (For many primary sites, the subscript "a," e.g., N1, may be used to indicate that metastasis to the node is not suspected, and the subscript "b," e.g., N1, may be used to indicate that metastasis to the node is suspected or proved.)
NX	Regional lymph nodes cannot be assessed clinically
Metastasis	
MO	No evidence of distant metastasis
M1 M2 M3	Ascending degrees of distant metasis, including metastasis to distant lymph nodes

Source: Reprinted with permission from the American Joint Committee for Cancer Staging and End Results Reporting, "Clinical Staging System for Carcinoma of the Esophagus," *Cancer*, March—April 1975, pp. 25-51.

SUMMARY

Cancer is a disease that begins on a cellular level and shows its effects throughout the body of the individual. This chapter has described the development of the normal cell and how it differs from the cancer cell. It is clear that while many advances in knowledge in these areas have been made, the total picture is as yet unseen. Mechanisms of dissemination have also been discussed; again the current level of knowledge precludes a comprehensive discussion of all the mechanisms involved. The difficulties in grading and staging have been discussed, and the most recent staging efforts have been presented.

It is emphasized to the reader that the information in this chapter cannot give definitive answers to all the questions that remain in the reader's mind, simply because the answers to these questions remain unknown. The current level of scientific knowledge does present a theory of cancer development and progression, but until the cause(s) of the disease are found and the methods for treatment become much more effective, some areas must remain unclear.

REFERENCES

1   Lowenstein, W. R., and Y. Kanno: "Intercellular Communication and the Control of Tissue Growth: Lack of Communication between Cancer Cells," *Nature*, **209**:1248–1249, 1966.
2   Foulds, L.: "Tumor Progression and Neoplastic Development," in *Cellular Control Mechanisms and Cancer*, London, Elsevier Publisher, 1964.
3   Baum, H.: "Konnen Lymphgefasse Direkt in das Venensystem Binmunden?" *Anat. Anz.*, **49**: 407, 1916

BIBLIOGRAPHY

American Joint Committee for Cancer Staging and End Results Reporting: "Clinical Staging System for Carcinoma of the Esophagus," *Cancer*, March–April 1975, pp. 25–51.
Bales, H. W., and J. D. Norante: "Head and Neck Tumors," in P. Rubin (ed.), *Clinical Oncology*, 4th ed., New York, American Cancer Society, 1974.
Billroth, S.: "Zur Entwickelungsgeschechte und Chirurgischen Bedeutung des Hodencystoids," *Virchows Arch. Path. Anat.*, **8**:268, 1955.
Braum, A. C.: *The Biology of Cancer*, London, Addison-Wesley, 1974.
Clark, W. H., L. From, E. A. Bernardino, and M. C. Mihm, Jr.: "The Histogesesis and Biologic Behavior of Primary Human Malignant Melanoma of the Skin," *Cancer Research*, **29**: 705–726, 1969.
Emerson, G., and C. Phillips: "Lung Cancer," in P. Rubin (ed.), *Clinical Oncology*, 4th ed., New York, American Cancer Society, 1974.
Ganong, W. F.: *Review of Medical Physiology*, 7th ed., Los Altos, Calif., Lange Medical Publications, 1975.

Griffiths, J. D., and A. J. Salsbury: *Circulating Cancer Cells,* Springfield, Ill., Charles C Thomas, 1965.

Richards, V.: *Cancer, The Wayward Cell,* Los Angeles, University of California Press, 1972.

Rigas, D. A.: "Purefication and Properties of the Phytohemagglutinin of Phaseolus Vulgaris," *American Journal of Medicine,* **10**:776, 1951.

Part Two

The Role of the Nurse in Cancer Management

Chapter 5

Nursing Assessment of the Oncology Patient

Diana L. Donley

Nursing assessments are a part of the nursing function. No one on the health care team spends more time with the patient than the nurse does. Therefore, nurses are in a unique position to assess the condition of the patient frequently, to observe small clues to changes in condition, and to intervene before a small problem becomes a major crisis.

All patients undergo changes from day to day and even from hour to hour. Some changes are expected and can therefore be planned for, so that minimal disturbance occurs to the patient's physiologic or psychologic equilibrium. The goal of nursing assessment is not to make medical diagnoses, but rather to differentiate the normal from the abnormal, to make nursing diagnoses, and thereby to plan effective nursing interventions. The nurse's observations are essential to aid the physician in distinguishing between effects of the cancer treatment, progression of the disease, and the identification of a new, recurrent, or coexisting illness.

Assessments are not limited to taking the history and physical examination or to the initial patient interview. Assessment is a process that is begun when the nurse first meets the patient and continues each time there is nurse-patient interaction, no matter how brief the interaction may be. Psychological assessments require the nurse's alertness to the verbal and nonverbal cues the patient gives and continues as an ongoing process as well.

This chapter will focus on the identification of problems specific to the cancer patient. The techniques of history taking and physical examination will be reviewed, and an introduction to differential diagnoses will be given. Since laboratory data often give valuable clues to the patient's condition and can indicate the nursing approach to be taken, this area will also be explored.

Although the nurse may study many texts and articles, these sources can only guide the nurse as to what states the patient may experience and are no substitute for direct patient observation. As Yogi Berra once said, "You can observe a lot by just watchin'." The cancer patient benefits from a lot of "watchin'."

THE NURSING HISTORY

The initial nursing history should include the chief complaint—that which caused the patient to seek medical advice or help. It should be followed by a brief sequence of events that seemed to occur with the appearance of the chief complaint. Most institutions provide a space for this information on their admission forms. Later, when the patient is more settled and the nurse is less rushed, a more detailed history can be done. It should be noted that not all the history needs to be done at the same time; as long as a brief admission history is recorded, this may suffice for a day or two. The rest of the data can be collected over a period of days. Doing this avoids taxing the patient's energy and taking a large block of the nurse's time as well.

The initial nursing history should include the chronological sequence of events that caused the patient to seek medical help. Closed-ended questions that lead to a yes-no answer should be avoided. Each complaint should be analyzed via seven dimensions, as listed below.

1 *Location:* Where is the pain?
2 *Quality:* What does the pain feel like?
3 *Quantity:* On a scale of 1 to 7, how strong is the pain?
4 *Chronology:* When did the pain first begin, and how long does it last?
5 *Setting:* What are you usually doing when the pain occurs?
6 *Aggravating or alleviating factors:* What seems to make the pain better or worse? (Stress? Relaxation? Eating? Analgesic?)
7 *Associated symptoms:* What accompanies the pain? (Dizziness? Weakness? Sweating? Vomiting?)

All positive *and* negative findings should be noted to provide a baseline for ongoing assessment.

THE PAST HISTORY

In exploring the past history, ask about the general status of health before this illness began, including childhood illnesses such as rheumatic fever, kidney infections, and mononucleosis as well as the usual infectious diseases. To explore adult health, include medical illnesses, surgery, and psychiatric or emotional disturbances. A brief obstetrical history and accidents, injuries, allergies, and immunizations should be included.

In exploring the family history, include health of the immediate family; age and cause of death of family members; and high-risk, hereditary, or familial diseases, such as tuberculosis, cancer, diabetes, cardiovascular diseases, or hypertension. Ask if any of the family members have had symptoms similar to the patient's in the past.

THE PERSONAL AND SOCIAL HISTORY

The personal and social history should include current life-style, such as home and family and present occupation, since certain occupations carry a higher risk for some diseases. People who work with aniline dyes, for example, are more likely to develop bladder cancer than is the general population. Ask about the economic status, social activities, leisure activities, and patterns of daily living. These include habits of smoking and drinking coffee and alcohol. Sleeping habits should be included. The patient may not have been able to sleep because of pain, dyspnea, or worry. A patient who is unemployed or is receiving some type of government financial assistance may have a diet that is inadequate in vitamins, minerals, and proteins, which could lead to malnutrition and an increased susceptibility to infections. Inquire about the patient's recent life changes and adjustments to them. An unplanned admission for the family breadwinner will cause concern for the economic impact of the illness on the family. Or there could be concern about who will care for the children in the patient's absence and how they will respond to the patient's not being at home. Ask about conflicts in the family. If the nature of the problem is known, the patient can be helped to ventilate instead of being labeled "uncooperative."

THE REVIEW OF SYSTEMS

The techniques used in the previous phases of the history might fail to reveal all-important symptoms, especially if they are remote in time or seem to be unrelated to the present problem. Uncovering these symptoms is one purpose of the review of systems. If a symptom has been dealt with in the previous section of the history, it need not be explored again. The possibility of pain in a system should be explored first, followed by disturbances in functioning. The problems suggested here are the ones more frequently seen in cancer patients.

General: Present weight (loss or gain, period of time, contributing factors), weakness, fatigue, malaise, fever, chills, sweats.

Skin: Pruritis, pigmentary and other color changes, tendency to bruising, lesions (locations), use of hair dyes and other possibly toxic agents (insecticides, etc.).

Head: Headache, head injury (how, when, where), dizziness, syncope.

Eyes: Pain, vision disturbances, diplopia.

Ears: Earaches, hearing disturbances, tinnitus, vertigo.

Nose and sinuses: Sinus pain, epistaxis, nasal obstruction, discharge.

Oral cavity: Mouth pain; soreness of bleeding of lips, gums, mouth, tongue, or throat; disturbance of taste; hoarseness.

Neck: Pain, limitation of motion, thyroid enlargement.

Nodes: Tenderness, enlargement, hardness.

Breast: Pain, lumps, discharge, operations. Does patient do self-exam, and how often?

Respiratory: Chest pain, pleurisy, cough, sputum (character and amount), hemoptysis, wheezing, shortness of breath, history of tuberculosis or recent contact with it, date of recent x-ray.

Cardiovascular: Precordial or retrosternal pain or distress, palpitation, exertional dyspnea, edema, nocturia, cyanosis, hypertension, anemia, date of last EKG.

Gastrointestinal: Heartburn, postprandial pain or distress, appetite, food intolerance, dysphagia (solids, liquids), jaundice, biliary colic, other abdominal pain, belching, nausea, vomiting, hematemesis, flatulence, character and color of stools (bleeding, melena, clay-colored diarrhea, constipation), change in bowel habits, rectal conditions (pruritis, hemorrhoids, fissures, fistual), ulcer, gallbladder disease, hepatitis, colitis, date of previous x-rays.

Genitourinary:

Urinary: Dysuria, frequency of urination, nocturia, polyuria, oliguria, micturation (hesitancy, urgency, narrowing of stream, dribbling, incontinence), hematuria, pyuria, kidney disease, albuminuria, facial edema, cystoscopy.

Male: Testicular pain, change in size of scrotum, blood in ejaculate, prostatic pain.

Female: Menstrual history if applicable; intermenstrual bleeding, vaginal discharge, complications of childbirth, date of last pap smear.

Sexual: Ask if patient has any concerns he/she would like to discuss. Change in libido; if female, contraceptive methods (type, how long used, problems).

Extremities:

Vascular: Intermittent claudication, thrombophlebitis.

Joints: Pain, stiffness, swelling (note location), gout.

Bones: Pain, fracture.

Muscles: Pain, cramps.

Back: Pain (location and radiation to extremities), stiffness, limitation of motion, sciatica, disc disease.

Central nervous system:

General: Syncope, loss of consciousness, stroke, convulsions.

Mentative: Emotional disorders, mood, orientation, memory disorders, change in sleep pattern, history of nervous breakdown, status of significant relationships.

Motor: Tremor, weakness, paralysis, clumsiness of movement.

Sensory: Radicular or neuralgic pain (head, neck trunk, extremities), paresthesias.

Hematopoietic: Bleeding tendencies (skin, mucous membranes), anemia and treatment, transfusion and blood reaction, blood dyscrasia, exposure to toxic agents or radiation.

Endocrine: Thyroid function, diabetes or its symptoms (polyuria, polydipsia, polyphagia).

PHYSICAL ASSESSMENT

The physical assessment of the patient can be accomplished using the head-to-toe approach. As with the nursing history, the physical assessment does not have to be accomplished all at one time. On admission, the nurse may examine only the areas in which the patient experiences discomfort. The remainder of the exam may be done at a later time as the nurse feels is appropriate. The nurse may easily incorporate many of the techniques into the daily routine by performing them at the time of the bath.

Psychological and Cognitive Functions

The cognitive function may be evaluated by observing if the patient is alert, normally cooperative, and oriented in four spheres (time, place, person, and purpose). If there is euphoria or depression, it will be evident. Mental capabilities may be evaluated as the nurse continues to communicate with the patient, and explanations can be given at the patient's level of understanding. If the patient is outgoing, friendly, withdrawn, or suspicious, these characteristics will be noticed. A later change in this status could be caused by a drug reaction, a reaction to the diagnosis, a change in electrolyte balance, or brain metastasis.

Skin

In examination of the skin, look for rashes or infections. While rashes could result from an allergy, they also could be due to chemotherapy or radiation or to emotional conditions. Persons who have severe rashes may have to have chemotherapy or radiation therapy postponed until the rash has cleared. Infections can indicate a depressed immune system and may mean that chemotherapy or immunotherapy will have to be postponed so that septicemia will not result.

Is the skin dry and flaky? Uremia and hypothyroidism are two conditions that could cause this type of skin. Are bruises or petechiae present? If so, these symptoms could indicate low platelet counts due to bone marrow suppression by cancer or its treatment, or they could mean that a liver disease is interfering with clotting mechanisms. There might also be a defect in capillary walls due to leukemia, vitamin deficiency, hemophilia, or low serum calcium. Abnormal skin sensations, such as itching, may be indicative of kidney or liver disease or may be symptoms of local pain. If the latter is true, scratching may relieve the pain as well as the itch. On occasions, pruritis is an unconscious attempt to relieve a deeper pain, whether physical or psychological. Other possible causes of pruritis may be eczema, hives, contact dermatitis, chickenpox, diabetes, leukemia, or Hodgkin's disease. The presence of these malignancies is usually accompanied by other symptoms, which will be discussed later in this chapter. Tingling or numbness of the extremities can be caused by drugs or can result from disruption of sensory fibers from the brain, as may occur in leukemic infiltration of the nerves.

Thinning of the skin is common in older patients, owing to the loss of collagen in the tissues, but for a young patient is a sign of malnutrition. Poor skin turgor is a sign of dehydration and indicates that the patient should not be started on the drug cyclophosphamide, since a dehydrated patient tends to have high concentrations of this drug in the kidneys and bladder for long periods. The cyclophosphamide crystals are irritating and can lead to hemorrhagic cystitis when concentrated in the bladder over an extended period. Patients on any type of cancer destruction therapy or those who have advanced disease may also have high uric acid levels, since uric acid is the end product of nucleic acid destruction. These patients should be carefully observed for dehydration, since prolonged episodes of high uric acid levels combined with dehydration tend to lead to uric acid stone formation.

Is the skin hot, as in fever, or clammy, as in shock? Is the skin clean? A person who usually maintains self-care measures but appears to have neglected personal hygiene for the first time could be undergoing a personality change due to disease progression. Conversely, such behavior could be an indication that the patient has become physically incapable of caring for himself or herself. If the person is usually cared for at home by relatives, a change in the home situation may have occurred; this situation will need to be investigated. It is possible that the person's needs exceeded the family's ability to provide care, and outside intervention may be indicated.

Face

What is the expression on the face? Are the emotions expressed there congruent with the verbal messages? Look at the muscle mobility. If it is not equal on both sides, the patient could have Bell's palsy or could have had a cerebrovascular accident (CVA). Persons who have had CVAs are poor risks to receive nitrogen mustard. The vomiting that can accompany this drug can be so severe as to cause a CVA if there is a tendency for this type of occurrence. If it is necessary to give this drug anyway, giving it at night after the administration of a hypnotic and an antiemetic will reduce these adverse reactions.

Eyes

Notice the presence of cataracts. Are the sclera yellow? The patient may have jaundice or simply may have been eating a great many carrots, as "prescribed" by some natural food anticancer diets. Are the conjunctiva red, as in inflammation, or white, as in anemia? Photophobia can result from diseases or from some drugs, such as fluorouracil.

Ears, Nose, and Throat

The nurse will by now know if there are any hearing defects, but should continue to assess for the presence of bleeding or infections of the external ear. Persons who have had allergic rhinitis for many years have thin, gray mucous membranes with a characteristic odor that the patient is unable to smell. If an odor persists after meticulous mouth care, reexamine the nose.

Examine the membranes of the mouth and pharynx. Again, pale colors indicate anemia. Bleeding gums can indicate leukemia, bleeding disorders, periodontal disorders, or vitamin deficiency and may be seen in pregnancy. What is the condition of the teeth? Are there sores in the mouth? Unless the lesions are caused by the cancer itself, as in leukemic infiltration, chemotherapy will not be started in the presence of mouth lesions if the side effect of the drugs to be used is stomatitis.

Neck and Lymph Nodes

Note the position of the trachea. A trachea that is deviated away from the midline could be pushed to the opposite side by a tumor or pulled to the same side by an atelectasis. Jugular venous distention indicates the presence of congestive heart failure and precludes the use of drugs that have this side effect. Palpate for masses in the supraclavicular area, along the sternocleidomastoid muscle, in the posterior cervical chain, and in the submandibular area. Enlarged nodes in the submandibular area are not always significant, as they can be caused by repeated sore throats, postnasal drip, frequent ear infections, etc. Enlarged nodes in the postauricular area are usually due to scalp pathology, while masses in the supraclavicular area usually indicate subclavicular pathology. Enlarged nodes in other areas are significant and may indicate infection or metastases. When enlarged nodes are present and are not due to infection, they will be measured weekly, or at every period of patient observation if the patient is an outpatient. Enlarged nodes in the inguinal region could be the result of repeated insect bites on the lower extremities or of repeated diaper rash as an infant, especially in the young patient. However, they still can indicate the presence of metastases. Enlarged nodes in the axilla may indicate a lymphoma or a breast cancer metastasis.

Heart

In examining the heart, listen for murmurs, gallops, and arrhythmias. Metastasis to the heart occurs rarely but has been seen, especially with melanomas. The symptoms of cardiac metastasis may vary from premature contractions to those of an infarction and are treated in the same manner as cardiac pathology from other sources.

Lungs

The lungs should be checked for rales, rhonchi, and wheezes. The best location from which to hear lung sounds is the back, as the only lobe that can be heard well indeed, the only one that can be heard at all from the front is the right middle lobe. A persisting cough without accompanying rales may signify that a tumor is pressing against a main-stem bronchus, it may mean that an enlarged right atrium is pressing against the recurrent laryngeal nerve, or it may be the first sign that pulmonary fibrosis is occurring. The state of oxygenation is important. Impaired oxygenation may be due to obstruction of a bronchus by a tumor, to a co- or preexisting illness such as emphysema, to occupation of the lungs by a tumor, or to fibrosis due to bleomycin, radiation or other types of therapy. Dyspenea can also occur because ascitic fluid is pressing against the diaphragm and reducing the breathing space.

Breasts

Check the breasts of both males and females, as cancer of the breast can occur in both sexes. Palpate for areas of tenderness. Observe for discharge from the nipples, retraction of the nipple, or orange-peel skin, all indicative of breast cancer. Thickened skin may result from radiation therapy. Even though a breast has been irradiated, cancer can still occur in the same area if the treatment dose was insufficient or can occur on the periphery of the previously treated field. Also, some patients feel unable to tolerate the full course of therapy and so decide to stop therapy before the full course is completed.

Abdomen

To examine the abdomen, first inspect it for girth, measuring it if distention is suspected. Look for obvious masses and pulsations. Next, listen for bowel sounds in all four quadrants. Bowel sounds typically occur at the rate of 5 to 30 per min. More frequent sounds indicate hypermotility, and diarrhea may be expected. If sounds are less frequent, bowel obstruction may be present, since bowel sounds are absent below the area of an obstruction. In addition, the absence of sounds could indicate paralytic ileus or absence of the bowel, as after a colostomy has been performed. A high-pitched whining sound may be indicative of a bowel obstruction.

Percussion is the third maneuver. A dull sound occurs over dense tissue masses and a more hollow one over gas- or fluid-filled areas. Using percussion, one can determine masses and the liver edge in a gas- or fluid-filled abdomen. To complete the examination of the abdomen, palpate, going lightly at first and then more deeply over the abdominal surface. If there is a known area of pain, palpate it last so the patient will not be splinting the abdomen to prevent pain during the examination. Remember to have the patient inhale deeply, with the knees drawn up, and then exhale. The muscles in the abdomen will then be more relaxed. Normally, masses will not be found in the abdomen.

The liver is normally at the margin of the ribs or cannot be felt at all. A liver felt more than two finger breadths below the costal margin could be enlarged because of tumor involvement, cirrhosis, or engorgement from congestive heart failure. The spleen is not normally felt in the abdomen; if it can be felt at all, this may indicate leukemic infiltration. Tenderness in the right upper quadrant may be due to biliary disease, stretching of the liver capsule, or presence of free air in the abdomen.

Genitourinary System

In the male, are the testes and penis normally developed for the patient's chronologic age? If not, an endocrine disorder may be present. Is there any swelling, sense of heat, or tender area? Normally the temperature of the testes is 1° to 2° lower than that of the body, so even moderate warmth may be significant. Is the foreskin easily retractible, or is phimosis present? Cancer of the penis tends to occur more often in uncircumcized males than in circumcized ones. Has incontinence produced irritated areas on the penis?

In the female, check for the presence or absence of a vaginal discharge or odor. A thin, watery discharge indicates trichomoniasis, and a beefy red appearance with a curdlike discharge indicates a monilia infection. Any external prolapse will be obvious. Vaginal and rectal exams are not usually done by the nurse unless the setting is a clinic where the nurse bears responsibility for this part of the examination.

Rectum

Although the rectal exam is seldom part of the screening physical examination performed by the nurse, it frequently is part of the ongoing assessment of the patient. If the ampulla, the area just past the sphincter of the rectum, is dilated in the absence of stool, the patient is usually impacted even if diarrhea, usually the overflow type, is present. External hemorrhoids will be obvious and may make it difficult for the examiner to find the anal opening. If a patient who normally has no problems with evacuation of stool begins to complain of constipation or, more frequently, of urinary difficulties, it may be the first sign of an impending spinal cord compression by a metastatic lesion. This is a surgical emergency, for the compression will result in permanent paralysis if not relieved immediately.

Neurologic Examination

To test gross motor function, ask the patient to move arms and legs. Observe the use of these extremities because the patient may have gross motor function but lack fine motor function because paresthesias or leukemic infiltration in the fingers have occurred. Observe the gait. A patient with a brain lesion will have a loss of function on the opposite side of the body from that of the lesion. Some gait disturbances may be observed as a result of vincristine therapy, since neurotoxicity is one of the drug's major side effects. Impotence can result from the use of this drug in the male patient.

For a more comprehensive discussion of the neurologic exam or of other parts of the examination, the reader is referred to one of the many books listed in the Bibliography.

NURSING DIAGNOSIS

The "nursing diagnosis" is the identification of actual or potential health problems that the nurse is capable and licensed to treat. These health problems include actual or potential disturbances of functions, life patterns or processes, and development. Nurses do not treat these health problems *medically* as do physicians (who perform surgery or initiate radiotherapy, chemotherapy, or immunotherapy). Rather, nurses identify the problem, make the appropriate referral, and initiate the health treatment recognized as beneficial by virtue of their education and experience. For example, nurses can prescribe proper cleansing techniques, use of emollients, and avoidance of irritating foods for the patient who develops stomatitis while on chemotherapy, while physicians prescribe changes in the dose of the chemotherapeutic agents, prescribe or delete other drugs from the treatment regime, and do further definitive studies as indicated.

Once these problems are identified, a nurse must decide when to refer the patient to a physician in accordance with the severity or significance of the sign or symptom. Throughout the course of this chapter, the term "diagnosis" will be used to refer to the nursing rather than the medical diagnosis unless otherwise stated.

Differential Diagnosis

To make the correct diagnosis, plan effective interventions, and make appropriate referrals, the nurse must have basic knowledge in the following areas:

1 Pathophysiology
2 The usual pattern and potential complications of the disease
3 The method of disease treatment to be used and its potential adverse reactions
4 The specific patient's history and assessment

In making a diagnosis, it is most helpful if the nurse can assess the patient as thoroughly as possible, review all possible causes of the sign or symptom, and then plan appropriate action. Actions may vary as the cause of the sign or symptom varies. For example, if the symptom is nausea, the nurse must be certain that anxiety about the effect of therapy is not the primary cause before deciding that an antiemetic medication will relieve the nausea. While use of an antiemetic is appropriate for the control of nausea regardless of its etiology, therapeutic conversation will be of much great benefit to the overly concerned patient than to the patient who has a physiologic reaction to treatment. If damage to the cells lining the gastrointestinal tract is the primary source of the nausea, therapeutic conversation will be of limited value in relief of the symptom.

Progression of cancer can occur in spite of therapy, and the patient can be assessed to determine if it indeed is occurring. By identifying the actual or potential problem, the nurse can point the way for further medical investigation of patient problems. The use of anticancer therapy, regardless of modality, does not preclude the development of a concurrent illness, the recurrence of a preexisting illness, or the progression of cancer, as occurs in cerebral metastasis. Some of the most difficult nursing decisions, therefore, focus on determining the type of observations to be made. Although it is essential for the nurse to be alert for all changes in patient conditions, few nurses feel they have enough time to thoroughly assess a patient's needs or levels of functioning. As a consequence, it may prove useful to consider other diseases or cancer progressions that could cause the observed sign or symptom or to know which area to observe most carefully. Table 5-1 shows the possible diagnoses of a sign or symptom related to the cancer itself, to the cancer therapy, or to the occurrence of a concomitant illness. For specific drugs that can cause each symptom see Table 16-2.

Some causes are more common than others. For example, tension is a much more common cause of headaches, even in the presence of cancer, than is cerebral metastasis. However, if the headache is persistent and is unrelieved by the usual analgesics, one should look further for its etiology. One symptom occurring by itself may not be significant, but its occurrence in a constellation of symptoms may be of increased significance. Each system will be discussed briefly to help the nurse identify the significant symptoms and the constellations in which they may appear. Possible causes of each symptom will be discussed in a descending order of probability of occurrence.

Central Nervous System

Headaches caused by tension commonly occur at the end of the day and persist for periods from several hours to several days. Pain is usually felt as a dull pressure in the frontal area. A brain tumor may cause well-localized pain and is often accompanied by personality changes, with convulsions occurring in nearly one-third of all patients. Confusion, delerium, and coma may occur. It is necessary to make sure that these symptoms are not due to electrolyte imbalance or to renal pathology with accompanying high blood-urea nitrogen levels.

Ears

Tinnitus is a frequent symptom and may be due to abnormalities in the ear, brain, or circulation; to the toxic effects of drugs, such as aspirin, quinine, quinidine, streptomycin, or digitalis; or to a brain tumor. Vertigo may be caused by Ménnière's syndrome or a brain tumor. The occurrence of these symptoms along may be insignificant, but their occurrence in conjunction with headache or sensory and motor disturbances may be indicative of a brain tumor.

Mouth, Nose, and Throat

Gingivitis causes swollen gums and some bleeding, but is seldom associated with pain. The most common causes of gingivitis are diabetes, deficiency of the C and B complex vitamins, and pregnancy. Gingivitis may also be caused by leukemia, which is associated with other symptoms, such as easy bruising, fatigue, anemia, and weight loss.

Table 5-1 Assessment Guide

| Sign or symptom | Cancer-Related Diagnosis | | Concomitant illness (in order of probable occurrence) |
	Cancer therapy	Disease progression	
Anorexia	Chemotherapy, radiotherapy, surgery	Hepatic involvement, advanced cancer. (Meat intolerance may be sign of gastric cancer.)	1 Anxiety 2 Depression 3 Infectious hepatitis 4 Cirrhosis 5 Alcoholism 6 Drug abuse 7 Acute illness 8 Uremia
Excessive thirst	Chemotherapy	Not usual unless there is pancreatic or cerebral metastasis.	1 Diabetes mellitus 2 Diabetes insipidus 3 Dehydration 4 Psychogenic polydipsia
Fatigue	Chemotherapy, radiotherapy, immunotherapy, surgery	Not usually seen until there is advanced stage of disease.	1 Anxiety 2 Depression 3 Chronic illness 4 Thyroid deficiency 5 Acute illness 6 Renal failure 7 Cirrhosis
Fever Acute	Chemotherapy, radiotherapy, immunotherapy	Recurrence of leukemia or lymphoma, especially meningeal leukemia; infections due to immunologic depression (from cancer, nutritional deficiencies, etc.).	1 Acute viral infection 2 Acute bacterial infection 3 Rheumatic fever 4 Phlebitis 5 Myocardial infarction 6 Pulmonary infarction 7 Drug reaction 8 Cerebrovascular accident 9 Transfusion reaction
Chronic or recurrent	Not usually seen	Recurrence of lymphoma, leukemia, or Hodgkin's disease; lung, kidney, liver, or brain metastasis; necrotic core of tumor.	1 Tuberculosis 2 Hidden abscess 3 Infectious mononucleosis 4 Subacute bacterial endocarditis 5 Brucellosis 6 Salmonellosis 7 Chronic phlebitis 8 Chronic infection

Sign or symptom	Cancer-Related Diagnosis		Concomitant illness (in order of probable occurrence)
	Cancer therapy	Disease progression	
Fluid retention	Chemotherapy	Protein deficiency due to advanced cancer, malnutrition, absorption defect; hepatic involvement; ovarian or mesenteric metastases; congestive heart failure; myocardial metastasis.	1 Birth control pills 2 Excessive salt/sodium intake 3 Hot weather 4 Congestive heart failure 5 Protein deficiency 6 Malnutrition 7 Renal failure 8 Cirrhosis 9 Pregnancy
Insomnia	Chemotherapy	Chronic pain, chronic cough, nocturia, orthopnia, thyroid involvement.	1 Anxiety 2 Depression 3 Chronic illness 4 Urinary tract disease (nocturia, pain) 5 Congestive heart failure (orthopnia, dyspnea) 6 Hiatus hernia 7 Drug reaction
Weight loss	Chemotherapy, radiotherapy (seldom seen with either), post-surgery	Hepatic involvement, gastric involvement, advanced cancer, thyroid cancer.	1 Diabetes mellitus 2 Hyperthyroidism 3 Renal failure 4 Emotional disturbance 5 Infectious disease 6 Chronic gastrointestinal disturbance

The tongue may become sore in response to chemotherapeutic agents, chemical or thermal irritants, deficiency of the C and B complex vitamins, anemia, prolonged use of antibiotics, or thrush (oral candidiasis).

Nosebleeds are caused most commonly by allergies due to changes in the oral muscosa), the common cold, trauma, or high blood pressure. A nosebleed may be the most obvious symptom of the bleeding tendency accompanying leukemia or thrombocytopenia. Usually when pathognomonic of the last two conditions the nosebleed will be accompanied by bleeding of the gums and/or

Chronic nasal discharge can accompany an obstruction of nasal passages by a foreign object, a nasal polyp, or infection. When such a discharge is caused by cancer of the nasopharynx or nasal membranes, it is often accompanied by bleeding and may or may not be painful.

While a sore throat is most often caused by viral or bacterial infections and can be caused by peritonsillar abscesses, infectious mononucleosis, or heavy smoking, it can also be caused by leukemia. In the latter situation, the sore throat will be accompanied by other signs of leukemia.

The white patch seen in the throat may be nothing more than an aphthous ulcer (canker sore) or thrush, but may also represent leukoplakia, which is frequently a precancerous lesion, or the white patch may be cancer.

Hoarseness may be due to laryngitis or to a benign vocal cord nodule, especially in younger persons. Persistent hoarseness may be indicative of cancer of the larynx.

Dysphagia is most commonly caused by anxiety, but may be seen with cancer of the throat or the esophagus or by diverticula of the esophagus.

Neck

Enlarged glands in the neck may be due to infection or a cyst or may be indicative of a metastasizing cancer.

Nodules in the thyroid may be benign even while causing symptoms of hyperthyroidism. A cancerous nodule in the thyroid may not be accompanied by symptoms of hyperactivity and may not be tender.

Heart

The heart is rarely involved by cancer, but metastasis to this organ can occur, usually from melanoma or by direct invasion from a lung or mediastinal lesion. The symptoms are those of a myocardial infarction, an arrhythmia, or a heart murmur. Cardiac tamponade due to pericardial effusion may occur. This condition is rarely diagnosed except by a postmortem examination.

Lungs

The cough caused by cancer or pulmonary fibrosis is chronic rather than acute in nature and may or may not be associated with hemoptysis, pneumonia, or pleural effusion. Lung sounds are frequently not heard over the area involved by cancer or fibrosis. Wheezing is not usually associated with cancer, unless there is an obstruction caused by advanced cancer of the larynx or tracheobronchial tree.

Breasts

Cysts of the breasts are neither reddened nor warm to the touch, as infected areas are, and may or may not be tender. Lumps caused by fibroadenomas are firm, nontender, and frequently irregular in shape. A cancerous lump is nontender in the early stages, but may cause pain as the size of the lesion increases. A cancerous lump is usually stony hard and may or may not be attached to underlying tissues.

Discharge from the nonlactating breast is a sign of an infection, an intraductal papilloma, or a cancerous growth. When cancer is the cause, the discharge may be clear or blood-tinged. "Orange-peel skin" (in which the skin dimples, resembling the peel of an orange) and dimpling of the skin (in one or more areas) are indicative of cancer.

Gastrointestinal System

Stomach   Dyspepsia is frequently caused by gastric hyperacidity and/or a peptic ulcer. Duodenal ulcers rarely if ever become cancerous, but there is a high rate of conversion of gastric ulcers to cancer. Ulcers are a much more frequent cause of dyspepsia than is cancer. Cancer of the stomach is frequently accompanied by meat intolerance. Weight loss and abdominal pain that is intractible to antacids accompany advanced cancer of the stomach. Infrequently, cancer of the large intestine may cause epigastric distress.

Eructation is most commonly caused by aerophagia from chewing, smoking, or drinking; by overeating; or by gallbladder disorders. Infrequently, the cause is gastric cancer.

Nausea and vomiting, while indicative of a reaction to radiation or chemotherapy, are most usually caused by viral gastroenteritis. Alternative causes could be drug intolerance (aspirin, codeine, Darvon, and digitalis being common offenders); an acute illness such as hepatitis, cholecystitis, or cholelithiasis; or peptic ulcers. The possibility of an anxiety reaction should be explored, and pregnancy should be considered in the younger female patient.

Hematemesis may occur as a result of a bleeding peptic ulcer, gastric cancer, acute gastritis, or ruptured esophageal varicies.

Upper abdominal pain may be due to cancer of the pancreas, but most usually it it due to viral gastroenteritis, cholecystitis, appendicitis, or a penetrating peptic ulcer.

Liver and Gallbladder   Pain in the right upper quadrant usually indicates cholecystolithiasis when the pain is severe and crampy in nature. Hepatitis may cause a dull ache in the right upper quadrant and is accompanied by anorexia, nausea, vomiting, fever, and jaundice. Pain caused by liver cancer, whether primary or secondary, is seldom accompanied by nausea or vomiting but is accompanied by jaundice, anorexia, weight loss, and occasionally fever.

Liver enlargement may be due to the presence of cancer within the organ. Irregular borders due to the tumor may be felt at the outer edges or on the surface when the organ is very enlarged. Other causes of an enlarged liver may be congestive heart failure, cirrhosis, hepatitis, or a liver abscess. Leukemia, lymphoma, or Hodgkin's disease may cause splenic as well as hepatic enlargement. The accompanying signs of these malignancies are enlarged lymph nodes, easy bruise formation, and fever.

Intestines and Rectum   Constipation, while usually due to inadequate fluid intake, not heeding the urge to defecate, sedentary habits including bed rest, or medications, may also be due to a mechanical obstruction of the bowel lumen by a large cancer. The obstruction may result in a decrease in the diameter of the stool or in alternating constipation and diarrhea. The solid wastes may become trapped above the obstruction, while the liquid wastes may seep around the constricted area.

Diarrhea may be caused by a viral infection, food poisoning, ulcerative colitis, food allergy, cancer of the colon, vitamin deficiency, or a reaction to radiation or chemotherapeutic drugs.

Lower abdominal pain may be due to viral gastroenteritis, diverticulosis, appendicitis, and, less frequently, to intestinal obstruction due to a tumor of the intestines. Cancer of other abdominal sites, pancreatitis, gallbladder disease, peptic ulcers, and diabetes are less common causes of lower abdominal pain.

Bloody stools are usually caused by hemorrhoids or a rectal fissure and usually appear as blood on the outer portion of the feces only. When bloody stools are associated with mucus, chronic constipation, thin and watery diarrhea, narrowing of the feces, or rectal pain, one must consider cancer of the rectum as a highly suspected source of the bleeding. Blood in the stool is a sign of a bleeding lesion higher in the gastrointestinal system. Reddish black or tarry stools are indicative of bleeding in the gastrointestinal system, while greenish black stools result when supplemental iron or a vegetable such as spinach is ingested. Beets and other reddish vegetables may cause red stools. A great deal of blood may be lost unnoticed from the gastrointestinal system through the stool, and anemia and fatigue may be the first symptoms that such a loss is occurring.

Hemorrhoids and cancer of the rectum can coexist, although this situation is not common. Melanomas may occur in the perianal region as well.

Kidneys and Bladder

Cancer of the bladder may first be noticed by a painless hematuria and frequency of urination. More common causes of frequent urination are infections, diabetes, an enlarged prostate—whether benign or malignant, or a bladder stone. An inability to urinate may be caused by an enlarged prostate. When hematuria is painless, cancer of the kidney and/or bladder must be considered.

Dysuria is seen in prostatitis, urethritis, and vaginitis and with bladder stones.

Reproductive Organs

Female   Discharge from the vagina may be due to trichomoniasis (a thin, watery, foul-smelling discharge), monilial infection (a thick, white, cheesy discharge), infection of the cervix (a thin, yellow-white discharge flecked with blood), gonorrhea (a thick, creamy discharge), or a cancer of the uterus or cervix (a bloody discharge of either brown staining or a heavy flow of blood). Senile vaginitis may be accompanied by a thin, watery discharge, sometimes with flecks of blood.

Frigidity may be due to emotional factors such as anxiety, inadequate sexual techniques, or painful sexual relations or to a reaction to some of the chemotherapeutic drugs used to treat cancer.

Male Penile discharges are rarely indicative of a malignant process, except in cancer of the penis. Discharges from the penis may be caused by a nonspecific urethritis (a thin, watery discharge), by gonorrhea or trichomoniasis (discharges appearing the same as the corresponding discharges in the female), or by acute prostatitis (a thin, watery discharge perhaps accompanied by blood).

Scrotal lumps are sometimes due to cancer of the testicle. The cancerous lump may be firm and irregularly edged and is usually not associated with pain, redness, fever, or dysuria. Scrotal lumps are more commonly caused by an inguinal hernia, hydrocele, spermatocele, variocele, epididymitis, or torsion of the testicle.

Impotence may be due to emotional factors, fatigue, chronic illness, multiple sclerosis, or diabetes, and may follow prostatic or lower abdominal surgery. It can also be caused by some drugs used to treat cancer, most notably vincristine.

Skin

Pruritis may be a symptom of local pain, and if so, scratching may relieve the local pain as well as the itch. Eczema, hives, contact dermatitis, chickenpox, and diabetes may also cause itching, as may leukemia and Hodgkin's disease. As previously noted, the presence of malignancies is usually accompanied by other signs.

Skin ulcers are usually due to impaired circulation or infected lacerations. Cancer of the skin forms a characteristic painless lesion in which the crater is rimmed by a raised, rolled edge and bleeding usually is also present.

Deeply pigmented areas are usually moles. If they appear in an older person, they may be senile keratosis, a benign lesion. A melanoma may arise spontaneously or from a preexisting mole. Therefore, moles subject to chronic irritation are usually removed as a preventative measure. The melanoma is dark brown to black in color. There may be a dark speckling or halo surrounding the lesion. Pain is rarely involved with early melanoma, and heat, redness, and swelling do not occur unless as a result of a secondary bacterial infection.

Musculoskeletal System

Joint pain, while due to osteoarthritis, rheumatoid arthritis, gout, joint infections, acute febrile illnesses, or lupus erythematosis most commonly (in descending order of occurrance) may also be due to leukemic infiltration of the joints.

Low back pain is caused usually by back strain, herniated nucleus pulposus, or arthritis. In the patient who has cancer, however, with no previous discomfort in the back, one should suspect metastasis to the spine. Multiple myeloma is frequently characterized by back pain, with radiation of the pain down one or both legs, mimicking disc disease. When cancer is the cause of the back pain, tenderness may be experienced over involved vertebra but redness and swelling are absent.

ASSESSMENT OF LABORATORY DATA

Nurses frequently miss important data about their patients because of the seeming incomprehensibility of laboratory data. Although the more common meanings of some of the lab values are widely understood, some of the less common but equally important meanings are not known. Table 5-2 presents the most commonly used laboratory examination and the conditions in which the results are increased or decreased. Not included are the electrophoretic examinations and the radioimmunoassays of hormones. The interested reader may find these in hematology or endocrinology texts.

One significant result may be sufficient to diagnose a pathologic process. For example, an elevated acid phosphatase is indicative of a perforated capsule of the prostate gland and occurs when cancer has caused the perforation. Some of the tests, however, are more nonspecific unless viewed in the context of other significant lab or clinical findings. The reader will be able to identify these tests by the number of conditions that affect the lab value.

SUMMARY

The nursing assessment is an essential process used to design effective patient care plans. It is composed of many parts: the nursing history, physical examination, review of patient and family interview data, review of previous patient records, and assessment of the laboratory data. Each patient should be approached with the firm conviction that this man or woman is a unique being in his or her life-style and problems. Yet the common thread of biologic and psychologic anatomy and physiology runs through us all. As normalities are identified the abnormalities will stand out much more clearly, and the nurse can make intelligent observations of how these abnormalities fit into a coherent pattern.

The amount of time spent in assessment at first glance may seem to leave the nurse time for little else. But if the nurse believes that knowledge is best gained and assimilated a little at a time, with adequate experience and supervision by a cooperative physician or a nurse skilled in these techniques, the nurse can gradually incorporate one technique at a time into his or her practice. As previously mentioned, an excellent time to assess the patient physically is during the period of morning care, the daily bath, or the evening care. Gradually the nurse's expertise in assessment will become an established fact and part of the daily routine.

Table 5-2 Assessment of Laboratory Values

Test	Serum chemistries	
	Increased	Decreased
1 Serum glucose	Phenochromocytoma, prednisone therapy, ACTH therapy stress, diabetes mellitus	Islet cell tumor; adrenal cancer; gastric cancer; fibrosarcoma; hepatic cancer, either primary or metastatic; postgastrectomy; gastroenterostomy; malnutrition
2 Blood urea nitrogen (BUN)	Impaired renal function, stress, increased protein catabolism, prerenal azotemia (due to decreased blood flow, e.g., congestive heart failure (CHF), salt and water depletion, shock), postrenal azotemia (obstruction of urinary tract)	Liver failure; low-protein, high-carbohydrate diet; long-term IV feedings
3 Uric acid	Gout, renal failure, increased destruction of nucleoproteins (leukemia, polycythemia, postradiation, resolving pneumonia, hemolytic anemia, antineoplastic treatment)	ACTH therapy, prednisone therapy
4 Cholesterol	Biliary obstruction (stone or cancer of duct, cholangeolitic cirrhosis) pancreatic disease	Severe liver damage, malnutrition, chronic anemia, ACTH therapy, prednisone therapy
5 Serum osmolality (freeze-point determination)	Excessive water loss or positive sodium balance, chronic renal disease (due to increased BUN and sodium)	Low serum sodium often combined with excess water; treatment with diuretic drugs; inappropriate secretion of antidiuretic hormone, as seen in bronchogenic cancer and cerebral tumors, trauma, and infections
6 Magnesium*	Renal failure, postadrenalectomy, antacid therapy with magnesium-based preparations	GI diseases showing malabsorption and abnormal loss of GI fluids (e.g., small-bowel resection, biliary and intestinal fistulas, abdominal irradiation, prolonged aspiration of intestinal contents), alcoholic cirrhosis, lytic bone tumors, diuretic drug therapy, long-term parenteral hyperalimentation

*Magnesium deficiency may cause apparently unexplained hypocalcemia and hypokalemia.

Table 5-2 Assessment of Laboratory Values (Continued)

	Serum chemistries	
Test	Increased	Decreased
7 Serum calcium	Bone tumor, primary or metastatic; acute osteoporosis hyperproteinemia (multiple myeloma)	Hypoparathyroidism (idiopathic or surgical); malabsorption of calcium and vitamin D (obstructive jaundice); hypoalbuminemia (cachexia); chronic renal diseases; inadequate calcium, phosphorus, and vitamin D ingestion as in starvation
8 Serum phosphorus	Hypoparathyroidism, bone disease (healing fractures, multiple myeloma, Paget's disease, osteolytic metastatic cancer of bone), myelogenous leukemia, highintestinal obstruction	Diabetes mellitus, hyperinsulinism
9 Alkaline phosphatase	Increased deposition of calcium in the bone (healing fractures, osteoblastic bone tumors such as osteogenic sarcoma or metastatic carcinoma, osteomalacia, ergosterol therapy): liver disease: any obstruction of biliary system (such as metastatic tumor, abscess cyst, sarcoid, leukemia, or carcinoma); hyperphosphatasia	Hypophosphatasia
10 Acid phosphatase	Carcinoma of prostate that extends through capsule, marked elevation of alkaline phosphatase levels	Not clinically significant
11 Serum amylase	Acute or exacerbated chronic pancreatitis, perforated or penetrating peptic ulcer, obstruction of pancreatic duct (stone, carcinoma, or drug-induced spasm of sphincter), acute alcohol ingestion, advanced renal insufficiency	Decreased levels are clinically significant only in occasional cases of fulminant pancreatitis
12 Serum lipase	Acute pancreatitis, perforating or penetrating peptic ulcer, obstruction of pancreatic duct (stone, carcinoma, drug-induced spasm of sphincter)	Not clinically significant

Test	Increased	Decreased
13 Serum glutamic oxaloacetic transaminase (SGOT)	Acute myocardial infarction, liver disease, acute pancreatitis, tissue injury (intestinal injury such as surgery, irradiation injury, cerebral neoplasms) *Falsely increased in* therapy with Prostaphlin, Polycillin, opiates, erythromycin	Not clinically significant *Normal in* angina pectoris, coronary insufficiency, pericarditis, congestive heart failure without liver damage
14 Lactic dehydrogenase (LDH)	Acute myocardial infarct, with/without CHF; congestive heart failure; hepatitis; untreated pernicious anemia	Not clinically significant
15 Creatinine phosphokinase (CPK)	Necrosis or acute atrophy of striated muscle, postoperative state	Not clinically significant

Hematology

Test (white blood cells) [WBC]	Increased	Decreased
1 Leukocyte	Acute infections, parenteral foreign proteins and vaccines, acute hemmorrhage, acute hemolysis of red blood cells (RBC), myeloproliferative diseases, (such as leukemia, leukemoid reactions of lymphomas, etc.), tissue necrosis (acute myocardial infarction [MI], necrosis of tumor, bacterial necrosis, etc.), emotional stress, recovery from agranulocytosis	Infections (overwhelming bacterial, viral, rickettsial, malaria, etc.), drugs and chemicals especially sulfonamides, antibiotics, analgesics, marrow depressants, arsenicals, antithyroid drugs, etc.), ionizing radiation, hematopoietic diseases (such as pernicious anemia, aleukemic, leukemia, aplastic anemia, hypersplenism), anaphylactic shock, cachexia
2. Lymphocyte	Cancer of stomach and breast, infections lymphocytic leukemia *Causes of atypical lymphocytes:*	Corticosteroid therapy Lymphocytic leukemia, viral infections
3 Basophile	Chronic myelogeneous leukemia, polycythemia, Hodgkin's disease, postsplenectomy, chronic hemolytic anemia, nephrosis, foreign protein injection	Period following radiation, chemotherapy, and glucocorticoids; acute phase of infection

Table 5-2 Assessment of Laboratory Values (Continued)

Hematology

Test (white blood cells) [WBC]	Increased	Decreased
4 Monocyte (absolute count more than 500)	Monocytic leukemia, other leukemias, myeloproliferative disorders, Hodgkin's disease and other malignant lymphomas, recovery from agranulocytosis, subsidence of acute infection, chronic ulcerative colitis, sarcoidosis, collagen diseases	Not clinically significant
5 Plasma cells	Plasma cell leukemia, multiple myeloma, serum reaction, infectious mononucleosis, benign lymphocytic meningitis	Not clinically significant
6 Eosinophile	Allergic reactions; some hematopoietic diseases, such as chronic myelogenous leukemia, polycythemia, Hodgkin's disease; postsplenectomy; ovarian tumors; tumors involving bone or serosal surfaces	Not clinically significant
7 Myelocyte	Infections (endocarditis, pneumonia), cancer of colon, embryonal cancer of kidney, acute hemorrhage and hemo lysis, recovery from agranulocytosis	Not clinically significant
8 Leukocyte alkaline phosphatase staining reaction†	Leukemoid reaction, lymphoma (including Hodgkin's reticulum cell sarcoma), acute and chronic lymphocytic leukemia, multiple myeloma, aplastic anemia, agranulocytosis, bacterial infections	Chronic myelogenous leukemia, nephrotic syndrome

Usually normal in lymphosarcoma *usually variable in* idiopathic thrombocytopenic purpura, acute myelogenous leukemia, acute undifferentiated leukemia |

†This test is clinically most useful to differentiate chronic myelogenous leukemia from leukemoid reactions.

Test	Increased	Decreased
9 Erythrocyte sedimentation rate (ESR)	Acute hepatitis; acute MI; significant tissue necrosis (especially neoplasms, such as malignant lymphoma and cancer of colon and breast); increased serum globulins (myeloma); decreased serum albumin; acute hemorrhage; nephrosis, renal disease with azotemia; dextran and polyvinyl compounds in blood	Uncomplicated viral diseases, angina pectoris
10 C-reactive protein	Neoplasm with widespread metastasis	Normally not detected in blood
11 RBC	Polycythemia vera, acute leukemia	Anemias, bone marrow invasion by cancer
12 Platelets	Postsplenectomy, polycythemia vera, chronic myelogenous leukemia	Anemias, dilantin therapy, antineoplastic therapy, bone marrow invasion by cancer, thymus tumors, radiation therapy, disseminated intravascular coagulation, acute leukemia, terminal chronic myelogenous leukemia
13 Reticulocyte	Blood loss of increased RBC destruction, metastatic carcinoma in bone marrow	Aregenerative crises, severe autoimmune type of hemolytic diseases

Spinal fluid

Test	Increased	Decreased
1 Proteins	Cord tumors, brain tumors, acute infections	Not clinically significant
2 Cell count	May be 100–150, but usually is 0–10	Not clinically signifcant

BIBLIOGRAPHY

Alexander, M., and M. Brown: "Physical examinations: part IV; the lymph system." *Nursing '73,* pp. 149–51. October 1973.
Essentials of the Neurologic Exam, Smith, Cline, and French, 1969.
Hobson, L: *Examination of the Patient,* McGraw-Hill, New York, 1975.
Jarvis, C.: "Vital signs." *Nursing '76,* **6**:4. pp. 31–37.
Murray, R., and J. Zentner: *Nursing Assessment and Health Promotion through the Life Span,* Prentice-Hall, Englewood Cliffs, N.J., 1975.
"Physical Assessment." A series in *Nursing '73–'76.*
Robinson, L.: *Liason Nursing: Psychological Approach to Patient Care,* F. A. Davis, Philadelphia, 1974.
Schwartz, L., and J. Schwartz: *The Psychodoynamics of Patient Care,* Prentice-Hall, Englewood Cliffs, N.J., 1972.
Sherman J., and S. Fields: *Guide to Patient Evaluation: History Taking, Physical Examination, and the Problem-Oriented Method,* Medical Examination Publishing Co., Flushing, N.Y., 1974.
Stevenson, I.: *The Diagnostic Interview,* 2d. ed., Harper and Row, New York, 1971.
Taylor, Robert: *A Primer of Clinical Symptoms,* Harper and Row, New York, 1973.
Wallach, J.: *Interpretation of Diagnostic Tests: A Handbook Synopsis of Laboratory Medicine,* Little, Brown, Boston, 1970.

Chapter 6

Nutrition and Cancer

Judi K. Shabert

Chemotherapy and radiotherapy must sometimes sacrifice the immediate nutritional well-being of the patient for the more urgent goals of controlling the spread of the neoplasm. The individual must contend with a loss of appetite and an increase in metabolic rate due directly to the disease process itself. To these stressful metabolic conditions are added the cancer therapies of surgery, radiotherapy, and chemotherapy, which often controls the growth of neoplasm but compromise the nutritional status of the individual. Insofar as secondary malnutrition is a result of current cancer therapy and the disease process, it is necessary for the nursing staff to be as knowledgeable as possible in the area of nutrition in order to control this condition. Doing this begins with an understanding of basic nutrition as it relates to cancer patients.

Nutrition has been underemphasized in the overall care of cancer patients. Only within the last few years has there been a rising concern about cancer nutrition, reflected in the literature and in the most progressive hospitals. However, there are still too many hospitals in which the nutritional needs of the cancer patient do not receive adequate attention. Because of the lack of concern elsewhere, the responsibility for the nutritional care of cancer patients often rests in the hands of the nursing staff.

This chapter is intended to provide nurses and other health professionals with an overview of nutrition of cancer patients as it relates to nursing care. It will begin with a review of essential nutrients and the research on their relationship to tumor growth. Next it will look at nutritional therapies commonly given to hospitalized patients with cancer. Lastly it will correlate the various cancer therapies and their effects on nutrition.

NUTRIENTS AND CANCER
Protein

Proteins are made up of amino acids linked together by peptide bonds. The breakdown of proteins begins in the stomach through a process of chemical and mechanical digestion. Completion of protein digestion and amino acid absorption take place in the small intestine.

The word "protein" is derived from the Greek word *protos*, which means "holding first place," and for the person with cancer it is indeed of prime importance. Studies done by Midler suggest that the tumor acts like a "protein trap." The individual may take in a seemingly adequate amount of protein and calories for his or her size, but as the tumor becomes increasingly enriched in protein, vitamins, and minerals, the individual loses weight and becomes cachexic.[1] Even if the individual is not eating or is not being given parenteral nutrition, the tumor grows at his or her expense. Because of this situation, there has been some investigation and research in the area of amino acid and protein manipulation in experimental animals and humans in an attempt to understand and thus control tumor growth.

Several investigators have tried methods to control neoplastic growth by starving the tumor of selected amino acids. In some instances the tumor size was reduced; however, the toxic effects were not selective to neoplastic cells alone, and the body tissue of the experimental animal was also depleted.[2]

There is still some debates as to the effects of force feeding calories and protein to patients with active neoplastic disease. In a study done by Waterhouse and Terepka,[3] the malignancies in some of the patients appeared to have accelerated during and after forced feeding. A more recent study by Souchon,[4] who administered hypertonic solutions of amino acids and carbohydrates to patients with gastric cancer receiving 5-fluorouracil, showed that there was an average weight gain of 8.7 lb in the adult patients on "total parenteral nutrition" (TPN) and an average total dosage tolerance of 7 g of 5-FU for the 13 days of therapy. The comparable group of orally fed patients lost weight during the same period of time and tolerated a total average dosage of 3.75 g of 5-FU. The patients on TPN tolerated a larger therapeutic dose of 5-FU, resulting in a response rate of 40 percent—greater than that usually reported. The responding patients were alive at least 1 year after therapy. The nonresponsive patients were dead within 6 months. The results indicate that there is a definite beneficial effect in administering calories and protein to cancer patients who are otherwise unable to eat.

This example is cited in order to convey the need on the part of the cancer care team to make a concerted effort at getting calories and protein into the patient whether it be by dietary adjustment or by supplemental protein and calories via TPN. Every attempt should be made on the part of the staff to manipulate the diet in order to bring optimum results to the patient.

Carbohydrate

The second group of calorie-donating nutrients is carbohydrates, or saccharides, which include sugar, starches, and cellulose. Carbohydrates are composed of oxygen, carbon, and hydrogen compounds linked together by glycosidic bonds. They are the bodies' primary source of calories. A major function of carbohydrates is to provide energy to body tissues for metabolic processes. Carbohydrates also serve to spare the breakdown of body protein. This function of carbohydrates can be served only if adequate calories are supplied to the body.

The carbohydrate lactose, which is found in milk, often raises havoc for the nursing staff working with cancer patients. One of the standard ways to increase protein intake in the diet of a cancer patient is to encourage the use of milk-fortified products. Milk does not have the same offensive taste to the cancer patient as meat does, and it can be ingested with little effort. However, the nursing staff should question the patient upon admission to the hospital about any adverse reactions to milk products. It has been found that 70 to 90 percent of all blacks and Orientals and 2 to 8 percent of all Caucasians[5,6] have an intolerance to lactose due to a deficiency in the enzyme lactase, which is responsible for the breakdown of lactose in the body. The symptoms of this enzyme deficiency are abdominal cramping, distension, gas, and diarrhea. A patient may not be aware of any adverse effects to milk products but his or her ethnic background should encourage the nurse to be cautious before administering large quantities of milk. Some individuals with lactase deficiency can tolerate milk if they drink it in small amounts at body temperature or if they are drinking milk with a meal. Dairy products such as cheese, yogurt, and cottage cheese are tolerated by lactase-deficient individuals because some the lactose has been fermented to lactic acid and other short-chain acids. A tasty substitute for milk, made from soybeans, is Ensure.

Fat

Fat is the most efficient and most concentrated form of stored energy. It yields 9 cal/g, compared with 4 cal/g for carbohydrate and protein. It serves as a source of and storage site for fat-soluble vitamins.

It has been found that early fat loss is common in patients having cancer. The amount of fat found in the muscles of cancer patients is half that found in a control group.[7] There is speculation that the loss of appetite and the apathy seen in cancer patients is due to lipid metabolites, which are a by-product of fat and lipid catabolism.

Vitamins

In the general practice of medicine and psychiatry, vitamin therapy usually means giving patients large portions of vitamins to treat an existing vitamin deficiency or to fortify the patient with megadoses of vitamins. Vitamin therapy in cancer research has been concerned with creating vitamin deficiencies rather than treating them. The assumption is, of course, that the tumor is rapidly dividing the needs the vitamins for cellular division and other metabolic processes. These vitamin deficiencies have been brought about in experimental animals and some human subjects by specific vitamin deprivation or by the action of a vitamin antagonist. Although a degree of tumor regression was seen in dietary-induced deficiences of pantothenic acid,[8] riboflavin,[9] and nicotinic acid,[10] the overall results suggested only transient improvements or marked weight loss in the host. There is also the danger of severe side effects, such as the grand mal seizures that resulted from giving patients a vitamin B_6-deficient diet along with an antimetabolite.[11] These factors make this type of therapy impractical and undesirable in most cases. More extensive experimentation needs to be done in this area.

The only work with vitamin deficiences which appears to be having considerable success is that done with Methotrexate,[12] a folic acid antagonist. Folic acid coenzymes are involved in the synthesis of important precursors of nucleic acids and proteins and are therefore critical to the metabolism of proliferating cells. The enzyme dihydrofolate reductase is involved in the synthesis of tetrahydrofolate, an active form of folic acid. Methotrexate acts by binding very strongly to this enzyme, thus preventing the synthesis of tetrahydrofolate and subsequent nucleic acids.

Vitamin C, ascorbic acid, deserves special consideration. It is well known that a variety of stresses increase the need for ascorbic acid in humans. Wound healing and therefore recovery time have also been shown to be enhanced by high doses of ascorbic acid. Other studies have shown that certain drugs, such as analgesics, sedatives, and antihistamines,[13] and smoking[14] further increase the need for ascorbic acid. Stress, wound healing, smoking, and the variety of other drugs are all important secondary considerations in the treatment of cancer patients. For this reasons alone, high doses of vitamin C are often prescribed in the treatment of cancer patients. Vitamin C is also known to be related to the proper functioning of the immune system and possibly related to the body's own defense against viral infections. Furthermore, vitamin C has been found to detoxify certain known carcinogens in rats.[15] These later findings underline the importance of vitamin C in the nutrition of cancer patients.

Vitamin A and its synthetic analogs, retinoids, have been the focus of recent studies as controlling agents for epithelial cancer, since epithelial tissue is dependent on retinoids to maintain normal cell differentation. In one such study[16] the tracheal epithelial tissue was deprived of retinoids; the tissue lost its normal ciliated columnar structure and developed lesions of squamous metaplasia. Addition of retinoids caused reversal of the process and replacement of abnormal squamous cells by ciliated mucous cells. Other work[17] showed reversal of epithelial lesions in prostate gland organ cultures. The retinoids were able to cause cellular repair of a pathological problem. The work in this area looks highly promising; however, natural retinoids (vitamin A), when given in the high doses required to reverse precancerous and cancerous lesions, are toxic to the body and show poor tissue distribution. Thus it would not be advisable for individuals to take vitamin A in excess of the amount required by the National Academy of Sciences, since this vitamin is fat-soluble and accumulates in the fatty tissue of the body.

After considering all the evidence related to vitamin therapy, one must come back to a practical consideration of the baseline of necessary vitamin intake for a cancer patient. It appears that neither of the two extremes, vitamin deficiency or vitamin excess, with the exception of vitamin C therapy, are beneficial in an overall perspective. This fact reflects a tragic irony in nutritional cancer therapy: that which is good for the patient is also good for the tumor, and that which is harmful to the tumor is ultimately harmful to the patient. Thus the only practical alternative available at this time is moderation, and the only guidelines available for vitamin intake are based on healthy individuals. Since it is known that many cancer patients are dealing with malabsorption syndrome or decreased food intake due to anorexia or obstructions, hospital personnel should aim to give at least the recommended amount of vitamins suggested by the Food and Nutrition Board, National Academy of Sciences, for healthy individuals until further information suggests otherwise. Because specific aberrations seen in cancer patients may prevent oral vitamin intake via food or vitamin pills, one may need to supply this recommended amount in a supplemental form by an injection or intravenous treatment.

Ingestion of excessive amount of vitamins is a popular practice today not only among individuals who may be considered food faddists but also among ordinary people who have been misguided by a current trend to think that one is unable to receive adequate nourishment in the food one eats. Taking surplus vitamins is encouraged by some people as the cure-all for every ailment. Cancer patients are easy targets for this misinformation. The nursing staff working with cancer patients should be wary of patients being involved in this type of faddism. From our present knowledge of high doses of vitamins, one suspects that with the exception of vitamin C, excess vitamins could cause a more deleterious effect than a positive one.

Fluid and Electrolytes

By far the most common causes of fluid and electrolyte imbalances in cancer patients are diarrhea, vomiting, and fistula drainage. Each of these problems results in losses of sodium, potassium, and chloride and concomitant loss of water.

Serum values of these electrolytes are frequently monitored as precise indications of the extent of the imbalances. Fluctuations in daily weights and intake and output are other indications of fluid disturbances. In the hospital setting, IVs are generally given to correct these conditions. For the patient at home, the only measures that one has to go by are the obvious signs of diarrhea and vomiting. A simple way of dealing with this condition is to suggest the use of Gatorade, which supplies sodium, potassium, chlorides, and glucose. Other drinks and foods high in sodium and potassium which one can suggest to the patient can be found in Table 6-1.

In some cases the tumors themselves secrete substances that cause electrolyte imbalances. Oat cell carcinoma and bronchiogenic cancer specifically cause an increase in antidiuretic hormone activity and produce a state of hyponatremia.[18]

The sudden and sometimes fatal onset of hypercalcemia may be brought about in bone or breast cancer due to the direct invasion of bone by tumor with destruction of bone mass and release of calcium into the blood.[19] Hypercalcemia requires urgent medical attention and may require a low-calcium diet (120 mg per day) that eliminates all milk products. One should be wary of well-intentioned family members and friends giving a child dairy products if the child has bone cancer and is on a low-calcium diet, unless these foods directly approved by the physician.

Edema may accompany advanced cancer. Daily weight may therefore be misleading as to the actual nutritional status of the individual. If inaccurate or no intakes and outputs are being done, one might possibly misinterpret a constant weight gain to mean the patient's condition is improving. Unfortunately, the opposite could be true. The nurse's evaluation of the situation could be very helpful in redirecting therapy.

NUTRITIONAL THERAPIES

IV Therapy

The carbohydrate (CHO) most well known to the cancer care team is glucose, or dextrose, the energy supply found in most IV bottles. A common practice in hospitals is to give IVs to patients post surgically or for dehydration, sometimes for extended periods of time. Because cancer patients on radiotherapy and chemotherapy are often plagued with vomiting and diarrhea, they are frequently placed on IV therapy. One should be aware that 1000 cc of 5% dextrose with water supplies a mere 200 kcal. An intake of 2 to 3 l—400 to 600 kcal—per day is

Table 6-1   Foods and Drinks High in Sodium or Potassium

Foods and drinks high in potassium	Foods and drinks high in sodium

Fruits and juices
  Cantaloupe, honeydew, dried peach, dried
  fig, apricot, raisin or date, banana,
  avocado, fresh apricot, peach, papaya,
	Canned soups, especially those made with
	  bouillon cubes
	Cheese
	Salted crackers
	Salted nuts, celery salt, table salt,

Vegetables
  Mushroom, white beans, lima beans,
  winter squash, potato, parsnip, chard,
  beet greens, spinach, kale, cowpeas,
  dandelion greens, artichoke, red beans,
  raw celery, carrot
	Worchestershire sauce, shoyu (soy sauce),
	  catsup
	Canned meats, fish, corned beef, bacon, ham,
	  sausages, salted and dried meat
	Peanut butter
	Tomato juice

hardly sufficient to supply the necessary calories needed by the body for maintenance. As mentioned previously, CHO spares the body from burning protein.
This is true only if adequate calories are being supplied to the body. With the
therapy of 5% dextrose with water, the body stores of protein are rapidly burning
up. Therefore, no cancer patient should be maintained solely on IVs for more
than 5 consecutive days at the most. Other methods of nutritional therapy are
available, and they should be used.

Tube Feedings

Tube feeding will be discussed here in a general manner and more specifically
under other headings. Perhaps the biggest obstacle to the use of tube feedings as
a therapeutic and necessary treatment for debilitated patients lies in the attitude
of the hospital staff. Often days are wasted before a feeding tube is inserted in the
hopes that a patient will initiate eating. There appears to be reluctance on the part
of staffs to tube feed a patient unless the patient is comatose. The attitude of the
staff needs to be positive, and they must be mindful of the far-reaching effects on
the patient in terms of recovery rather than the immediate concerns of inserting a
feeding tube and administering food in such a manner. Using a positive approach
and an accurate account of the previous day's calorie and protein intake, one can
usually persuade a patient that a tube feeding temporarily placed can do much for
the patient's future health and recovery.

Because of the invention of thin polyethylene tubing, feeding tubes are no
longer as physically irritating as they once were. The patient feels little discomfort, and there is no damage to the mucous membranes of the gastrointestinal
tract, as there was with rubberized tubing.

There are numerous tube-feeding liquids available, and one should carefully
consider the physical condition of the patient before initiating a particular type of
feeding. If the patient has exhibited any lactose intolerance, one should use a
tube feeding that is lactose-free. Patients who have had impaired digestion for
whatever reason should be started on the tube feeding slowly. Liquid formulas
that have a high osmolality are more prone to cause diarrhea in these patients. As
a precaution, half-strength formula should be used, and only 150 cc or less of
formula per feeding can be given at 2-hour intervals the first day. This amount
can be increased to full strength by the third day. On the fourth day the feedings
should be given every 3 hours, and the quantity should be increased by 50 cc per
day up to 300 cc or more per feeding as the patient can tolerate it. Isocal, both
lactose-free and iso-osmotic, is tolerated by most patients with no difficulty.
Generally, when a tube feeding is increased by the method just stated and no
lactose is being given, there is little likelihood of diarrhea. If diarrhea does occur,
one may add regular apple sauce, banana puree, guava juice, or pureed carrots to
the tube feeding.

Patients being discharged from the hospital may be instructed how to make
their own feeding formula. By far, this is the least expensive method for the
patient. In addition, it enables many patients to feel as though they are contributing to their own care. It also gives them the opportunity to put whatever food

they want in the formula, which is psychologically of benefit to them. The dietitian along with the occupational therapist can be helpful in this area by showing the patient how to make the formula prior to discharge.

Elemental Diets

The term "elemental diet" refers to liquids, chemically refined products such as Vivonex and Flexical, that are made up of nutrients in a form most easily absorbed by the body. Carbohydrates are given as mono- and oligosaccharides. The protein portion has been hydrolyzed to amino acids. If fats are present in the formula, they are in the form of medium-chain triglycerides. The philosophy behind the use of elemental diets stems from the ease with which the gastrointestinal tract can absorb these basic nutrients across the mucous membrane. There is minimal digestion and little or no residue.

For patients who have fistulas or obstructions, these formulas are ideal. The absorption of elemental diets is done almost entirely in the upper bowel, in the jejunum and the duodenum. Therefore, adequate calories and protein can be supplied and absorbed to aid in wound healing while little stress is placed on the gastrointestinal tract. With no residue in elemental diets, the complications due to the undigested portion of a normal diet are eliminated.

There is a definite place for elemental diets during the treatment of cancer. Both 5-FU and radiation therapy are known to cause mucosal changes in the gut that appear to hinder the absorption ability of the cells. Damage occurs to the surface epithelial cells of the mucosa in patients who have received 5-FU therapy. Radiation causes diarrhea and enteritis. The experiments[20,21] using elemental diets versus regular diets done on both human subjects and rats have shown very positive results. On biopsy, the mucosal cells were much more nearly normal in those subjects who were given elemental diets than in the controls. A stable weight was seen throughout the testing period, and the appetite resumed more quickly for those on elemental diets.

Because of the basic composition of elemental diets, patients sometimes object to their taste, especially the taste of those products that are higher in amino acid content. Some of the companies are putting out flavor packets with the diets, which when used in combination (orange and vanilla) appear to be more acceptable to the patients. Using a fruit juice of the patient's choosing is another effective method to make the product more acceptable. Elemental diets made into slushes or popsicles may also work. If the patient is entirely averse to the taste of the product, a feeding tube can be inserted as a last resort. Elemental diets are nearly clear and of a watery consistency, so a small #8 French nasogastric tube is all that is necessary. This tube causes less discomfort to the patient than a larger tube would.

One need always be aware that the recovery of a nutritionally wasted patient will take much longer than the recovery of a patient who has been given the chance to maintain a stable weight. Elemental diets should be highly considered as a dietary treatment because of their uniqueness in being able to supply easily assimilated calories and protein as well as allowing the gut to rest and recover from chemotherapy and radiation treatment.

Total Parenteral Nutrition

Total parenteral nutrition, the technique of supplying a hypertonic solution of glucose, amino acids, vitamins, and minerals to the general circulation via the subclavian vein, is indicated for individuals who are unable to maintain adequate nutrition by any other means. Since only a limited degree of malnutrition can be tolerated by the human body, TPN should be initiated when other methods of feeding, such as the oral route, tube feeding, or elemental diets, are unable to adequately supply calories, protein, minerals, and vitamins. Specific situations include obstruction in the gastrointestinal tract, radiation enteritis, and abdominal fistulas. TPN is also recommended to augment feeding for patients unable to eat due to cancer of the head and neck.

There has been a higher response rate to 5-FU therapy for patients who are receiving TPN than for those on oral feeding.[4] Gastrointestinal complications of 5-FU may include mucosal ulcerations, nausea, vomiting, and diarrhea. Maintaining adequate nutrition during these periods of therapy is limited. With TPN the bowel experiences no mechanical or chemical stimulation, so it can rest and heal. (This technique has been called a "physiologic colostomy" and *may* obviate the need for a temporary surgical colostomy in selected patients.)

Much of the work using TPN on cancer patients has been done by Dudrick and Copeland. The criteria they use to assess the need for TPN include having a weight loss of 10 lb, being 10 percent below ideal or normal body weight, and having serum albumin concentrations below 3.4 g/100 ml. Most of the patients in their studies who were chosen to be put on TPN had previously not been candidates for cancer treatment merely because of the fear of complications due to their state of malnutrition, which is frequently infection. The results of their work showed that of 70 surgical patients put on TPN, 68 percent were able to undergo major curative resections. There was an operative mortality rate of only 4 percent.[22]

Copeland et al. have reported weight gains of 13 to 17 lb in patients during radiotherapy treatment to the head and neck area while on TPN. In another series of patients with cancer of the head and neck area, seven out of eight patients who received TPN prior to surgery showed no postoperative complications although surgery for removal of the cancer was extensive.[23]

The usefulness of TPN in the treatment of cancer patients is being recognized more frequently. Optimal wound healing usually comes about through optimal nutrition, and it is apparent that a well-nourished patient will have a better response rate to healing than will a malnourished patient. TPN is able to restore lost nutrients and promote weight gain in many patients who are seriously debilitated.

TPN is not without complications, of which an important one is sepsis. Administration of TPN requires skillful management. The cancer care team should be thoroughly knowledgeable in all aspects of administration of this hypertonic solution and in the care of the catheter site before attempting this type of nutritional therapy.

TREATMENT MODALITIES
Surgery

Preoperative Concerns   Any patient about to receive surgery should be in an optimal nutritional state. Wound healing and recovery time are shortened in individuals whose nutritional status is stable.

Outpatients who will be preparing their own diets must be adequately instructed in the importance of proper nutrition prior to surgery. The anxiety and anticipation of the pending hospitalization and scheduled surgery may cause some patients to lose their appetite. Given information that stresses the necessity of a well-balanced diet, most people will make a conscious effort to eat. Above all, a high-protein intake should be encouraged for enhancement of wound healing.

Some patients are admitted to the hospital for surgery in a malnourished state and display overt nutritional deficiencies that may or may not be caused by the neoplastic growth. One cannot expect to restore significant amounts of body tissue in a few days, but surgery can usually be delayed for a week of so until some measures can be taken to correct electrolyte, fluid, vitamin, and mineral problems. During this period of time, it may be necessary to tube feed the patient if oral feeding has become too laborious. If the nutritional status is extremely poor, one may find total parenteral nutrition to be necessary as an adjunct to oral feeding.

A state of malnutrition in a newly admitted patient may also be caused by an obstruction in the digestive tract due to tumor growth, stenosis from radiotherapy, or adhesions from previous surgery. Presurgically, intervention to improve the nutritional state may not be possible except through the use of a highly nutritious liquid feeding, an elemental diet, or total parenteral nutrition. As long as the patient can still swallow liquids in spite of an obstructive tumor in the head and neck region, the patient can be given a high-calorie, high-protein liquid det. Bowel obstructions that prevent digestion and absorption in the jejunum and lower bowel necessitate the use of elemental diets. In the case of a total obstruction above the jejunum, only TPN can make significant improvements in the patient's nutritional status. The physician must weigh the risk of taking the patient to surgery for the removal of the obstruction or using TPN for a while prior to surgery to improve the surgical risk.

Surgery of the digestive tract usually entails some type of radical change either in mastication, swallowing, digestion, or excretion. It is imperative that patients know prior to surgery what they will be confronted with when the anesthesia wears off. A patient who has been told she or he is to have a "mandibulectomy" is a long way from a patient who understands that this means a large portion of her or his face will be removed, a tube will be inserted for feeding, and eating will be a drawn-out, tedious process involving foods of a very foreign texture. These same types of concerns hold true for gastrectomy, ostomy, and pancreatectomy patients. Time and careful teaching have to be given presurgically with the intent of making the procedure easier for the patient to accept. One can expect to elicit a great deal more cooperation in feeding and caring for oneself if the patient has been well informed of the results of surgery before surgery takes place.

Surgeries of the Head and Neck   Surgical excision of tumors in the head and neck area may call for radical changes in food ingestion. For example, in a partial glossectomy, mandibulectomy, or resection of the hard or soft palate, the patient is left with difficulties in mastication and swallowing. It is extremely frustrating for such a patient to try to manipulate a bolus of food in his or her mouth. Drooling and difficulty in keeping food in the mouth are experienced. Swallowing is also impaired. The staff can aid the patient in overcoming these difficulties by leading him or her through a steady progression in the diet from liquid foods to semisoft foods.

A tube feeding may be given initially following head and neck surgery. The extent of the surgery and the patient's rate of recovery will govern how long it will be kept in place. When surgery to the head and neck area requires that a feeding tube be placed permanently or kept in for an indefinite period of time, instruction for self-feeding should begin 2 or 3 days postoperatively. A patient progressing to oral feedings begins with a liquid diet that should not be too extreme in temperature or too spicy in order to prevent irritation of the suture line. The patient will usually find it easiest to sip such a diet through a straw. The patient can then advance to pureed foods. Freshly pureed (blenderized) foods are by far more desirable than commercially prepared pureed foods, which patients usually find unpalatable. A patient who tolerates this diet well should be advanced to a diet of chopped and semisoft foods. It is best that each mouthful of food be of only one texture. Soups with both liquid and solids require greater manipulation in the mouth and in swallowing than do either liquids or solids alone.

Milk, as well as causing gastrointestinal upsets for lactose intolerate individuals, also causes excessive mucus production in some people. For patients on a liquid diet following head and neck surgery—where phlegm is a real problem—milk substitutes might be the answer. These products generally do not cause allergic reactions. A decrease in mucus production in the esophagus is apparent following their ingestion.

A great deal of concern for the presentation and appearance of food should be given to patients who have had surgery in the head and neck area, especially glossectomy and laryngectomy patients. Not only are they faced with mechanical problems in the ingestion of food, but often also their senses of taste and smell aare impaired. Food that is presented in an attractive and appealing manner by a staff member who is pleasant and supportive will do much for the acceptance of that food by the patient. Patients should be encouraged to request any kind of food, and their requests, however unusual, should be honored. Desserts need not always be pureed fruit; for example, one patient was fond of dates, figs, and nuts blended together with a little milk and canned fruit. It was extremely high in calories and was far more interesting to eat than the pureed fruit the patient had been taking.

Surgery of the Esophagus The largest percentage of tumors of the esophagus are found in the middle and lower thirds of the esophagus. An esophagectomy is the usual method of treatment. Nutritional problems that arise following this surgery include malabsorption of fat, which is thought to be due to the vagotomy done during the surgical procedure. Steatorrhea may be controlled by the use of commercially prepared medium-chain triglycerides (MCT Oil). Recipe booklets and materials on how to use MCT Oil are available from the manufacturer and should be given to the patient and the family if any success is to be expected from this approach. Esophageal fistula formation may necessitate the need for a new feeding site, such as a gastrostomy, which will aid in the healing of the fistula by bypassing the source of irritation to permit adequate nutrition. This will allow wound healing to take place. Obstructions of the esophagus found to be inoperable have been treated in a palliative manner by the formation of a gastrostomy feeding site.

Surgery of the Stomach Nutrition in patients who have had a total or subtotal gastrectomy has two goals of prevention, namely, to prevent dumping syndrome and to prevent vitamin B_{12} and iron deficiencies. Dumping syndrome shows symptoms of weakness, sweating, and palpitations and is seen following mealtime in some but not all patients who have had gastric resections. It results from a rapid emptying of ingested material from the stomach into the small intestine.

If a patient is experiencing dumping syndrome, an appropriate diet is one that decreases the amount of concentrated carbohydrate in the diet to 150 g per day, reduces the size of the meal, and limits liquids taken at mealtimes. The diet should contain a large amount of protein. An outline of the diet can be found in Table 6-2. All candies, jellies, chocolates, and sugars should be eliminated. If hypoglycemia develops in gastrectomized patients, dietary treatment is the same as that for dumping syndrome.

Stomach size is decreased, so the patient has a feeling of fullness after eating very little food. Hence, with time, gastrectomy patients tend to show significant yet gradual weight loss. They need to be reminded that even though they feel full, their stomach capacity is not as great and they are not taking in as many calories. They must eat more frequently, usually six small meals per day to obtain as many calories as they had taken in when they were able to eat normally.

Both vitamin B_{12} and iron deficiencies due to malabsorption have been shown to develop within a few years following gastrectomy surgery. Occasional testing for serum levels of B_{12} and plasma levels of iron and administration of these substances when their levels fall slightly below normal will prevent overt deficiencies.[24]

Table 6-2 Sample Diet for Postgastrectomy Dumping Syndrome

Breakfast	g CHO	Lunch	g CHO	Dinner	g CHO
1/2 cup fruit juice	10	1/2 sandwich with 2 oz		3 oz meat, fish, or	
2 scrambled eggs		meat	15	poultry, gravy	
with 1 oz cheese		Lettuce salad with		1/2 cup potatoes or 1/3	
1 piece toast	15	diced chicken (2 oz)		cup rice	15
Butter or margarine		Oil and vinegar		Cooked green beans	
	25	dressing		1/4 cantaloupe	10
		1/2 cup water-packed			25
		fruit			
			10		
			25		

Snack		Snack		Snack	
1/2 cup milk	4	1/2 cup baked custard	18	5 soda crackers	19
Sugar-free cereal	15	with cream	2	2 oz cheese	
2 hard-cooked eggs		1/2 cup water-packed		Butter or margarine	
	19	or fresh fruit	10		19
			30		

Ileostomy   Postoperatively, the diet given to ileostomates is advanced from liquids to low residue until such time as the physician feels sure that there will be no possibility of obstruction and a normal diet may be instituted. For 10 or so days immediately following the formation of an ileostomy, larger amounts of fluid and sodium are lost which must be monitored and replaced if necessary. The intestine quickly adjusts to this situation, and soon losses are in the range of only 300 to 600 ml per day of water, 40 to 100 meq per day of sodium, and 2.5 to 20.0 meq per day of potassium.[25] It is unnecessary to encourage the use of a large increase in fluids or electrolytes in ileostomates since the kidneys make necessary adjustments for the losses from the ileostomy.

Diarrhea presents problems that should be recognized and dealt with immediately. Some patients again find that Gatorade, taken when diarrhea symptoms first appear, alleviates the need for hospitalization. Foods that may be given for K^1 replacement are bananas, potatoes, and orange and tomato juices.

Dietary adjustments to control stool formation are generally unwarranted since the stools are liquidlike no matter what the patient eats. As surprising as it may seem, marshmallows are an exception. The gelatin in the marshmallows provides consistency and formation to the stool. One should not suggest the use of marshmallows to a patient who is overweight.

Colostomy   The postoperative progression diet for a colostomy follows the same course as the diet following an ileostomy by going from liquids to a regular diet. The colon differs from the small intestine, however, in its ability to compensate for fluid losses by increasing the absorptive capacity in the remaining segment of colon so that stools are formed. This situation has dietary implications primarily in regard to odor and to gas production. The patient feels embarrassed and uncomfortable socially when unable to control odor and gas. Generally, the nursing staff tell the patient that the foods that were troublesome before the colostomy will affect him or her after the colostomy is formed. Each person is different, and what may work for one person will not work for another. There are foods the patient should be aware of because they have a greater tendency to cause gas and odor than others do. These foods are listed in Table 6-3. These foods should be introduced one at a time to test the effects they have on the patient. Some foods, such as beer, prunes, and high-fat foods (nuts, olives, butter), may cause diarrhea and should be used with caution.

The nutritional information most useful to a colostomy patient is to eat a well-balanced, calorie-controlled diet at regular times each day so the body can develop a pattern for digestion and elimination. Most individuals, even those with a normal bowel, are affected adversely by overeating and eating non-nutritional food. The colostomate is no exception.

Surgery of the Pancreas   Following pancreatic surgery for removal of cancerous tissue, patients will experience a loss in both exocrine and endocrine function. There is a reduction in pancreatic enzymes which necessitates extopic administration of therapeutic doses of these enzymes to aid in digestion. Diabetes mellitus may also develop, calling for the use of a diabetic diet. Should malabsorption of fats be a problem, the use of MCT Oil may be necessary.

Chemotherapy

The success of chemotherapeutic drugs stems from their ability to inhibit growth of neoplastic tissue. One category of chemotherapy drugs, the antimetabolites, function by blocking one step in intermediary metabolism during celluar division. Their most dramatic effect is on rapidly growing cells, which include cancer cells and some rapidly reproducing cells, some of which are found in the gut mucosa. It is no wonder that gastrointestinal upsets are frequent side effects of antimetabolite drugs. Some of the other chemotherapy drugs, the alkylating agents, and the antibiotics also cause nausea, vomiting, and diarrhea, and vinca alkaloids can cause constipation.

Table 6-3   Foods that May Cause Gas or Odor in Colostomy Patients

Gas		Odor	
Legumes	Nuts	Eggs	Cauliflower
Carbonated	Green peppers	Beer	Spinach
beverages	Cauliflower	Legumes	Asparagus
Beer	Melons	Onions	Parsley
Bran cereals and	Sauerkraut	Cabbage	Sauerkraut
breads	Highly seasoned	Broccoli	Fish
Cabbage	foods		
Broccoli	Corn		

One finds little in the literature concerning nutritional therapy for patients taking chemotherapeutic drugs. This lack can best be explained by the fact that to date, few measures have been found that help in reducing the side effects of nausea and vomiting that accompany treatment. The best approach to nutritional therapy requires practicality and common sense to ease the discomfort of the problems created by these drugs. Thorough assessment of dietary intake is essential to obtain baseline information on the prior eating habits of the patient. The diet should at all times conform to the patient's established patterns, although one should keep in mind that hospitalized patients tend to eat better in the morning, when they are rested. In the evening patients are weary from the hospital routine and the numerous tests they may have taken.

Whenever possible, chemotherapy drugs that cause nausea and vomiting, such as nitrogen mustard, 5-fluorouracil, methotrexate, and bleomycin, should be given late in the day. Common practice is to give them early in the morning, thus the side effects cause the patient to lose his or her appetite for two or three meals. If the drug can possibly be injected late in the afternoon, the effects of nausea and vomiting will cause the patient to lose the evening meal, but he or she may regain some appetite by morning. For even less dietary influence, medications can be given in the evening.

The appetite of a nauseated patient receiving chemotherapy is very fragile. To bring such a patient a tray laden with food may only further diminish the patient's already weakened appetite. The patient may become overwhelmed at the sight of so much food and may completely lose his or her appetite. Therefore, try to make the tray as simple as possible, using small plates with smaller than average servings of food. It is then possible to give between-meal snacks that supply the additional calories and protein the patient needs. A word of caution: dietary departments are infamous for serving between-meal snacks with little nutritional value, such as jello and cookies. Be specific when ordering six small meals for the patient. Request high-calorie, high-protein snacks, such as milk or milk substitutes along with a half a sandwich and custard.

An important consideration for patients on 5-FU, Adriamycin and certain other drugs is that they may possibly have alterations in taste sensation. The aversion is most pronounced in protein-type foods such as meat products, chicken, and fish. An effective way to work around this aversion is to diminish the taste of the protein food by offering the foods as a cold entree. Chicken or ham in a salad or roast beef in a cold sandwich can be more acceptable than these meats served hot, since the odor of the food will not be as trong. One might also rely more heavily on dairy dishes, such as cottage cheese and fruit plates, and macaroni and cheese casseroles, which have a less noxious taste or aroma.

A pharmacological approach to reduce nausea and vomiting has been tried with effectiveness. Antiemetic agents were given to patients with colorectal cancer as a prophylaxis during 5-FU therapy. The antiemetics found to be effective were Compazine, Dartal, and Torecan. Ineffective antiemetics were Tigan, Cinnerazine, and pentobarbital.[26]

Alkylating agents and antimetabolites can also cause oral ulcerations or irritation, which are aggravated by acidic and highly seasoned food. Therefore, seasoning should be kept at a minimum. Even though house diets are generally ordered for hospitalized cancer patients on chemotherapy, the nurse should feel free to request bland types of food to supplement this menu. Because of their acidity, juices such as orange and grapefruit are less acceptable to the patient than are the more bland nectars, such as pear and peach. Because of the numbing and cooling effect they have on the mouth, popsicles relieve some oral discomfort.

Radiotherapy

The full-course radiation therapy of 6 weeks takes a huge toll on the nutritional well-being of a cancer patient when it is being administered to the neck, thoracomediastinal, or abdominal region. It is known that nutritional deficiencies arise because of swelling, irritation, or mucosal changes in the gastrointestinal tract. Chronic changes, such as ulceration, fat malabsorption, and intestinal stricture, also appear following radiation to the abdomen. Yet the long-term effects of radiation therapy on nutrition appear to receive little attention either in the literature or in the hospital setting.

Radiation to the Head and Neck A typical case of radiation to the nasopharynx area follows a course of increasing irritability to the esophagus. Following the first week of therapy, there is discomfort upon swallowing. The second week it becomes more difficult to swallow highly textured foods, and by the third week only soft or liquid types of food will pass through the esophageal area. During the last three weeks of therapy and for a period of time after the conclusion of radiotherapy, the patient may not eat at all. An individual who is fighting neoplastic growth and possibly recovering from recent surgery will surely be put in acute negative nitrogen balance. The patient will be in a depleted metabolic state, which prevents rapid recovery and intensifies the patient's already weakened condition. There is a solution to this problem which is rather simple but frequently overlooked. A nasogastric feeding tube can be inserted just prior to radiation therapy, and the patient can be maintained on a highly nutritious, high-calorie, high-protein diet for the full course of radiation therapy. If the patient is prepared and well informed of the anticipated side effects of radiation, he or she will probably consent to the tube feeding with little objection. It takes a staff member who is both convinced of the necessity for optimal nutrition and concerned enough about the patient's welfare to encourage this particular therapy.

Sometimes the person best skilled at passing a nasogastric tube is the anesthesiologist. If the tumor makes passing a regular-size feeding tube difficult, a smaller tube should be passed and a clear, elemental diet given.

If the physician with whom one works is averse to tube feeding a patient who will be given radiation to the head and neck area, the only alternative is to inform the patient of the expected consequences of the radiation treatment. Encourage the patient to eat as much as possible prior to therapy, with the understanding that after 2 to 3 weeks of therapy, eating solids will be nearly impossible. This approach is hardly the most desirable, but until nasogastric tube feeding therapy is given routinely and is seen as a successful route to optional nutrition, it is the only one available.

A word of caution about the type of liquids given during radiation to the head and neck area: citrus juices are irritating to the mucosal lining of the esophagus, as are spicy liquids such as tomato juice.

Commonly occurring side effects of radiation therapy to the head and neck region include destruction of salivary glands and loss of taste sensation. Because of the loss of salivary secretion, dental decay may become a problem. This difficulty is compounded by the trismus frequently seen in people with head and neck cancer. There are difficulties in removing teeth following radiotherapy, so a thorough dental screening should be done prior to treatment to remove any tooth that could give rise to problems.

Large amounts of liquids and foods with gravy and sauces should be offered at mealtime to patients who have diminished salivation. The degree of trismus and the number of teeth extracted will influence the particular type of dietary modification. Some patients with trismus are able to open their mouths wide enough to eat soft foods such as cheese casseroles, tuna casseroles, or dried chopped beef with cream sauce. Others are able to take pureed foods. For those severely affected by trismus, a tube feeding is often the only answer. Along with the already mentioned soft foods or blenderized, pureed foods, one can offer the patient soft-cooked eggs, soft scrambled eggs, cooked cereal with an egg added for protein, soups, juices, and milk substitutes. Given the opportunity, patients will often think of rather ingenious ideas for foods. This opportunity should be given often.

Gastrointestinal Radiation   A patient may be irradiated in the abdominal region for testicular cancer or carcinoma of the bladder. Whatever the reason for abdominal radiation, the effects to the gut are generally similar and differ only in the degree of radiation and the length of treatment. The gut sloughs off all new cells being produced. The acute symptoms are cramping, gastrointestinal upsets with nausea and vomiting, and diarrhea with subsequent loss of electrolytes and fluids. The chronic problems seen following treatment include ulcerations, enteritis, fat malabsorption, and abdominal strictures.

Therapy often includes antidiarrheal agents and antiemetics. These appear to have little or no effects on the ability of the gut to absorb nutrients. They do minimize some of the side effects of radiation, however.

Diet therapy aims at reducing the amount of irritable substances going through the gastrointestinal tract. A low-residue diet is generally ordered. One may also try to curb diarrhea through the use of constipating or stool-forming (high-residue) foods. These includes cheese, pureed carrots, guava nectar, bananas, and apple sauce. Coffee, tea, and prune juice should be avoided because of the stimulating effect they have on the gut. A milk substitute might be given in preference to milk because of the lactose.

During radiation the gut is sloughing off all newly formed cells and is unable to digest complex food stuffs found in normal diets. Recent studies indicate that elemental diets may be of use to abdominally radiated animals because the diets can be absorbed directly across the cell membrane.[20]

NUTRITION AND THE CANCER CARE TEAM

Nutrition is one of the few areas in which nearly all members of the cancer care team can contribute substantially to the care of the patient. The quality of care can be increased when the expertise of the whole team is identified and well coordinated. For example, the speech pathologist is generally not utilized in the nutritional care of patients. However, the speech pathologist can be a tremendous asset in teaching a patient with a glossectomy or a mandibulectomy how to eat and swallow once again. The occupational therapist can contribute by evaluating the limitations the patient may have following radiotherapy or surgery. Where trismus may be a complication for an individual with cancer in the head and neck area, the occupational therapist can teach the patient how to make foods modified in consistency which are tasty and appealing as well as nutritionally sound. Where dining out may eventually be a source of discomfort for the patient who has coordination problems due to a brain tumor or other problems, the occupational therapist can work with the patient in areas of socialization.

The tremendous financial burden placed on hospitalized patients can be alleviated somewhat through the efforts of the social worker. Often an individual who has never had to seek financial assistance would not know what assistance can be obtained. The patient may be eligible for food stamps and other governmental assistance. The social worker can identify the areas of need and contact the agencies that might be able to help. For example, the American Cancer Society sometimes lends blenders to patients who have to make tube feedings. Various community organizations contribute food to needy families at the holiday season. Meals-on-Wheels is a service that brings meals to people who are physically unable to leave their homes. Homemaking services that send people into homes to cook and clean may be available for certain patients. The coordination of these services by the social worker is highly valuable.

Prolonged bed rest has the effect of diminishing an individual's appetite. Because of the periods of time a cancer patient may have to spend in bed as well as the effects of some of the cancer treatments, there is a loss of protein mass in the body. The physical therapist can develop exercises for the patient to use to strengthen his or her body. The important overall effect may contribute to the patient's feeling of well-being, may stimulate the appetite, and may increase food intake. The physical therapist also has the expertise to evaluate the physical home environment. If the patient lives alone and will be doing his or her own cooking, the physical therapist can determine what kinds of special equipment are necessary and what the limitations of the living environment are for tasks of daily living. The knowledge that the entire cancer care team is concerned about his or her nutritional status is of great psychological benefit to the cancer patient and may often stimulate him or her to greater effort in the preparation and/or consumption of a nutritionally sound diet. It will also impress upon the patient the importance of such a regime.

The nurse's aide is often the person on the team who is with the patient at mealtimes. The nurse's aid may be the one who delivers the food tray or feeds the patient. The role of the nurse's aide may be crucial in the actual ingestion of food by the patient. A calm, pleasant, reassuring manner is necessary to encourage the patient to eat. The nurse's aide may also be the one who records the intake and output of the patient. This record is one key way in which the dietitian collects data and determines the necessary nutritional plan.

Besides collecting data on the hospitalized patient, the dietitian must obtain the baseline nutritional history and make an assessment of the patient's nutritional needs. With this information, the dietitian makes recommendations to the doctor and nurse concerning the nutritional aspects of the care plan for the patient. The dietitian works with each team member individually concerning her or his area of involvement with the patient. Fundamental here is the relationship between the dietitian and the nurse. The time the dietitian has available to spend with each patient is limited, especially at mealtimes. However, the nurse is with the patient all day. The actual coordination and execution of the care plan rests with the nursing staff. For example, the dietitian can teach the patient's family the required diet only if informed by the nurse when the family arrives. Also, the nurse is available to evaluate the quality of the feeding technique a nurse's aide is using. The nurse knows first-hand if a tube feeding is causing an adverse reaction in a patient. The nurse's role in the nutritional care of a cancer patient is paramount. As do many other members of the team, the dietitian relies on the nurse as the source of information on the daily routine and concerns of the patient.

SUMMARY

The nurse should be aware of the nutritional status of the patient at all times. Nutritional problems may be evident from the onset of neoplastic growth, or they may appear at any time throughout the course of the illness. As discussed above, some nutritional therapies, such as 5% dextrose with water, have limitations. Treatment modalities, such as chemotherapy or radiotherapy to the head and neck area, may also complicate the nutritional picture. Indeed, secondary malnutrition is often seen in cancer patients. However, with the use of elemental diets, total parenteral nutrition, and the ingenuity and coordination of the cancer care team, there is much more hope for the cancer patient's nutritional status.

REFERENCES

1   Midler, G. B., "Some Aspects of Nitrogen and Energy Metabolism in Cancerous Subjects: A Review," *Cancer Research,* **11**:821, 1951.

2 Sugimura, T.; Birnbaum, S. M.; Winitz, M.; and Greenstein, J.F., "Quantitative Nutritional Studies with Water-Soluble Chemically Defined Diets VIII. The Force Feeding of Diets Lacking in One Essential Amino Acid." *Archives of Biochemical Biophysics,* **81:**439, 1959.

3 Terepka, R. A., and Waterhouse, C., "Metabolic Observations during the Forced Feeding of Patients with Cancer," *American Journal of Medicine,* **20:**225, 1956.

4 Souchon, E. A.; Copeland, E. M.; Watson, P.; and Dudriek, S. J., "Intravenous Hyperalimentation as an Adjunct to Cancer Chemotherapy with 5-Fluorouracil," *Journal of Surgical Research,* **18:**451, 1975.

5 Bayless, T. M., Paige, D. M., and Ferry, G. D., "Lactose Intolerance and Milk Drinking Habits," *Gastroenterology,* **60:**605, 1971.

6 Welsh, J. D., "Isolated Lactase Deficiency in Humans: Report on 100 Patients," *Medicine,* **49:**257, 1970.

7 Costa, G.; Samal, B. A.; Brennan, J.; and Pickren, J. W., "Changes in the Composition of Human Muscle during the Growth of Malignant Tumors," *Proceeding of the American Association of Cancer Research,* **6:**12, 1965.

8 Morris, H., and Lippincott, S., "Effects of Pantothenic Acid on Growth of the Spontaneous Mammary Carcinoma in Female C3H Mice," *Journal of the National Cancer Institute,* **2:**47, 1941.

9 Lane, M.; Alfrey, C. P.; Mengal, C. E.; Doherty, M. A.; and Doherty, J., "The Rapid Induction of Human Riboflavin Deficiency with Galacto Clavin," *Journal of Clinical Investigation,* **43:**357, 1964.

10 Cowan, D. H., and Alison, R. E., "Evaluation of 6-Aminonicotinamide in the Treatment of Metastatic Hypernephroma," *Cancer Chemotherapy,* **54:**175, 1970.

11 Gellhorn, A., and Jones, L. O., "Pyridoxine Deficient Diet and Desoxypyrodoxine in the Therapy of Lymphosarcoma and Acute Leukemia in Man," *Blood,* **4:**60, 1949.

12 Cline, M. J., "Pharmacologic Basis of Cancer Chemotherapy," *Cancer Chemotherapy,* vol. 21, W. B. Saunders Philadelphia, 1971.

13 Burns, J. J.; Connel, A. H.; Dayton, P. G.; Evans, C.; Martin, G. R.; and Taller, D., "Observations on the Drug-Induced Synthesis of D'Glucuronic, L-Gluonic and L-Ascorbic Acids in Rats," *Journal of Pharmaceutical Experimental Therapy,* **129:**132, 1960.

14 Peletier, O., "Vitamin C Status of Cigarette Smokers and Nonsmokers," *American Journal of Clinical Nutrition,* **23:**520, 1970.

15 Warren, F. L., "Aerobic Oxidation of Aromatic Hydrocarbons in the Presence of Ascorbic Acid; The Reaction with Antracene and 3-4 Benzpyrene," *Biochemical Journal,* **37:**338, 1943.

16 Sporn, M.; Dunlop, N.; Newton, D.; and Smith, J., "Prevention of Chemical Carcinogenesis by Vitamin A and Its Synthetic Analogs (Retinoids)," *Federation Proceedings,* **35:**1332, 1976.

17 Chopra, D. P., and Wiloff, L. J., "Inhibition and Reversal of Carcinogen-Induced Lesions in Mouse Prostate in Vitro by All Trans-Retinoic Acid," *Proceeding of the American Association of Cancer Research,* **16:**35, 1975.

18 Vorherr, H.; Massry, S. G.; Utiger, R. D.; and Kleenan, C. R., "Anti-diuretic Principle in Malignant Tumor Extracts from Patients with Inappropriate ADH Syndrome," *Journal of Clinical Endocrinology,* **28:**162, 1968.

19 Chopra, D., and Clerkin, E. P., "Hypercalcium and Malignant Disease," *The Medical Clinics of North America,* **59:**441, 1975.

20   Pagean, R., "Effects of Feeding an Elemental Diet during Abdominal Irradiation," *Strahlentherapie,* **149**:318, 1975.
21   Bounous, G., Gentile, J. M., and Hugon, J., "Elemental Diet in the Management of the Intestinal Lesion Produced by 5-Fluorouracil in Man," *Canadian Journal of Surgery,* **14**:312, 1971.
22   Dudrick, S. J., and Copeland, E. M., "The Role of Nutrition in the Treatment of Cancer," *Nutrition and the M.D.,* **2**:1, 1976.
23   Copeland, E. M.; MacFadgen, B. V.; MacComb, W. S.; Guillamondegui, O.; Jesse, R. H.; and Dudrick, S. J., "Intravenous Hyperalimentation in Patients with Head and Neck Cancer," *Cancer,* **35**:606, 1975.
24   Rodgers, A, C.N., and Steyn, J. H., "Vitamin B_{12} Absorption in Patients with Ileal Resections," *British Journal of Urology,* **46**:625, 1974.
25   Smiddy, F. G.; Gregory, S. D.; Smith, I. B.; and Golighter, J. C., "Faecal Loss of Fluid, Electrolytes, and Nitrogen in Colitis before and after Ileostomy," *Lancet,* **1**:14, 1960.
26   Moertel, C. G., "Nutrition and Chemotherapy of Cancer," *Workshop on Diet and Nutrition in the Therapy and Rehabilitation of the Cancer Patient,* National Institutes of Health, Washington, D.C., March 26, 1975.

BIBLIOGRAPHY

Burkitt, D. P., "Cancer of the GI Tract: Colon, Rectum, Anus, Epidemiology and Etiology," *Journal of the American Medical Association,* **231**:517, 1975.
Cowan, G. J., and Scheetz, W., *Intravenous Hyperalimentation* (London: Henry Kimpton, 1972).
DeWys, W., "Abnormalities of Taste as a Remote Effect of a Neoplasma," *Annals of the New York Academy of Science,* **230**:427, 1974.
Faulk, W. P., Demaeyer, E. M., and Davies, A. J., "Some Effects of Malnutrition on the Immune Response in Man," *American Journal of Clinical Nutrition,* **27**:638, 1974.
Gailani. S., Ohnuma, T., and Rosen, F., *Cancer Medicine* (Philadelphia: Lea & Febiger, 1973), 872–888.
Goodhart, Robert S., and Shils, Maurice E. (eds.), *Modern Nutrition in Health and Disease,* 5th ed. (London: Henry Kimpton, 1975), 981–996.
Lipsett, M. B., "Hormones, Nutrition and Cancer," *Cancer Research,* **35**:3359, 1975.
Nutrition and Cancer (New York: American Cancer Society, 1972).
Peters, J. A., "National Cancer Institute Programs on Nutrition and Cancer," *Cancer Research,* **35**:3544, 1975.
Wynder, E. L., "Overview: Nutrition and Cancer," *Preventive Medicine,* **4**:322, 1975.

Chapter 7

Surgical Approaches to Cancer Management

LoRaine Carlson

Surgical removal of malignant tumors is the oldest form of treatment for this condition. Surgery has retained its leading role for centuries and is still the treatment of choice in a high percentage of cases. Because of recent advances in other treatment modalities, surgery is increasingly becoming only a part of the wider interdisciplinary treatment approach. Therefore the surgeon is less often solely responsible for treating a cancer patient, and surgeon, radiotherapist, chemotherapist, immunotherapist, and nursing staff as a team often make decisions regarding the treatment of cancer.

Surgery is indicated in other than radical removal of cancerous tissue. It may also be required in the course of cancer therapy for taking biopsy specimens, for palliative measures, for modifying the hormonal status by removal of enocrine glands, and for suppressing pain by neurosurgical procedures.

DIAGNOSTIC SURGICAL TECHNIQUES

It is now universally accepted that few types of cancer can be properly treated unless the histologic type has been correctly identified. The histologic diagnosis cannot always be established before an operation; for example, when cancer of the colon, of the retroperitoneal regions, or of the kidneys is involved, the histologic diagnosis is established during surgery. However, in the majority of cases, the histology can be determined before surgery is attempted. In esophageal, gastric, oral cavity, pharyngolaryngeal, rectal, bladder, and bronchial tumors, histologic diagnosis can be based on very small biopsy specimens obtained by use of a suitable instrument during endoscopic investigations.

Biopsy Technique

Although a biopsy often involves only minor surgery, it is extremely important that it be performed properly, since a badly performed biopsy may yield a false negative diagnosis and delay treatment of the disease. When lymph nodes are removed in cases of suspected lymphoma, a large quantity of tissue, usually more than one node with its capsule, should be taken so the diagnosis can be based on extensive evidence. Dissection of healthy tissue surrounding the tumor should be included whenever the excision technique makes doing this possible. This procedure may produce extreme anxiety in the patient, for when the results are positive, patient and family are forced into a more critical decision, especially when radical or extensive surgery is recommended. Considerable support from the oncology team is vital.

The surgeon will usually observe the following guidelines for specimen removal: (1) the line of incision must be such that it can easily be included in a wider excision of the entire tumor, if necessary, without danger of local recurrence along the biopsy scar; (2) the surgical instruments used for the biopsy itself must not be used to continue an operation without being sterilized, because of the risk of contamination with tumor cells; (3) when a lesion is clinically doubtful, the surgeon must not be satisfied with a single negative tissue biopsy, whether done during or after operation, since it is sometimes necessary to take three, four, or even five specimens before a positive result is obtained. When a frozen-section biopsy is to be taken from a tumor on a limb in the course of an operation, a tight tourniquet should be applied above the biopsy incision to prevent venous and lymphatic cellular dissemination; then if the limb is to be amputated, the incision will be made above the tourniquet. If after the frozen section the pathologist has the remotest doubt regarding malignancy, removal of the remainder of the mass must not be undertaken until the definitive microscopic specimen has been prepared. An important detail in cases of frozen-section examination is that the surgeon should not embark on resection until receiving the written diagnosis signed by the pathologist. A diagnosis given by word of mouth or by telephone in large centers with several operating theaters carries the risk of making an error and attaching a diagnosis of cancer to the wrong patient.

Needle Biopsy   A useful way to obtain significant material without unduly injuring the patient is by needle biopsy. It demands great care and skill. Some technical aspects of the procedure include positioning the needle in such a way that the entry hole can easily be included in the area of skin that would be excised or irradiated and cauterizing the needle course when possible to prevent the dissemination of tumor cells. It is unwise to take needle biopsies from tumors of highly vascularized organs, such as the thyroid, because of the risk of insidious bleeding. The possibility of insidious bleeding must be recognized by the nursing staff regardless of the location of the biopsy, and direct pressure should be applied for an appropriate amount of time, observing the site for bleeding and changes in the vital signs. One general complaint about needle biopsy is that if positive it is useful, but if negative it affords no guarantee whatsoever that cancer is not present, since the cancer itself might not have been biopsied.

One of the hazards of any biopsy is the dissemination of neoplastic cells. There are no quantitative data on this point to determine the potential harm of such dissemination (see Chapter 4, "Pathophysiology of Cancer"). However, there are no means of ensuring that neoplastic cells have not escaped. Excision does not rule out the possibility that the knife has passed through tissues containing cancerous cells which are often present within a band of some centimeters around the macroscopic tumor margins, or that these cells, given the speed of venous and lymphatic drainage, could have been carried to distant organs within a matter of minutes or even seconds.

Diagnostic Laparotomy   Laparotomy for diagositc investigation has been a fairly general practice in the past few years. This operation is necessary whenever an abdominal syndrome of suspected neoplastic origin cannot be diagnosed with the usual radiologic or endoscopic investigations. It also has been advocated for excluding occult intraperitoneal, lumboaortic, or liver metastases before such major surgery as hemipelvectomy for sarcoma, pneumonectomy for bronchial carcinoma, or esophagectomy for esophageal carcinoma, especially in view of the high frequency of occult liver or intra-abdominal metastases that occur with these malignancies. Perhaps the most frequent indication is to aid in the staging of malignant lymphoma, particularly Hodgkin's disease.

PREOPERATIVE EVALUATION

No appropriate surgical intervention can be undertaken without a preliminary assessment of (1) the exact extent of the disease, (2) the biologic aggressiveness (growth rate) of the tumor, and (3) the patient's general condition. The extent of the disease must be defined by means of diagnostic aids that allow for detection of the size of the primary tumor, the extent of any regional lymph node involvement, and the presence of any blood-borne metastases. Clinical examination must include (1) the appropriate radiographic investigations, some of which (namely lymphoangiography and angiography) have recently revealed unexpected diagnostic potential; (2) radioisotope investigations; and (3) endoscopies. Colonoscopy and duodenoscopy now often permit accurate preoperative diagnosis with histologic documentation of cancer of the large bowel, duodenum, and ampulla of Vater and occasionally the pancreas. Another promising field of investigation is enzymatic and immunologic diagnosis.

The biologic aggressiveness (growth rate) of the cancer is usually estimated from the extent of the disease, the patient's general condition, and previous negative studies if any, of the organ involved. Assessment of the patient's general condition is highly important. A patient with a visceral cancer usually experiences some type of repercussion from the cancer. The most common examples of this are anemia due to prolonged blood loss; electrolyte imbalance due to vomiting, diarrhea, or defects in intestinal absorption; hypoalbuminemia due to malnutrition; and toxic signs, including fever, due to reabsorption of degraded matter produced by the tumor. All must be corrected as much as possible before surgical treatment is begun. There is increasing evidence that the patient's immune status correlates inversely with the extent of the disease. Therefore it is probable that immunologic tests will be performed routinely in the near future, although this approach is now investigational, in an effort to define the prognosis of the disease and thus its susceptibility to curative surgery.

THE PLANNING OF TREATMENT

A surgeon who is preparing to treat a patient with a malignant tumor must always be aware that he or she cannot provide rational treatment in isolation. A coopera-tive effort with the pathologist, radiotherapist, chemotherapist, im-munotherapist, and oncology nursing team can ensure that the patient gets the best treatment. The importance of the interdisciplinary approach, both formal and informal, and in both the strategic and tactical aspects of patient manage-ment, cannot be overemphasized. In all hospitals in which cancer is treated, there should be a standing oncology committee of clinical oncologists, including the nurse oncology clinicians, to oversee and coordinate the plans of treatment and care for cancer patients. Such committees exist in cancer centers, and their tasks are to draft treatment protocols, detail plans of treatment for the most frequent conditions, and yet allow the individuality of each patient's feelings, family, and very special needs.

MULTICENTRIC TUMORS

Multicentric lesions of the same organ or system may occur when the entire tissue of the organ is subjected to carcinogenic stimulus. Paired organs such as breasts, testes, and ovaries raise special problems. The risk of carcinoma in the contralateral breast after mastectomy has been calculated to be 10 to 20 times greater than the breast cancer risk in the general female population.[1] Systematic preoperative mammography has demonstrated a high incidence of bilateral breast cancer, as it detects occult carcinomas that cannot be found by palpation. The high frequency of bilateral mammary carcinoma has led some surgeons to perform a precautionary simple mastectomy of the contralateral breast whenever they do a radical mastectomy for carcinoma. To avoid disfigurement, careful subcutaneous dissection of the mammary tissue plus insertion of pros-thesis has been proposed. Without going to these lengths, one should certainly keep a close check on the contralateral breast after mastectomy by frequent clinical examination and mammography. Ovarian carcinoma is bilateral in 40 to 50 percent of cases, and hence bilateral oophorectomy is mandatory. Bilaterality is a less frequent problem in tumors of the testes, as the incidence is only 2 or 3 percent.

RATIONALE OF RADICAL CANCER SURGERY

Most malignant tumors arise from one or more foci in the same organ and are confined to that organ for a variable length of time. Although tumor cells may escape early from the primary focus, they are unlikely to "take" in distant organs unless they adhere in emboli of some size. The chances of successful surgical treatment depend on the technical feasibility of removing the primary tumor with a reasonable margin of surrounding healthy tissue and the absence of metastatic foci. When these two conditions are satisfied, radical surgery is indicated. It may be contraindicated in one of the following circumstances: (1) if the operative mortality is too high in relation to the chances of cure, (2) if the mutilation would be too severe, (3) if there is a risk of inducing a deterioration in the course of the disease, and (4) if similar results can be obtained from conservative or nonsurgical treatment.

Operative Mortalities

Current techniques of anesthesia, resuscitation, and postoperative care have reduced operative mortality to such a great degree that it hardly constitutes a problem. Some radical operations, such as those involving the esophagus or pancreas, continue to carry a high operative mortality, especially in elderly or debilitated patients. One must make the decision on an individual basis, bearing in mind that cancer is a fatal disease and that if the surgery affords a reasonable chance of cure, it should be offered even if the operative risk is high. The patient and the family should participate in this decision if it is at all possible.

Undue Mutilation

Another contraindication for radical surgery is undue mutilation. The surgeon must assess what "undue" means to a given patient when compared with the degree of relief and the chance of cure that the operation offers. The patient's psychologic reactions, social and family environment, and need and fitness for employment must be carefully considered. The decision for or against radical surgery must depend on a careful analysis of the complex life situation with regard for the quality of life that can be offered as well as its duration. The surgeon and the oncology team must strive to be objective and free from environmental and contingent psychologic pressures from within. This is no time to be influenced by fear of criticism from colleagues or the public. In deciding against a major operation, the surgeon must be sure of not being unfair to a patient in denying the patient even a small chance of cure, if this is what he or she desires. The oncology team may need to approach those colleagues who have special expertise in a particular area.

The possibility that a surgical procedure may accelerate the course of cancer has long been the subject of debate. Dissemination of cancerous cells owing to manipulation of the cancer must have more intensive study to confirm or deny that this condition affects the prognosis. Rough or clumsy manipulation of cancerous tissue does carry a potential risk in the operative field. The effects of surgery, psychologic and physical stress, anesthesia, and the interruption nutrition all have an effect on the physiologic processes and the immune system. The total effect of surgery and its accompanying factors may differ greatly from patient to patient and therefore are not easily subject to sweeping generalizations.

Palliative Surgery

Palliative surgical treatment of cancer is treatment without the prospect of cure. Elimination of the most burdensome symptoms, prevention of complications, prolongation of life, and psychologic uplift are some of the aims of palliative surgery. Much of cancer surgery may be considered palliative given the fact that occult spread of the disease before treatment is great in a high percentage of cases. The limitations are far greater than is the case with curative or radical surgery, as palliative surgery does not attempt a cure but simply an improvement of the patient's condition. A high operative risk may reasonably be faced when there is a prospect of cure, but is not justified in the case of palliation.

Indications   The indications for palliative surgery are less well defined than those for radical surgery. In a number of cases, notwithstanding the presence of distant metastases, the primary tumor may be the chief cause of suffering; therefore a palliative operation is indicated. A frequently occurring example of this situation is a large, ulcerated, and painful limb sarcoma that is beyond the range of radiotherapy or chemotherapy and for which the only acceptable solution is amputation of the limb. This operation may insistently be demanded by the patient. Another example of palliative removal is the simple mastectomy performed because of extensive cancer of the breast when the organ is ulcerated and is a source of bleeding and infection. While the surgery is not curative, it affords the patient relief of symptoms.

Relief of Obstructions   A fairly important part of palliative surgery is the clearing of obstructions produced by the presence of a large cancerous mass. Obstructions may occur in the alimentary tract, the urinary tract, the bile ducts, or the blood vessels, whether venous or arterial. While obstructions of the traceobronchial tree are occasionally subject to surgical restoration of patency, ordinarily they require removal of bronchial and distal pulmonary tissue. Lymphatic obstruction usually represents advanced disease or effects of prior therapy and is rarely approached surgically.

Alimentary tract obstructions are the ones that most often require surgical intervention. The most frequent sites of obstruction are the esophagus, the stenosis of which can often be remedied by the insertion of an intracavitary prosthesis; the pylorus, easily bypassed by creation of a gastroenteric anastomosis; and the large intestine, especially the distal portion. When the intestines are occluded, simple bypass may possibly solve the problem, or a colostomy may be necessary. Obstruction of the small bowel is common in carcinomatosis of the peritoneal cavity, especially when the primary is ovarian cancer. With small-bowel obstruction, surgical procedures are rarely helpful for long periods and may be technically very difficult. Decompression with a long tube may restore functionally adequate patency and seems preferable to the more complex surgical procedure. *Obstruction of the ureters* is not uncommon in pelvic tumors; resolution of the obstruction depends on whether it is unilateral or bilateral and on the extent of the disease. The ureters can be diverted into the large intestine. However, construction of a urinary diversion may give rise to a urinary problem with which the patient may not be able to cope, and the patient may have more time to suffer much pain both psychologic from the urinary diversion and physiologic from the pelvic cancer. Therefore, if there is no prospect of the success of a major operative procedure, the patient may experience a relatively painless death when uremia from the ureteral obstruction is permitted to proceed to that terminal phase.

Surgery for perfusion or infusions as a means of placing tubes or catheters for the administration of chemotherapeutic agents requires a delicate procedure. The goal is to convey drugs in high concentration to a cancer that is confined to a single anatomic region, thus sparing the rest of the body the harmful effects of these drugs. To perfuse an extremity it is necessary to connect arteries and veins of the limb to extracorporeal circulation equipment. For infusion of an organ, the artery selected must be defined and prepared, and a small catheter is then inserted into its lumen. This can be accomplished percutaneously as well as through an open incision.

Hormonal Manipulation

Surgical alteration of the endocrine status of a patient with hormone dependent cancer constitutes a special area of cancer surgery. The most common operation of this kind is an oophorectomy in the treatment of breast cancer of premenopausal patients. It brings about clinical regression of the tumor in 30 percent of patients, especially those with skeletal and soft-tissue metastases, and improvement with retardation of tumor growth in another 20 percent. The best results are obtained in patients between the ages of 35 and 45; the response is less good and less frequent among those under 30 years of age.[2] Another common endocrine operation is orchiectomy in patients with prostatic cancer; the operation produces long remission in a high percentage of cases. The adverse psychologic effects of orchiectomy can be partially overcome by the use of testicular prostheses. Orchiectomy is also successful in an uncommon condition, metastasizing breast cancer in the male.

Reconstructive Surgery after Extensive Surgical Resection

The need to remove an ample margin of apparently healthy tissue around the visible borders of a tumor sometimes involves extensive surgical resection with considerable functional impairment and disfigurement. It is therefore essential for the surgeon to call on a good plastic surgeon who is able to mitigate the adverse effects of extensive surgery. The surgical procedures that most frequently require reconstructive operations are those of the head and neck, breasts, and superficial tissues of all sites. The type of reconstructive surgery chosen depends on many factors: the site and extent of previous surgery; the loss of subcutaneous tissue; the chance that the primary surgery achieved a permanent cure; the age and general condition of the patient; and the availability of free skin grafts, cartilage grafts, and tube grafts. Reconstruction may be immediate and permanent; immediate and temporary, usually with free grafts for the purpose of emergency biologic integration pending permanent measures; or delayed for safety reasons until suitable graft tissue can be prepared and transferred.

SURGICAL PAIN CONTROL MEASURES

The pain that accompanies neoplastic disease may exceed the endurance of the patient because of its duration and severity. This creates a different problem for both the patient and those who care for him or her. Most procedures for palliation of pain in cancer do not change the course of the disease. Control of intractable pain by neurosurgical intervention should be undertaken relatively early, while the person's condition is good enough to tolerate general anesthesia and while anticipated survival is sufficiently long to justify the period of postoperative pain and limited activity. Prevention of drug addiction is another argument for early intervention. Generally speaking, when life expectancy is less than 3 months, nonoperative procedures are the best therapy.

Cordotomy

Cordotomy for relief of pain in cancer can be expected to provide adequate relief in 70 to 80 percent of cases. The sites chosen most frequently for surgical interruption of the spinothalamic tracts lie within the spinal cord, for the treatment of pain in the extremities; the thoracoabdominal region; or the pelvic region. The preferred site for interruption of the spinothalamic tracts is dictated by two considerations: the level of analgesia desired and the level of the cord at which impulses from the painful area enter. There are a number of conditions associated with cancer in which anterolateral cordotomy may fail to relieve the complaint of pain despite the adequacy of the procedure. The most frequent is addiction to narcotics, in which the request for drugs is equated with pain. Depression and emotional disturbances in patients with cancer require careful evaluation, as pain may be a manifestation of the emotional disorder and not a reflection of the disease. Hence a cordotomy will fail.

The single most frequent complication of cordotomy is urinary retention. Bilateral cordotomy is associated with a higher incidence of urinary retention and often requires an indwelling catheter. The possibility of urinary tract infection must be considered. Either unilateral or bilateral cordotomy may compromise potency as well as sexual sensation. Bilateral cordotomy affects sexual sensation in both sexes. The effects on sexuality should not be considered as a minor drawback to the physician, for they may well be a major factor to the patient, and should not be disregarded, especially when the patient is young.

Pelvic Exenteration

Pelvic exenteration, often called "pelvic evisceration" or "pelvic sweep," is a surgical procedure indicated for carcinomas that are radioresistant or incurable by less radical surgery, that are destructive locally and capable of growing to a great size, and that do not tend to metastasize. Figures 7-1 and 7-2 show the stages of cancer of the cervix. Pelvic exenteration would probably be performed only in stage IV, shown in Figure 7-2. The inevitable outcomes, if the tumor is allowed to grow, are extensive local destruction, enteric and/or urinary obstruction, sepsis, pain, hemorrhage, and death. Pelvic exenteration, a surgical procedure that mutilates body structure and changes body excretory and sexual function, is performed on both sexes and for adults in all age ranges. Because none of the pelvic organs are essential to life and because they are anatomically suitable for en bloc dissection, the procedure is considered reasonable.

According to Brunshwig,[3] pelvic exenteration was first performed in 1948 and consisted of en masse resections of the bladder, vagina, uterus, adnexae, lower ureters, pelvic colon, and pelvic cellular tissue to include lymph nodes with denudation of the sciatic nerve roots. Urinary and fecal diversions were carried out by one of several methods: (1) formation of a wet colostomy with ureters implanted 8 to 12 cm proximal to the end colostomy; or (2) construction of a separate urinary diversion by isolation of a lower segment of ileum and implantation of the ureters into this loop, the distal end of which is brought out as a urinary stoma in the right lower quadrant of the abdomen; an ordinary colostomy is fashioned in the left lower quadrant. As experience increased with these patients, it became evident that under certain instances, the neoplasm extended forward into the bladder but not backward into the rectum, and the operation was carried out removing bladder, vagina, and uterus, sparing the rectum. The

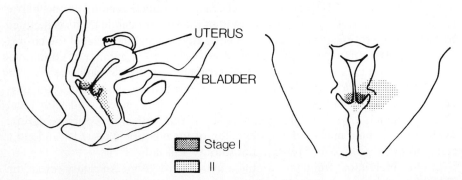

Figure 7-1 Early stages of carcinoma of the cervix. *Stage I:* Carcinoma is confined specifically to the cervix and may be subdivided into stage Ia or stage Ib. *Stage II:* Carcinoma extends beyond the cervix but not onto the pelvic wall and involves the upper two-thirds of the vagina.

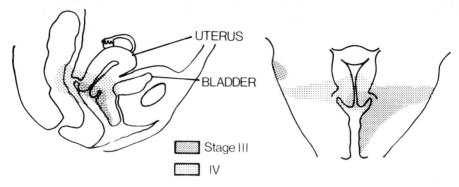

UTERUS

BLADDER

Stage III

IV

Figure 7-2 Late stages of carcinoma of the cervix. *Stage III:* Carcinoma has extended onto the pelvic wall, allowing no cancer-free space between tumor and wall. The lower one-third of the vagina is involved. *Stage IV:* Carcinoma extends beyond the true pelvis or involves the mucosa of the bladder or rectum.

ureters are implanted into an isolated segment as described or into the intact colon. This partial exenteration is known as an "anterior pelvic exenteration" (see Figure 7-3). In situations in which the cancer extends backward into the rectal colon, there is excision of the rectum, vagina, uterus, adnexae, and pelvic nodes, necessitating a permanent colostomy, but there is an intact urinary tract. This procedure is known as a "posterior pelvic exenteration" (see Figure 7-4). "Total pelvic exenteration," consists of the en masse removal of the rectum, distal sigmoid colon, urinary bladder, distal ureters, internal iliac vessels and their lateral branches, all pelvic reproductive organs, and lymph nodes (see Figure 7-5). The entire pelvic floor and peritoneum, levator muscles, and

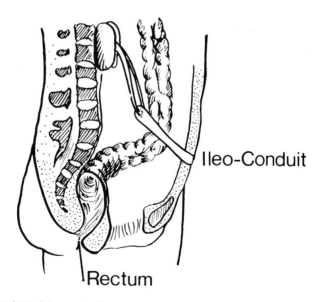

Ileo-Conduit

Rectum

Figure 7-3 Anterior pelvic exenteration.

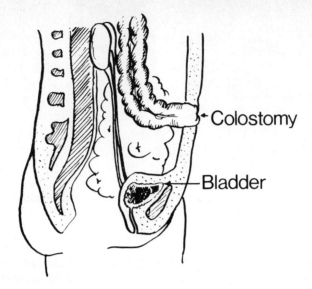

Figure 7-4   Posterior pelvic exenteration.

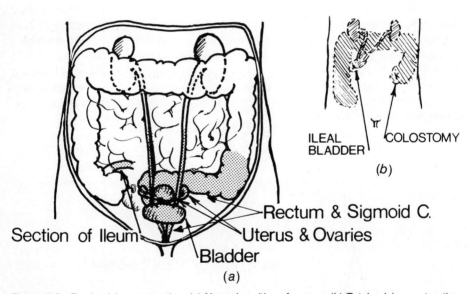

Figure 7-5   Total pelvic exenteration. (a) Normal position of organs. (b) Total pelvic exenteration.

perineum are also excised in women. Urinary and fecal diversion are performed via an ileal conduit and a colostomy.

Indications for Pelvic Exenterations   The indications for pelvic exenterations in advanced cancer of the cervix, whether new or recurrent cancer, are (1) actual invasion of the bladder, rectum, or both by cancer of the cervix; (2) such close extension to bladder, rectum, or both that separation of one or both would lead to difficult removal of all neoplasms, so sacrifice of one or both adjacent organs is consistent with wide resection of cancer; (3) hydronephrosis of one or both kidneys or nonvisualization of one or both kidneys on preoperative pyelograms; (4) the surgeon's assessment that the patient can tolerate psychologically and be rehabilitated from this type of radical surgery.

Contraindications The contraindications are (1) metastases outside the pelvis; (2) swelling and sciatica-type pain in one or both legs; (3) psychosis; and (4) when, at exploratory laparotomy, it is determined that a plane of separation cannot be developed between the cancerous pelvic mass and the sides of the pelvis, so that if the exenteration were to be carried out, neoplastic tissue of necessity would be left behind.

Hamilton and Schlapper[4] report that approximately 20,000 new cases of cervical carcinoma, not including cancer in situ, will be diagnosed in 1976. Radioresistant or recurrent carcinomas of the cervix are the most frequent indications for pelvic exenteration: cancer of the cervix metastasizes to adjacent organs and along lymphatic pathways to regional lymph nodes. There is a tendency for cervical neoplasms of the squamous cell variety to remain localized in the pelvis for long periods as they grow along the planes of least resistance and in continuity with surrounding tissues despite the metastatic spread. This characteristic of squamous cell carcinoma makes en block dissection possible.

Cancer of the endometrium has a high cure rate with primary treatment as well as a low incidence rate, so radical surgery is not frequently done. There is a higher incidence of vaginal adenocarcinoma among adolescent women whose mothers received diethyestilbestrol during their first trimester of pregnancy than among the general population.

Exenteration is the alternative to a lethal disease. The person faced with such massive surgery must have the desire to cope with altered methods of such basic needs as urinary and fecal elimination as well as sexual intercourse. Thus, psychological evaluation is as essential as physical evaluation. Hamilton and Schlapper provide an excellent postoperative care plan.[4]

Complications Previous radiation may pose some problems since it causes damage to healthy living tissue and some necrosis of all tissues. Thus when x-ray therapy has been given preoperatively, intestinal obstructions may occur in the postoperative period, or enteroperineal and colorectal fistuals may develop. Irradiated tissue has decreased vascularity, does not regenerate normally in response to injury, and is more susceptible to necrosis if infected or traumatized. Fistulas, which are generally treated conservatively, form in this sequence: there is first a dependent bowel segment in the pelvis which becomes partially obstructed; edema, ischemia, and ulceration follow; perforation through the perineal scar finally appears. For a patient with this type of surgery, the perineal floor is relatively thin and is composed of skin, subcutaneous tissue, and scar tissue. Therefore, some degree of herniation will be experienced as perineal bulging during standing or coughing. Necrosis of the ileal segment may occur if that section of the bowel was previously in an irradiated field. The ongoing renal status is evaluated by means of periodically repeated intravenous pyelograms and ileograms.

A physiologic and psychologic crisis occur with a pelvis exenteration; diligent nursing and medical care are needed. Those who hope to be therapeutic agents to any person faced with pelvic exenteration must deal with their own feelings concerning mutilation. The long-term survival rate reveals that the procedure, although radical, is justifiable. According to Brunschwig,[3] pelvic exenterations, complete, or partial, are difficult operations, and the postoperative care presupposes thorough training in abdominopelvic surgery in the broadest sense. Collaboration between surgeon, gynecologist, and urologist is important for the benefit of the patient. As collaboration progresses, each individual specialist in turn may assume the major responsibility for the group's procedure, although radical, is justifiable. According to Brunschwig,[3] pelvic these operations is a spirit of defeatism and lack of appreciation of what can be done. The most serious and unfortunate factor is the habit of procrastination until such time that the opportunities for benefit to the patient are greatly reduced, to the point that the situation becomes hopeless.

Brunschwig has reported the following results of pelvic exenteration when performed for cancer of the cervix (new and recurrent cases combined). The number of patients operated on from September 1947 through December 1957 was 430. Ninety-one (31.6 percent) were living and well without cancer 5 years later.

HEAD AND NECK SURGERY

Cancer of the head and neck can lead to deforming radical surgery that can be devastating in its effects. In the past this was primarily a disease of males, with a male/female ratio of 4:1. Women are now increasingly affected, and the ratio is closer to 2:1.[5] Malignant tumors of the buccal cavity, pharnyx, and larnyx contributed to 4.5 percent of the deaths among males and 1.4 percent of the deaths among females from cancer in the United States in 1967.[6] Unlike the incidence of lung cancer, the incidence rate of squamous cell cancer of the head and neck region has been comparatively stable in recent years. One reason for the difference in the incidence of these two types of cancer could be that the patients who smoke and develop lung cancer are mainly cigarette smokers, while squamous cell cancers of the mouth, pharynx, and extrinsic larynx are more often related to cigar and pipe smoking. Cancer of the vocal cord, like cancer of the lung, seems to be related to cigarette smoking.

Early attempts at cures of head and neck cancer by surgical excision began during the nineteenth century. They were mostly unsuccessful. Radium and roentgen rays were discovered at the beginning of the twentieth century, and radiation therapy was added to the treatment of head and neck cancer. The results still left much to be desired. In the 1940s, surgical techniques became more sophisticated and were more successful as an alternative to or conjunct therapy with radiation.

Cancers of the head and neck are extremely significant to the patient because many of these tumors and their subsequent treatment are readily visible to others. In contrast, carcinoma of the abdominal cavity may be fatal without changing the patient's appearance or acceptance by society. Therapy of patients with head or neck cancer requires that patients feel presentable to family, friends, and peers, or they will feel life to be not worth living.

The head and neck region has several essential functions. One of these functions is the preservation of a clear airway for respiration. Another function is swallowing and the conduction of food and liquids into the gastrointestinal tract. Although the latter function can be short-circuited by gastrostomy, the loss of taste is a serious loss, for taste can be one of life's greatest pleasures. Speech is a third important function. While a patient can speak in the absence of the larnyx by learning esophageal speech or by having a mechanical connection between the airway and the mouth so that the lips and tongue can be used for articulation without the larnyx, the larnyx is still essential for normal speech.

Treatment of cancers of the head and neck calls for a multidisciplinary team approach. Oncology subspecialties need to be well developed and integrated to provide the best patient care. Survival results reflect only the length of life, not its quality. Quality and quantity of survival are influenced by all cancer therapists in a team approach. The surgeon and the radiotherapist are the essential nucleus, while the general, plastic, otologic, and oral surgeons should be consulted at various times.

In a significant portion of patients with oral cancer, the initial clinical presentation is unfortunately unfavorable. Extensive infiltration at the primary site plus invasion of adjacent structures lessen the chance of local control of the disease by either irradiation alone or surgery alone. Clinical evidence of regional lymph node spread indicates a poor prognosis. In the recent past, radical surgical excisions has seemed to give the most promising answer to the problem. The combined operation of neck dissection plus mandibulectomy and excision of the primary lesion has given considerable success where other treatment methods have failed. However, the long-range effectiveness of radical surgery is limited since the incidence of recurrence is high. Therefore the prognosis for the patient with oral cancer remains discouraging, despite increasingly radical operations and more sophisticated irradiation techniques.

The choice of treatment method should be based on which surgical operation or irradiation technique is most likely to cure the individual patient or, failing this, which will achieve maximum palliation. Many factors, such as age, general condition of the patient, the anatomic site of involvement, the state of the disease, and the availability of experienced personnel, all influence the decision. For early cancer, the short-range cosmetic and functional advantages of irradiation are apparent, though surgery may be equally effective, less painful, and less time-consuming. For the patient with advanced disease, radical excision has advantages. The chief deterrent to its choice is the natural reluctance to advise mutilating operations without the certainty of cure. This attitude must be balanced by the fact that the disfigurement and loss of function following radical surgery seldom equal that caused by unrestricted cancer growth.

The majority of oral cancers are squamous or epidermoid in type. The basic surgical principle in their management is to obtain adequate wide excision of the primary lesion plus removal of regional lymph node metastases when and if they appear. Lip cancers have a tendency to remain localized. Their surgical management is chiefly concerned with adequate removal of the primary growth, usually accomplished by a simple V-type incision. Neglected infiltrative lesions and those recurring after prior treatment usually require more extensive excisions combined with plastic repair utilizing neighboring tissues.

Buccal mucosa cancers tend to run an agressive course. Since they may be encountered at the commissure of the mouth, along the occlusal plane of the teeth, or at the retromolar area, surgical management is complex. Invasion of either the upper or the lower gingival gutters is often seen, and trismus is not an uncommon finding. To be effective, through and through excision is often required in advanced cases, and an associated neck dissection is usually advisable. Plastic reconstruction should immediately follow. This is complicated procedure, requiring the use of forehead, shoulder, or neck flaps. Removal of the mandible may be necessary, and this will interfere with teeth occlusion and support of the tongue while impairing swallowing and breathing and producing a cosmetic deformity. Several techniques have been recommended to handle this problem. The procedure used depends on how much mucous membrane lining is available for closure. If the resection is small and a limited amount of mucous membrane is bone are removed, immediate replacement may be obtained by bone graft and the teeth may be wired in occlusion. Unfortunately, in most cases there is a major mucous membrane deficit, and soft-tissue replacement can be accomplished only by a skin flap. Stainless steel wire can be used to stabilize the mandibular fragments; the wire is removed later and replaced with bone grafts.

Following hemiglossectomy the remaining portion of the tongue may be reconstructed to a small, flat structure by means of a suture of the tip to the side of the tongue. This is preferable to suturing it into the buccal area. Free skin grafts can be applied to small posterior, denuded areas. Even a small but mobile tongue is helpful in speech and swallowing.

When the facial nerve has been sacrificed, immediate transfer of a portion of the masseter muscle to the corner of the mouth is helpful in restoring oral function.

Cancers of the hypopharynx and larynx are unique. These tumors produce symptoms early, and the area of tumor involvement can usually be visualized at the initial examination. Hoarseness is the primary symptom of laryngeal cancer. A dilemma arises because the symptoms produced by cancer are similar to those produced by benign conditions. As a result, patients who have cancer of the larynx and hypopharynx are frequently treated for benign conditions, which delays detecting the correct etiology. To detect cancer of the larnyx and hypopharynx early, an indirect laryngoscopy should be done. Biopsy may be performed by direct laryngoscopy with the use of local or general anesthesia.

Lesions that involve the membranous portion of the true vocal cord and extent to involve the anterior commissure and 25 percent of the opposite cord or within 1 cm subglotally are treated by hemilaryngectomy. Cancers involving only the supraglottis (epiglottis and false cords) can be treated by partial laryngeal surgery (supraglottal resection), thereby preserving laryngeal function without decreasing survival.

MASTECTOMY

Cancer of the breast is the leading cause of death from cancer in women. It is no wonder that there has been great interest in identifying precancerous or presumably curable lesions. The pathologic recognition of noninvasive (in situ) cancer has been fairly well established. The identification of lesions that are regular and predictable precursors to invasive and metastasizing cancer has been the subject of many investigations. Chronic cystic mastitis has been considered precancerous by some authorities but not by others. There are three benign breast lesions—fibrocystic disease, fibroadenomas, and intraductal papillomas—that have the potential for malignant transformation and so are considered to be premalignant. Most of these lesions, however, do not change. Only two of the seven distinct types of fibrocystic disease—duct epithelial hyperplasia with atypia and apocrine metaplasia with atypia—seem to have a true malignant transformation potential.

The minimum requirement of management for a patient with one of the truly precancerous variants of fibrocystic disease would be very careful follow-up examinations and diagnostic aids. Serious consideration must be given to some definitive surgical procedure in patients who are exhibiting signs of severe emotional stress or who have other epidemiologic factors placing them in an even higher risk group for developing breast cancer. Since these lesions are commonly bilateral and multicentric, any surgical procedure would entail a complete removal of both breasts if absolute protection is to be obtained. This can best be accomplished by bilateral complete mastectomies and breast reconstruction. Bilateral subcutaneous mastectomies offer a better cosmetic result, but it is doubtful whether all breast tissue can be removed with this technique. Fibroadenomas are treated by simple excision, which is best accomplished through incisions made along the natural dynamic wrinkle lines. Intraductal papillomas are best managed by complete excision of the central ducts with preservation of the nipple and areola. As this operation precludes future nursing of infants, it is not ideal for young women anxious to have and nurse children.

Subcutaneous mastectomy is the surgical treatment for minimal breast cancer. According to some authors, the idea that subcutaneous mastectomy might not remove the entire cancer can be held only by those individuals who cannot conceive of the completeness of the various techniques of subcutaneous mastectomy. These techniques allow resection of the entire breast and even an axillary dissection, with removal of the areola, subareola, and all of the ductal tissue, leaving only preplanned skin flaps for reconstruction. Preplanning is the key to the modern surgical approach to noninvasive or minimal cancer. Subcutaenous mastectomy has been used successfully in central tumors of the breast.

At the time of surgery a frozen section of the tissue is examined under the microscope. If the tumor is malignant, the first incision is closed. Drapes, instruments, and gloves are changed in an attempt to prevent possible spread of cancer cells, and the more extensive operation is then performed. If there are no gross signs of extension of the carcinoma, the surgeon does a radical mastectomy, consisting of removal of the entire breast, pectoral muscles, axillary lymph nodes, fat, fascia, and adjacent tissues in one piece. The surgeon must determine the amount of overlying skin that can safely be left to cover the defect. If it is insufficient, a skin graft may be done. Preoperatively the surgeon may order the anterior surface of a thigh shaved and prepared surgically in case need for a graft should arise. If the lesion is located in the medial quadrant of the breast, particularly the upper medial quadrant, an extended radical mastectomy may be performed; this procedure includes removal of the parasternal lymph nodes. Lesions in the medical quadrant tend to metastasize to the internal mammary chain of lymph nodes. The surgeon may expose nodes by splitting the sternum or by dividing the coastal cartilages of the second through the fifth ribs. Following the removal of the breast and adjacent tissue, a stab wound may be made near the axilla, and a catheter is inserted and attached to negative suction. The purpose of the catheter is to remove blood and serum that may collect under the skin flap. The collection of this debris would prevent healing and predispose to infection. There usually is very little drainage from the incision when a catheter is inserted, and an extensive dressing is not always necessary.

Silastic silicone rubber has achieved fairly wide acceptance for reconstruction after simple mastectomy for benign disease. Numerous papers on augmentation after subcutaneous mastectomy can be found in the surgical literature. Prosthetic augmentation following mastectomy for malignant diseases has only recently been considered. There seems to be a natural reluctance to make further assault where a tissue already is so seriously traumatized or where the prognosis is so uncertain. The resultant heavy scar tissue and lack of skin cover following a radical mastectomy, along with the post radiation damage usually done when breast cancer is this extensive, make the prospect of reconstructive procedures less desirable.

There are some procedures in use today for the correction of the chest deformity created by a radical mastectomy. If the opposite breast is large, it can satisfactorily be used in part for reconstruction in some instances. This procedure still does not correct the upper-chest deformity, nor does it eliminate the possible danger of using a breast in which another malignancy may develop. Synthetic implants can be inserted under the skin and scar. The implants may be of solid type, or they may be one of the inflatable prostheses. It should be noted that one prosthesis often used has Dacron patches that encourage the formation of fibrosis to envelope the prosthesis. If this prosthesis is used, it is recommended that it be overfilled to prevent wrinkling. This is to prevent erosion of the thin skin overlaying a wrinkled implant. The breast may be reconstructed also by the use of a large abdominal-tube pedicle with nipple replacement by graft either from the labia minora or from the opposite areola and nipple.

COLORECTAL SURGERY

Surgical treatment of obstruction of the colon due to cancer was slow to evolve, because of the fixation on the mechanical approach, while the complications of anemia, malnutrition, and dehydration raised insoluble problems for the early surgeons. Peritonitis was also a constant problem. Rankin developed the simplest and most direct method of resection of the lesion from the extraperitoneal position.

The functions of the lower part of the intestinal tract are those of absorption, storage, and evacuation. Any interference with these functions by a lesion that irritates, ulcerates, and obstructs will cause vital changes in the health of the individual. Indigestion, malnutrition, change in bowel habits, anemia, and local discomfort and pain may be present to some degree as the growth develops. More acute manifestations, such as obstruction, peritonitis, and hemorrhage, usually come later and will cause death unless the lesion is well treated.

In any body area, early recognition of cancer is most important in relation to the possibility of successful treatment. With the diagnostic means now available, cancer of the colon and rectum may be detected in a high percentage of the cases if one gives heed to the rather indefinite but recognizable symptoms that may indicate the presence of lesions early in the onset of the disease. The diagnostic methods are simple: a digital examination, the sigmoidoscopy, and the barium enema. Surgery offers the only hope of cure, but it promises an excellent hope if the presence of cancer is detected at an early stage. The progression of cancer in the large bowel is not rapid, but in unfortunate cases in which cure cannot be hoped for, comfort and palliation may be offered. Studies of the problem show that the weak spot of the attack against cancer of the colon and rectum is due in large part to procrastination on the part of the patient and/or physician and to misuse of the simple and effective diagnostic measures now available. Many cancers of the rectum and colon originate in adenomas of polyps. These precancerous lesions may give rise to symptoms, or they may be silent for a long time. They can often be found on careful routine examination. Of all cancers that commonly affect humanity, cancer of the colon and rectum has the best prognosis if the lesions have remained local.

Although treatment by surgical methods evolved slowly, many clinical studies of patients have clarified diagonstic procedures and have improved the methods of treatment. The advances in the auxilliary sciences along with growing understanding of the chemical and physiological abnormalities of the patient have brought about a simplification of surgical techniques. For example, multiple operations have nearly become obsolete. Primary resection with immediate anastomosis is now routine (see Figure 7-6). There has been a fall in the mortality rate for the treatment of large-bowel obstructions. In the period from 1916 to 1919 the rate was 66 percent, and in 1970 only 4 percent. The mortality rate for resection of cancer of the rectum was 20 percent in 1920 and fell to 3 percent in 1970.

Symptoms of Colorectal Carcinoma

The symptoms of carcinoma of the colon depend on a number of factors, such as the anatomical location of the lesion, its size and stage of development, and the presence of complications such as perforation, obstruction, and hemorrhage. In the absence of complications, certain general symptoms are often evident: (1) dyspepsia or ill-defined abdominal discomfort or pain that tends to persist, (2) the presence of blood in or on the stool, (3) occasionally a palpable mass in the abdomen, and (4) alteration in bowel habits which may be manifested as constipation alternating with diarrhea. Frequently the diarrhea consists of the passage of much mucus along with some blood or clots.

Lymphatic System

Many operations that fail to cure the person when the expectation for a cure is high do so because involved lymph nodes are not removed (see Figure 7-7). The flow of lymph usually traverses each group of nodes from the epicolic nodes (located closest to the colon itself) to the principal nodes located along the lymphatic vessels near the mesenteric arteries. Grinnell has reported that occasionally, especially in the hepatic flexure and sigmoid regions, the flow bypasses

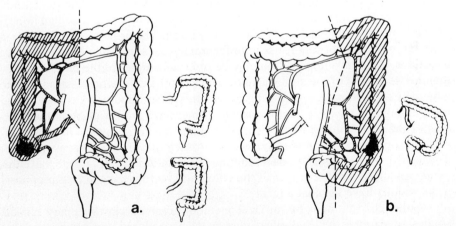

a.   b.

Figure 7-6 Sections of the colon and blood vessel network that should be resected for cancers in two locations. Anastomosis is indicated in each example. (*a*) Cecum and lower ascending colon. (*b*) Descending colon and upper sigmoid.

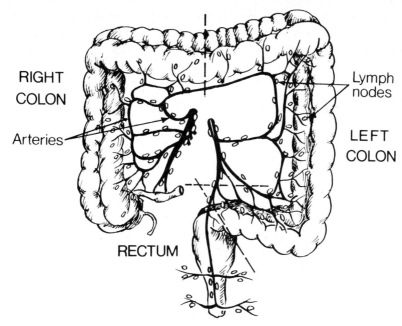

RIGHT
COLON

Lymph
nodes

Arteries

LEFT
COLON

RECTUM

Figure 7-7   Arterial blood supply and lymphatic drainage of the large intestine.

the epicolic and paracolic nodes and goes directly to the intermediate or even principal nodes.[7] Blockage of the main channels by tumor may thus result in upward or downward (retrograde) flow through the paracolic nodes. Therefore the necessity for removing wide segments of the colon with the accompanying lymphatic vessels in cancer operations becomes obvious.

Preoperative Preparation

Preparation of the patient preoperatively should be designed to enable him or her to be in the best physical and mental condition possible. This may mean the patient should be admitted to the hospital a few days before surgery. Although no amount of preoperative care will make curable the lesion that has been neglected, many patients who would have been considered inoperative in the past because of their poor physical condition can now undergo major operative procedures. Most people with carcinoma of the colon or rectum will have suffered a significant weight loss and consequently will have a low level of body protein beside depleted stores of carbohydrate and fat. It is not necessary that a patient return to normal weight before the operation, but it is important that sufficient hepatic glycogen be provided to support the patient during the stress of anesthesia, the surgery, and convalescence. Having a positive nitrogen balance before surgery is very desirable, since protein is essential for wound healing and important to other phases of the stress reaction.

Much has been written about local preparation of the bowel for surgery. Sterilization of the bowel has been so stressed that it almost appears that an anastomosis will not be successful in its absence. It is true that preoperative bowel sterilization with antibiotics has lowered the morbidity rate and probably the mortality rate of colonic surgery. However, the literature indicates that the anastomosis heals not because it is in a sterile field but because it has been subjected to minimum trauma, has a good blood supply, and is not under undue tension.

The operation of choice for cancer located below the peritoneal reflection is a one-stage combined abdominoperineal resection with the establishment of a permanent abdominal colostomy. In women past the menopause, bilateral oophorectomy is indicated as part of the operation for cancer of the colon and rectum because of the high incidence of subsequent carcinoma of the ovary. The actual technique of restoring continuity of the bowel after resection varies among surgeons. A satisfactory anastomosis will be obtained provided there is normal blood supply to the ends, the serosa is accurately inverted and approximated, the suture line is not under tension, and tissues are gently handled. Closed anastomoses can be performed, but an open anastomosis provides more accurate approximation of layers.

In the combined abdominoperineal resection for carinoma of the rectum, the end of the descending colon is brought through a separate stab wound in the abdominal wall in the left lower quadrant above the primary incision. The surgeon should be assured that the colostomy has sufficient blood supply as demonstrated by free bleeding from the end. If there is any question concerning the adequacy of the blood supply, the descending colon should be resected to the point of free bleeding before the colostomy is established. The colostomy is closed with a catgut purse-string suture to be opened approximately 24 hours after the operation. Close attention should be directed to complete closure of the pelvic peritoneum so as to prevent postoperative herniation of the small bowel and subsequent small-bowel obstruction. Closure of the abdominal wall is accomplished with interrupted stitches of stainless steel wire in the peritoneum and fascial layers and continuous wire in the subcutaneous tissue and skin. The subcutaneous and subcuticular wires are pulled out when healing is complete after a period of 7 to 10 days. This method of closure, using the strongest suture material and the one causing the least tissue reaction, is not likely to be complicated by wound infection or disruptions. The healed wound leaves an abdominal wall in which incisional hernia rarely develops.

Care of the Colostomy

People who undergo combined abdominoperineal resection are faced with the presence of a permanent abdominal colostomy and often feel they can never return to an active, productive existence. This should not be. Many thousands of people with colostomies engage in normal activities and learn that the presence of the colostomy in no way makes a person an invalid. In the majority of cases a colostomy will adjust itself so that evacuation occurs once or twice a day at a regular time. Most people have a warning a few minutes before the movement occurs. The nursing team must not make the person so colostomy-conscious that he or she can think of nothing else. A carefully constructed colostomy will shrink to a small opening on the abdominal wall, not unlike a rosebud, with a few months after the operation. Using a few squares of gauze to absorb the small amount of mucus secreated by the exposed mucosa is all that is necessary. It is very helpful to the person to have a receptacle made of plastic or synthetics that can be held in place by an elastic belt around the body. This receptacle can be used for protection at times when it may be impossible to give attention to the colostomy should an unexpected evacuation occur. The dome should not be large enough to be obvious when the patient is clothed; it should never be made of rubber because a fecal odor is most difficult to remove from rubber. Appliances with a diameter so large as to exert pressure some distance from the colostomy are prone to cause herniation. It is not necessary to use an ointment to protect the skin surrounding the colostomy, as is the case with an ileostomy. Gentle cleansing with mild soap and water after each movement will keep the skin in good condition.

Routine enemas or irrigations through the colostomy are seldom necessary any more than they are for the person whose rectum is intact. Occasional episodes of constipation may necessitate the instillation of a small quantity of water into the colostomy through a soft rubber tube, but normally any constipation can be relieved by mild laxatives. If it becomes necessary to irrigate the colostomy, great caution must be exercised in inserting the rubber tube. It should never be advanced against resistance, since perforation of the bowel by the tube is a real danger in this situation.

Digital dilation of the colostomy is not usually necessary as a regular procedure. Sometimes over a period of months slight constriction tends to develop at the stoma. If it does, gentle dilation with the gloved and lubricated finger will be helpful. If dilation is necessary it should first be performed by the physician, who instructs the patient in the proper technique as the procedure is performed. After this the person can dilate the stoma when necessary.

The difference between the consistency of the fecal matter in the sigmoid colon and that normally in the rectum is not great, so special diets are not necessary for proper functioning of a colostomy. A patient finding that some foods result in undue diarrhea or constipation should avoid them just as anyone would.

PSYCHOLOGICAL ASPECTS OF CANCER SURGERY

People who undergo any type of major surgery for cancer fear social rejection and have concomitant anxiety in all social relationships, especially when the surgery involves deformity and reconstruction. Since the family is the institution in which primary social interaction takes place, the kind of emotional response the individual experiences within the family after undergoing surgery becomes an important factor in the patient's efforts to restore social function and self-esteem. In the case of the person who interprets the surgery as something that has reduced his or her value and acceptability, the emotional response of the spouse will play a critical role in the patient's adaptation. The oncology nursing team must have a theoretical understanding regarding identity, self-concept, body image, and sexuality to support, explore, and identify problems the person and family have when the patient faces surgery. Cancer and its treatment pose a threat to an individual's sense of self, body image, and sexuality. The manner in which physical care is given says a great deal since it indicates the acceptance of the patient as a whole or partially functioning person by the staff. Interpersonal competence is the ability to produce desirable and valued outcomes to one's transactions with people, and this must be a priority for both staff and patient.

The attitude of the person's family is so very important in shaping the person's self-image. The patient may create negative attitudes by excluding the family from his or her confidence. This situation will create tensions that will increase unless interrupted. There may be actual rejection on the part of the marital partner and an expression of disgust at the sight of the surgical results. The problems that arise in marital relations may be due to lack of understanding or lack of information. The partner may fear injuring the operative site(s), and the result will be avoidance of reestablishing a satisfactory relationship without an explanation. For example, the colostomy may be used by either partner as an excuse for abstinence from sexual relations when there is a desire to avoid relations for other reasons. Both partners need to know that sexual relations can be resumed without fear unless they are otherwise advised by the physician. For the patient who has undergone a pelvic exenteration, sexual relations should be resumed only when permitted by the physician.

Much misunderstanding is prevented if the partner is included in the plans for recovery. If a colostomy is involved, the couple must learn what the colostomy is and what limitations, if any, will ensue. The family members can best assist by showing understanding of the person's new situation and thoughtful provision of privacy. Unrequested assistance, although accepted, not only may not be appreciated by the person but also may create bigger problems by placing the person in a dependent role, thus causing self-rejection and despair. The person who has had cancer surgery, extensive or otherwise, is a family member, a partner, an adult and does not want to perceive himself or herself as a child. Therefore he or she should be encouraged and allowed to make decisions and to participate as freely in the care as able.

SUMMARY

Surgery is a valuable tool for combating the effects of cancer. Although it is not the only tool, it is one that can give the patient the best chance for cure provided early and accurate diagnosis and treatment are also given. Many types of surgery for cancer eradication are termed "radical," and several have been extensively described both in this chapter and elsewhere in the literature. The bibliography provides further information.

The cancer patient undergoing surgery needs holistic care so that not only the physical adjustments can be accomplished, but the sexual, psychological, body image, and social adjustments can be made as well. This will enable the patient to return to his or her family and community with conditions being right for optimum rehabilitation as a person and as a fully functioning member of society.

REFERENCES

1   Robbins, G. F., and S. W. Berg. "Bilateral Primary Breast Cancer: A Prospective Clinico-Pathological Study," *Cancer,* **17**:1501, 1964.
2   Grattarola, R. "La Ovariectomia nel Carcinoma Mammario," in *Atti Corso Oncologica Clinica,* C. E. A. Milano, 1971
3   Brunschwig, A. "What Are the Indications and Results of Pelvic Exenteration?" *Journal of the American Medical Association,* **194**:3, October 18, 1965.
4   Hamilton, M., and N. Schlapper. "Pelvic Exenteration," *American Journal of Nursing,* **76**:2, 266–272, February 1976.
5   Thomas, B. J. "Coping with the Devastation of Head and Neck Cancer," *RN,* October 1974, pp. 25–30.
6   Wynder, E. L. "Etiological Aspects of Squamous Cancers of the Head and Neck," *Journal of the American Medical Association,* January 1971, pp. 452–453.
7   Grinnell, R. S. "Lymphatic Metastases of Carcinoma of the Colon and Rectum," *Annals of Surgery,* **131**:494–506, 1950.

BIBLIOGRAPHY

Arons, M. S., H. Wexler, S. M. Sabesin, and N. Mantel. "Effects of Cortisone and Amputation on Metastasis," *Cancer,* **15:**227, 1962.
Avery, W., C. Gardner, and S. Palmer. "Vulvectomy," *American Journal of Nursing,* **74**:3, 453–455, March 1974.
Balewski, N., D. Geronemus, and H. Seigel. "Hemipelvectomy: The Triumph of Mrs. A," *American Journal of Nursing,* **73**:12, 2073–2077, December 1973.
Behren, J., et al. "Laryngectomy: Paving the Way to Successful Rehabilitation," *Nursing '74,* **4**:60–66, June 1974.
Branson, H. K. "The Nurse and Mutilation Reaction," *Bedside Nurse,* **3**:26–28, September 1970.
Chedumbrum, S. P. "Nursing Care Study: Carcinoma of the Tongue," *Nursing Mirror,* **135**: 33–43, August 1972.
Christopherson, V. A., P. R. Couler, and M. O. Wolanin, *Rehabilitation Nursing: Perspectives and Applications.* New York: McGraw-Hill, 1974.
Crichton, C. "Nursing Care Study: Carcinoma of the Cervix in Pregnancy," *Nursing Times,* **70**: 906–906, June 1974.
Daley, K. M. "Don't Wave Goodbye," *American Journal of Nursing,* **74**: 1641, September 1974. [about a hemiglossectomy]

Davis, R. W. "Care of the Patient with a Laryngectomy," *Bedside Nurse,* **3**:13–17, November 1970.

Devlin, H. B., J. A. Plant, and M. Griffin, "Aftermath of Surgery for Anorectal Cancer," *British Medical Journal,* **3**:413–418, August 1971.

Druss, R. G., et al. "Adjustment to a Permanent Colostomy," *Archives of General Psychiatry,* **20**: 419–427, April 1969.

Grinnell, R. S., "Lymphatic Metastases of Carcinoma of the Colon and Rectum," *Annals of Surgery,* **131**: 494–506. 1950.

Hickey, R. C. *Palliative Care of the Cancer Patient,* Boston: Little, Brown, 1967.

Holland, J., and E. Free III. *Cancer Medicine,* Philadelphia: Lea & Febiger, 1973.

International Association of Laryngectomies, *First Aid for Neck Breathers,* International Association of Laryngectomies, 1973.

Jamieson, C. W., "Advances in Treatment of Breast Cancer," *Nursing Times,* **69**: 1369–1371, October 1973.

Jensen, V. "Better Techniques for Bagging Stomas: Part I: Urinary Ostomies," *Nursing '74,* **4**: 60–64, July 1974.

———. "Better Techniques for Bagging Stomas, Part II: Colostomies," *Nursing '74,* **4**: 30–35, August 1974.

———. "Better Techniques for Bagging Stomas, Part III: Ileostomies," *Nursing '74,* **4**: 60–63, September 1974.

Leis, H. P., and S. Pilnik. "Breast Cancer: A Therapeutic Dilemma," *Association of Operating Room Nurses Journal,* **19**: 813–820, April 1974.

Leonard, B. J. "Body Image Changes in Chronic Illnesses," *Nursing Clinics of North America,* **7**: 687–695, December 1972.

McCorkle, M. R., "Coping with Physical Symptoms in Metastatic Breast Cancer," *American Journal of Nursing,* **73**: 1034–1038, June 1973.

McDuat, F. "Acoustic Nerve Tumors: Diagnosis, Surgical Management and Nursing Care," *Journal of Neurosurgical Nursing,* **6**: 20–26, July 1974.

Paletta, F. X. "Composite Operations and Reconstruction," *Journal of the American Medical Association,* July 1971, pp. 459–460.

Read, C. R. "Comeback after Cancer," *Family Health,* **6**: 22–23, March 1974.

Richardson, D. K. "Malignant Change in Benign Tumor," *Nursing Times,* **70**: 339–340, March 1974.

Ritter, B. "Breast Surgery Demands Sympathetic Care," *Nursing Care,* **7**: 26–29, August 1974.

Robbins, G. F. "High Cancer 'Cure' Rates Create Human Problems—Rehabilitation," *Journal of the American Medical Association,* **222**: 418–421, October 1972.

Robert, M. M., et al. "Simple versus Radical Mastectomy," *Nursing Digest,* **2**: 85–88, May 1974.

Rosillo, R. H., M. J. Welty, and W. P. Graham. "The Patient with Maxillofacial Cancer. Part II: Psychologic Aspects," *Nursing Clinics of North America,* **8**: 153–158, March 1973.

Searcy, L. "Nursing Care of the Laryngectomy Patient," *RN,* October 1972, pp. 35–41.

Secor, S. M. "Colostomy Rehabilitation," *American Journal of Nursing,* **70**: 2400–2401, November 1970.

Shedd, D. P., et al. *The Nurse's Role in Rehabilitation of Cancer Patients with Facial Defects.* New York: The American Cancer Society, 1974.

Sparberg, M. *Ileostomy Care.* Springfield, Ill.: Charles C Thomas, 1971.

Stitt, A. "Coping with Colostomy," *Emergency Medicine,* **2**: 85–90, February 1970.

Trowbridge, J. "Caring for Patients with Facial or Intra-Oral Reconstruction," *American Journal of Nursing,* **73**: 11, 1930–4, November 1973.

University of Texas, M. D. Anderson Hospital and Tumor Institute, *Rehabilitation of the Cancer Patient,* Chicago: Year Book Medical Publishers, 1972.

Welty, M. J., W. P. Graham, and R. H. Rosillo. "The Patient with Maxillofacial Cancer. Part I: Surgical Treatment and Nursing Care," *Nursing Clinics of North America,* **8**: 137–151, March 1973.

Chapter 8

Radiotherapy, Cancer, and the Nurse

Sharon S. Ogi

Radiotherapy is an important modality in the treatment of cancer. As is surgery, radiotherapy is utilized in the treatment of localized disease, while chemotherapy and immunotherapy are applied in the treatment of systemic disease. Since the discovery of x-rays by Wilhelm Conrad Roentgen in 1895 and the discovery of their radioactivity by Marie Sklodowska Curie in 1898, radiotherapy has progressed, achieved, and proven itself as a mainstay in cancer management.

This chapter is designed to give the nurse an overall understanding of the following things:

1 Characteristics of radiations
2 Radiation units
3 Uses of radiations
4 Goals of radiotherapy
5 Methods of treatment in radiotherapy
6 Physiologic effects of radiotherapy
7 The nurse's role in radiotherapy

The purpose of this chapter, therefore, is to present a broad overview of the many facets of radiotherapy. With such knowledge, the nurse will be better able to guide the nursing care delivered to radiotherapy patients and their families.

CHARACTERISTICS OF RADIATIONS

The radiations being considered in this chapter consist of electromagnetic energy (waves) and subatomic particles. These radiations have the ability to knock electrons out of their orbits around an atomic nucleus, producing the process called "ionization." Atoms in the path of these rays, such as living cells, become ionized, physical and chemical changes occur in the cells, and biological effects result. There are two kinds of ionizing rays: waves and particles.

Electromagnetic Waves

In nature, there exists a broad spectrum of rays of varying wavelengths (Figure 8-1). The varying wavelengths give the rays their characteristic properties. In radiotherapy, rays of shorter wavelength, specifically x-rays and gamma rays, are used.

Particles

Chemical elements existing in nature are characterized by the number of protons and orbital electrons each maintains. When a neutron(s) is added to the atomic nucleus of an element, an isotope is created. While most isotopes are stable, some are unstable; i.e., the nucleus undergoes a spontaneous change. When this change occurs, the isotope emits ionizing radiation known as "radioactivity." An example of naturally occurring radioactivity is radium. Artificial radioactive isotopes can also be produced by bombarding chemical elements with neutrons in a nuclear reactor.

Whether radiation is from natural or artificial radioisotopes, it emits one or more of three kinds of particles: alpha, beta, and gamma. Alpha rays (or particles) are composed of two protons and two neutrons. These rays are easily absorbed and have minimal penetration capacity; a sheet of paper can stop them. The alpha rays do not penetrate skin surface, but can be damaging if the radioisotope that emits them is located within tissue.

Beta rays are actually fast-moving electrons whose penetrating power varies with the particular radioisotope. Beta rays have a greater penetrating power than do alpha rays, being able to penetrate thin metal foils and soft tissues for distances of small fractions of a millimeter to approximately a centimeter. Along their pathway, beta rays produce ionizations. Scattering of beta rays can be prevented by shielding the beta emitting isotope with layers of metal.

Gamma rays are the same as the more penetrating x-rays. When the source of the ray is a radioisotope, it is called a "gamma ray," and if it comes from electrical machines, it is called an "x-ray." Gamma rays have a greater penetrating power than do alpha or beta rays. They can reach deep tissues as well as go through the whole body; thus they are of great value for treatment purposes.

Radioisotopes are constantly changing, constantly giving off energy and decaying to a more stable element. "Half-life," the term used to indicate the rate of decay, is the amount of time needed by the radioisotope to decay to half its original activity level. The half-lives of radioisotopes vary. For example, radium has a half-life of 1600 years whereas radiocobalt has a half-life of 5 years and radioiodine a half-life 8 days.

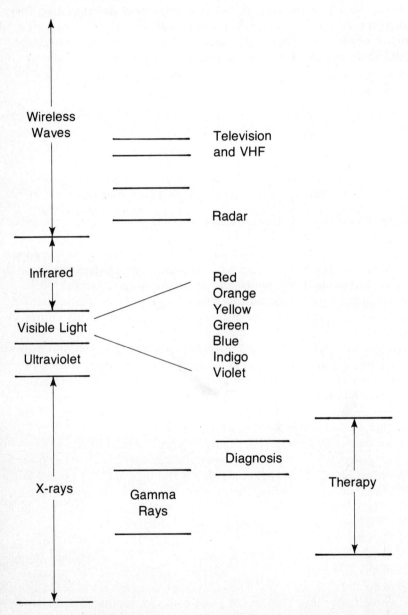

Figure 8-1 The electromagnetic spectrum of waves and wavelengths. (*Reprinted with permission from J. Walter, "Electromagnetic Spectrum of Waves and Wave Lengths," Cancer and Radiotherapy, Churchill LIvingston, London, 1973, p. 48.*)

RADIATION UNITS

Roentgen (R)

X-rays and gamma rays are measured in terms of the roentgen. This is the amount of energy in a beam of rays as it is delivered—as it emerges from the generating source.

Radiation Absorbed Dose (rad)

Rad is the term used to define the measurement of the absorbed dose of ionizing radiation, i.e., the amount of energy that is absorbed by the issue. This is an important unit measure for the nurse who cares for the patient receiving radiotherapy because the radiotherapist will list the treatment dose in rads.

Roentgen Equivalent Man (rem)

The rem is an important unit of measure when one is concerned about safety. The rem measures the amount of any ionizing radiation that has the same biological effectiveness as 1 rad of x-rays. This is of importance as some radiations are more effective in producing biological effects than others are. The National Council on Radiation Protection and Measurements recommends that a person receive no more than 1250 mrems (millirems) to the entire body every 3 months or no more than 100 mrem per week. Mrems are measured with the use of film badges or pocket dosimeters. The film badges are read approximately every month and thus are practical for people who work in radiology, radiotherapy, or nuclear medicine departments. The pocket dosimeter has the advantage of immediately determining the amount of radiation received. As a consequence it is ideal for nurses who care for patients receiving internal radiotherapy, since they are exposed to the radiation only when in the patient's room.

USES OF RADIATIONS

X-rays from machines and gamma rays from radioisotopes are of great value in both cancer diagnosis and cancer therapy. Diagnostic x-rays are quite familiar to nurses and include chest x-rays, skeletal surveys, upper gastrointestinal examinations, barium enemas, etc. Such studies are usually done in the diagnostic radiology department and can reveal numerous forms of anatomical irregularities.

Diagnostic radioisotope studies are generally carried out in the nuclear medicine department of a hospital and can reveal functional (physiological) irregularities. All isotopes, whether radioactive (unstable) or stable, behave chemically in the same manner. Biologically, the body's processes cannot distinguish between stable and radioactive substances of the same elements. This fact has led to the development of radioactive tracer studies. The individual being tested receives a very minute diagnostic dose of a radioactive substance, whose uptake by the body is recorded by various types of highly sensitive machines. Examples of common nuclear medicine studies are thyroid scans, bone scans, liver scans, and brain scans.

"Radiotherapy" consists of the treatment of certain diseases by radiation. The overall purpose of radiotherapy is to destroy or contain tumor cells in vivo without producing excessive destruction of normal tissue. Although nonmalignant conditions may be treated with radiotherapy, the majority of radiotherapy patients have malignant disease.

GOALS OF RADIOTHERAPY

When ionizing rays are used for cancer treatment, the goal may focus on cure or on palliation.

Cure

The curative goal can be achieved by (1) radiotherapy alone, (2) combination with surgery preoperatively and postoperatively, (3) combination with chemotherapy, (4) combination with immunotherapy, or (5) any combination of the above modalities. Radiotherapy can be the sole treatment modality in cancer when used with a curative intent. The relative radiosensitivities of malignant tumors are listed in Table 8-1. Radiotherapy used with a curative intent seeks to destroy malignant tissue in vivo and has cure rates equal to those of surgery for many malignancies.

When radiotherapy is used in combination with surgery preoperatively, there are two objectives: (1) to reduce the incidence of metastases by killing the peripheral, well-oxygenated cells that are most likely to metastasize and (2) to

Table 8-1   Relative Radiosensitivities of Malignant Tumors (listed in order of decreasing radiosensitivity)

1   Malignant tumors arising from hemopoietic organs (lymphosarcoma, myeloma)
2   Hodgkin's disease
3   Seminomas and dysgerminomas
4   Ewing's sarcoma of the bone
5   Basal cell carcinomas of the skin
6   Epidermoid carcinomas arising by metaplasia from columnar epithelium
7   Epidermoid carcinomas of the mucous membranes, mucocutaneous junctions, and skin
8   Adenocarcinomas of the endometrium, breast, gastrointestinal system, and endocrine glands
9   Soft-tissue sarcomas
10   Chondrosarcomas
11   Neurogenic sarcomas
12   Osteosarcomas
13   Malignant melanomas

Source: Juan A. del Regato and Harlan J. Spjut in L. V. Ackerman, *Cancer: Diagnosis, Treatment, and Prognosis,* 5th ed., C. V. Mosby, St. Louis, 1977, p. 101.

shrink the tumor and make it surgically resectable. This combined approach is usually used for moderately advanced cancers of the head and neck and cancers of the rectum, lung, bladder, and esophagus.

Radiotherapy can also be used in combination with surgery postoperatively. Radiotherapists generally prefer to irradiate the patient preoperatively rather than postoperatively. This preference is due to the fact that surgery reduces the blood supply of tumors, hence their oxygen content, and tumor cells that lack oxygen are much more resistant to irradiation. In addition, there may be the risk of spreading the tumor cells during surgery by handling of the tumor. Nevertheless, postoperative radiotherapy is often used when the surgeon is unable to remove all of the tumor and/or when the surgeon is unable to remove or reach lymph node areas.

Palliation

Palliative radiotherapy is given primarily to provide relief of symptoms and to prevent complications. When the goal is palliation, the patient may have disseminated disease, but radiotherapy is used to a specific, local area to provide relief of symptoms, e.g., relief of painful bone metastases or of neurological symptoms due to brain metastases. Prevention or treatment of pathologic fractures of the bone, due to bony metastases, may be another use of palliative radiotherapy. Prolongation of life and/or psychological uplift for the patient may be secondary gains with this form of therapy.

METHODS OF TREATMENT IN RADIOTHERAPY

The two basic types of treatment approaches with radiotherapy are the external and the internal methods.

External Radiotherapy

External radiotherapy consists of treatment that uses various machines to produce the x-rays or gamma rays. Most machines are electrical, but some utilize radioactive substances such as cobalt 60. These machines are divided into two types: orthovoltage, and megavoltage or supervoltage. They are primarily classified by their penetrating power, which, in turn, depends on the wavelengths of the rays they produce.

Orthovoltage machines are low-voltage (100,000 to 500,000 V). They produce rays of comparatively long wavelength and result in large doses delivered to and absorbed by the skin. Until 10 to 15 years ago, these machines were considered the "old workhorses" of a radiotherapy department. With the development of new machines and voltage capacities, the low-voltage machines are less frequently used. Orthovoltage machines, however, still maintain a role in the management of skin lesion or lesions in which the maximum effect must be obtained close to the skin surface.

Megavoltage or supervoltage machines (1,000,000 V or more) produce

x-rays, resulting in significantly greater penetration power than with the orthovoltage radiations. Megavoltage machines have what is called a "skin-
sparing" effect; i.e., the maximum reaction of the beam takes place beneath the
skin surface. The radiocobalt (^{60}Co) machine is a megavoltage machine that
delivers an amount of gamma rays equivalent to the amount of x-rays emitted by
4 million eV machine. It must be remembered that the radioactivity is continuous
and that the half-life of ^{60}Co is 5 years. Therefore, the radioactive source for the
^{60}Co machine has to be replaced or the treatment time extended over a period of
years in order for the same dosage to be delivered all the time. Other common
megavoltage machines used today are the linear accelerators. These machines
are available in the range of 4 to 45 million V or 4 to 45 MV or MeV (million
electron volts). The linear accelerator operates from an electrical source, so
there is no loss of radiation. Consequently, in contrast to the ^{60}Co machine, the
linear accelerator requires no source replacement. Also, because of the higher
energy level used, treatment time is shorter with the linear accelerator than with
the ^{60}Co machine.

The mainstays of a radiotherapy department today are the ^{60}Co machine and
the linear accelerator. However, other forms of external radiations, e.g., electron therapy and neutron therapy, are being used. The electron beam that
produces x-rays can be used by itself as a form of external therapy. The advantage of using electrons for treatment is that they have a maximum range in tissue
depending on their initial energy. All the tissues deeper than the maximum range
of the electrons are effectively spared from receiving any significant amount of
radiation.

The neutron beam form of external radiotherapy is primarily experimental.
Its clinical value has yet to be assessed. It is thought that neutron beam therapy
may be useful in treating the otherwise radiation-resistant tumors, i.e., tumors
that have an oxygen deficit or have anaerobic metabolism.

Effects on Normal Tissues   Skin   Skin reactions are of great importance in
external radiotherapy regardless of the site of the malignancy. The characteristic
skin effect is erythema (reddening of the skin). In the past, appearance of
erythema was used as a gauge for determining the dosage level to be delivered.
However, with current megavoltage equipment and its associated skin-sparing
effect, erythema, while still of importance, is not a primary limiting factor in
radiotherapy. Erythema usually occurs near the second week of treatment, and
the resulting radiodermatitis may be acute or chronic. An acute reaction usually
occurs when a patient receives a large dose in a short period of time. Acute
reactions are divided into four degrees of severity that correlate with increasing
dosages:

   1 *First degree (epilation dose):* Brings about destructive effects on hair
roots. The hair can be pulled out painlessly or falls out spontaneously. It occurs
approximately 18 days after a dose is delivered. The hair grows again in 2 to 3
months.
   2 *Second degree:* Consists of the bright red erythema that occurs in the
localized irradiated area. Sweat glands are inhibited and may be permanently

destroyed. Hair falls out and may or may not grow back. When the erythema subsides, there is often a residual pigmentation that resembles a sunburn and may be permanent. Usually the patient experiences some itching and peeling of the skin (dry desquamation).

3 *Third degree:* The erythema is deeper and purplish. Blisters appear and burst to form ulcers that exude serum (moist desquamation). Healing is usually complete in 2 to 3 weeks. Sweat glands are destroyed, and hair loss is permanent.

4 *Fourth degree:* Known as "radiation burn." This severe effect should not be seen, whereas the first three degrees may be seen. In this case, the erythema is deep and of intense color. The blisters go deeper, and the entire skin surface sloughs offs, resulting in a very painful condition. Healing may occur but usually takes weeks or months due to blood vessel destruction. This reaction represents a technical mistake or an error in judgment.

Chronic reactions can occur after months or years and are a result of receiving small doses over a long period of time. People who work with radiation in industry, as well as patients, may experience chronic radiation reactions but may not experience an acute reaction phase.

Skin sensitivity varies from person to person. As with sunburns, fair-haired and fair-skinned people are usually more sensitive than dark-haired and dark-complected people. Skin sensitivity also varies with anatomic location. The more sensitive areas include the axilla, groin, vulva, and anus; their sensitivity is due in part to friction and moisture. The back of the hand, heel, sole of the foot, midline of the back, and bony prominences are sensitive because of relatively poor blood supply and scattering of radiation.

Sequelae to skin reactions may include ischemia, pigmentation, atrophy, thickening, telangiectasia, late ulceration, and malignancy. With the advent of megavoltage machinery, many of these reactions occur with less frequency.

Mucous Membranes   The gastrointestinal lining (mucosa) is extremely sensitive to radiation because of the rapid cellular turnover rate characteristic of the tissue. When a cancericidal dose of radiation is delivered to this area, some of the reactions that may occur are ulceration, diarrhea, and bleeding. In addition, the patient is subject to a high risk of morbidity as well as mortality. For this reason, cancers located in the stomach or colon are not treated by radiation. Radiation reactions of gastrointestinal mucosa lead to inhibition of the functioning of mucous and salivary glands. As with skin reactions, the superficial ulceration of the mucosa creates a whitish membrane composed of fibrim that originates from the mucosa creates a whitish membrane composed of fibrin that originates from the exudate (mucositis). As healing occurs, the white mucositis becomes

When the mouth, pharynx, or esophagus is treated with radiation, the patient experiences dryness of the mouth, loss of taste, sore throat, and dysphagia. When the abdominal or pelvic cavities are treated, gastrointestinal spasms, diarrhea leading to dehydration, and bleeding may occur. With intracavitary internal radiotherapy in cervical cancer, the rectum receives some radiation that can result in proctitis, tenesmus, passage of mucous, and occasionally passage of blood. Late effects of radiotherapy on mucosa may appear weeks, months, or years after the cessation of treatment. These late reactions may include adhesions, fibrosis and stenosis leading to obstruction, ulceration, fistula formation, bleeding, and malabsorption syndrome. Treatment of late reactions may be prophylactic and/or symptomatic depending on the reaction anticipated and/or present.

Hematopoietic Tissue   The bone marrow and lymphoid tissues are especially sensitive to radiotherapy. Usually the reaction is apparent in the leukocytes, lymphocytes, and platelets. Since the life span of the red blood cells is about 4 months, they are less radiosensitive than other blood cells are. The effect on the patient's blood count varies with the size of the area treated and the amount of bone marrow irradiated. One will usually see a decrease in the white blood cell and platelet counts.

Reproductive Organs   In males, sperm production can be inhibited by doses as low as 50 rad, and permanent sterility can result with 1000 rad. Androgenic hormonal production is not changed drastically. In females, however, hormonal effects are more obvious and tend to be more significant. Ovarian hormonal production can be reduced or abolished, leading to a temporary or permanent cessation of menstruation. Genetic mutations may occur with low doses of radiation. For this reason, radiotherapy to female reproductive organs is used with extreme caution.

Eyes   If the eye is irradiated, several reactions may occur. With the exception of the conjunctiva, the eye is rather radioinsensitive. Following irradiation to the lens of the eye, with a dose ranging from 750 to 1000 rad, a cataract may develop depending on the patient's age. When the lacrimal duct is irradiated it may become obstructed, and if the obstruction is not relieved it can be permanent. When areas close to the eye are being treated, the eye is usually spared by the use of shielding or tangential fields to minimize the dosage to the visual apparatus.

Kidney   Renal blood vessel damage or degenerative changes may result with irradiation of the kidneys. One may see increased blood pressure and acute or chronic nephritis with elevated blood-urea nitrogen levels, renal failure, and uremia. The marginal safety level for renal radiotherapy is 2000 rad.

Brain and Nerve Tissue   Nervous system tissues are usually quite radioresistant, although reactions may occur with high dosages. The reactions are usually due to damage of vascular supply leading to degenerative changes.

Bone and Cartilage   With high doses of radiation to bone, vascular damage may occur and result in necrosis and fracture. If growing bone is radiated in the epiphysis and damage occurs, there can be retardation of bone growth with shortening of the limb or spinal scoliosis.

Lungs   When lung tissue is irradiated, one gets an inflammatory reaction (radiation penumonitis) that may lead to fibrosis. Fibrosis prevents proper expansion of lung tissue and leads to a decrease in vital capacity. In addition, the patient becomes more susceptible to pulmonary infections.

Radiation Sickness   A generalized illness can occur during a course of radiotherapy, with the severity depending on the body part and volume of tissue irradiated. The patient usually experiences nausea, fatigue, malaise, and weakness. Radiation sickness can be attributed to the increase of breakdown products in the bloodstream due to cellular death and is treated symptomatically. The incidence of radiation sickness has decreased because of improved patient care and radiation therapy techniques.

Internal Radiotherapy

Internal radiotherapy utilizes various radioactive substances and application techniques to treat cancer from within the body. The three major subdivisions of internal radiotherapy are systemic, interstitial, and intracavitary therapy. In addition, the sources of ionizing radiations for internal radiotherapy can be divided into two forms: those that are enclosed completely in a metal container (sealed sources) and those that are in liquid solution form (unsealed sources).

There are many small sealed sources. Some of the more familiar include radium, cobalt, cesium, radon, gold, and iridium. These substances are found in various kinds of applicators, such as needles, beads, seeds, ribbons, etc. This form of therapy delivers local radiation to a limited amount of tissue. Unsealed sources are designed to deliver radiation either systemically, throughout the body via the normal vascular pathways, or intracavitarily in serious cavities.

Systemic therapy can be given either orally or intravenously. Systemic therapy is commonly seen in the use of radioiodine (^{131}I) for hyperthyroidism or for certain kinds of thyroid cancer.

Interstitial therapy consists of the placement of an applicator directly into the malignant tissue. Common radioactive substance and their methods of application include cobalt beads into a buccal mucosa carcinoma, radium needles into a lesion in the head and neck tissue or the mandible, iridium ribbons into head and neck lesions, and gold seeds into lung lesions.

The placement of radioactive substances into a body cavity such as the chest cavity, abdominal cavity, or vaginal vault is known as "intracavitary therapy." Either sealed or unsealed sources may be used with this form of therapy. An example of intracavitary therapy is the radium applicator used in the treatment of cervical carcinoma. Examples of the use of unsealed sources in intracavitary therapy are the placement of radiophosphorus (^{32}P) into the chest cavity for malignant pleural effusions and its placement into the abdominal cavity to treat abdominal seeding of a malignant tumor. Table 8-2 lists the various radioisotopes and their therapeutic uses in internal radiotherapy.

PHYSIOLOGIC EFFECTS OF RADIOTHERAPY

As previously stated, ionizing radiations (waves and particles) have the ability to affect living cells create to biological effects. All cells, both normal and malignant, go through the cell cycle (Figure 8-2). The cell cycle consists of gap 0 (G_0: resting/functioning phase), gap 1 (G_1: metabolizing phase/commitment to reproduce), synthesis (S: phase during which the DNA content is doubling), gap 2

Table 8-2 Radioisotopes and Their Therapeutic Uses

Radioisotope and symbol	Kind of internal radiotherapy	Uses	Half-life	Emissions		
				Alpha	Beta	Gamma
Cobalt 60 (^{60}Co)	Interstitial (beads)	Buccal mucosa carcinoma	5 years			X
Iodine 131 (^{131}I)	Systemic (p.o. or IV)	Primary and metastatic thyroid carcinoma (papillary and follicular carcinoma), hyperthyroidism	8 days		X	X
Phosphorus 32 (^{32}P)	Systemic (IV), intracavitary (instillation)	Polycythemia vera, palliative treatment for CML and CLL, metastatic breast and prostate carcinoma, bone cancer, malignant pleural effusions	14 days		X	
Radon 222 (^{222}Rn)	Interstitial (seeds)	Cancers of the tongue, neck, etc.	4 days			X
Radium 226 (^{226}Ra)	Interstitial (needles)	Oral Cancers	1600 years			X
	Intracavitary (applicator)	Cervical/uterine cancers	1600 years			X
Iridium 192 (^{192}Ir)	Interstitial (seed, wire)	Head and neck cancers	75 days			X
Gold 198 (^{198}Au)	Intracavitary (instillation)	Palliative management of malignant ascites and pleural effusions, bladder cancers	3 days		X	X
Cesium 137 (^{137}Cs)	Interstitial, intracavitary	Cervical/uterine and head and neck cancers	30 years			X

(G$_2$: building of energy reserves), and mitosis (M: cell division). Radiotherapy does the most damage to cells during the synthesis and mitosis phases of the cell cycle, as more essential cell material (i.e., the DNA) is exposed during these times. Rapidly dividing, undifferentiated cells are most sensitive to radiotherapy, while nondividing, highly differentiated cells are most resistant. Usually, most malignant cells are rapidly dividing and undifferentiated, while normal cells are nondividing and highly differentiated. The oxygenation and nutritional status of cells also influence the effectiveness of radiotherapy. For example, a large tumor's outer edges are more radiosensitive than its sometimes necrotic core because of the better vascularization, oxygenation, and nutrition of

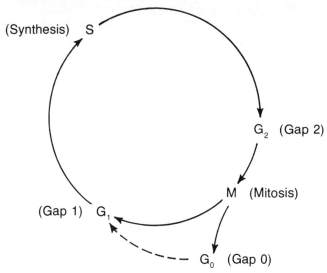

Figure 8-2 The cell cycle.

the outer edges. However, the ionizing rays cannot distinguish between normal or malignant cells, so they affect all cells. Normal tissues that divide fairly rapidly and thus are radiosensitive include lymphatic tissue, bone marrow, intestinal epithelium, the germ cells of the ovaries and testes, and epithelial tissue of the skin. Normal tissues that are radioresistant include fibrous, muscle, bone, and nerve tissue. Because of the nonselectivity of cells by the ionizing rays and the radiosensitivity of normal tissues, the patient experiences side effects of radiotherapy.

The ionization of living cells leads to physical and chemical changes within the cell. The energy absorbed by the nucleus of the cell can lead to chromosomal damage (mutations), cessation or temporary suppression of cellular reproduction (mitosis), the blockage of immune responses, and cell membrane damage resulting in a breakdown of oxygen and nutrient supply. As stated earlier, ionizing rays cannot distinguish between normal or malignant cells, thus both are affected.

The effect of radiation is always destructive, although the damage may be great or small. If there is minimal destruction, the cell may recover and return to normal functioning, but if maximal damage occurs, the cell will either die or be unable to reproduce itself. Usually, actively dividing (growing) cells are killed outright when irradiated. Other cells may die in the process of trying to divide (which is the most important mechanism of radiotherapy) or by premature aging of the cell in which mitosis is halted.

Acute effects of radiation are a function of the dose delivered and the volume of tissue treated. Also, there is some dependence on the rate of delivery. Physiological reactions result primarily from the depletion of actively reproducing cells, which creates an imbalance in the cellular homeostatic mechanism.

This imbalance leads to the acute effects observed clinically. Normal tissues usually involved in acute reactions are those of the gastrointestinal tract, bone marrow, and skin. The clinical reactions observed are those of mucocitis, gastrointestinal upset, bone marrow depression (usually of white blood cells), epithelitis, and alopecia due to epilation. Treatment of the reactions is usually symptomatic and will be covered in succeeding areas of this chapter. Acute reactions to radiotherapy usually disappear shortly after the daily dose is decreased or the radiation treatment course is completed.

Intermediate radiation effects are related to the fractionization of the dose as well as the total dose delivered. These reactions are thought to result from injury to slowly reproducing cell-renewal systems, possibly the endothelium or connective tissue. Some of the more important effects are pneumonitis and pericarditis. Pneumonitis from radiation usually develops 2 to 3 months after treatment if the lungs or portions of the lungs were irradiated. Radiation pneumonitis is usually asymptomatic but may be associated with a dry, hacking cough and mild exertional dyspnea. The lung's tolerance to radiation is volume-dependent; i.e., smaller volumes of tissue can tolerate higher doses of radiation and large volumes tolerate much smaller doses of radiation. If the heart is in the irradiated field, one may see radiation-induced heart disease, usually manifested as acute pericarditis, within a year after treatment. The signs and symptoms are usually pleuritic chest pain, pericardial friction rub, electrocardiogram abnormalities, and enlargement of the cardiac silhouette. These effects are also treated symptomatically.

Late-appearing effects of radiotherapy are also directly related to fractionization of the dose and the total dose delivered to the surrounding normal tissues in the treatment field. These reactions can occur as early as a few months or as late as several years after radiation treatment. These effects, such as tissue necroses, fistulas, or dense fibroses, are chronic, unlike the acute and intermediate reactions and may not bear any relation to prior acute or intermediate reactions. The management of late effects depends on the location but is usually treated conservatively.

THE NURSE'S ROLE IN RADIOTHERAPY

The remainder of this chapter will focus on the nursing implications in the care of the radiotherapy patient and the patient's family. Emphasis will be placed on nursing implications in the care of a patient receiving external radiotherapy and one receiving internal radiotherapy.

Nursing Implications with External Radiotherapy

The present section focuses on total patient care rather than on listing specific nursing actions for each patient need. Patients receiving external radiotherapy must be assessed on various parameters in order for the nurse to make accurate judgments and plan the patients' care.

Initial parameters for patient assessment include the following:

1 Histologic diagnosis and staging
2 Extent of the treatment field
3 Treatment goal
4 Daily and total dosage
5 Duration of treatment
6 Patient's nutritional status
7 Patient's resources and liabilities

In addition, before you begin working with radiotherapy patients and their families, it is vital that you be aware of your own attitudes, fears, and philosophy about radiotherapy and cancer. You must also have a baseline of knowledge of what radiotherapy entails, how it works, what the biologic responses are, and what the treatment goals are. It is advisable that you visit the radiotherapy department where the patients will be going for treatment in order to observe the physical layout and the routine and to get to know staff members. With this knowledge and familiarity, you will be better able to care for your patients. You will be better able to understand and interpret the patients' comments about their experiences and will be able to establish good communication lines between the nursing unit, radiotherapy staff, and patient and family.

Nursing implications for these patients and families lie within three distinct time frames, that prior to treatment, that upon initiation of treatment and during treatment in the hospital, and that after discharge from the hospital.

Pretherapy Considerations Prior to the initiation of radiotherapy, it is advisable that you spend some time counseling the patient and the family. By exploring with the patient and family what their comprehension of radiotherapy is and what the treatment is going to do for the patient, it is possible to correct misconceptions, identify potential problem areas, and reinforce the radiotherapist's explanation of the treatment. At the same time, the patient's apprehension may be eased when you are able to give accurate information about the treatment experience, e.g., where the department is located, how the patient gets from the nursing unit to the department, what routines are followed in the radiotherapy department, what equipment is used, and what the attitudes and practices of the staff are. You must also explain to the patient and family the following:

1 The radiotherapist may mark the treatment portal with indelible ink (or gentian violet), which the patient is not to wash off.
2 The patient should feel no sensation during the treatment.
3 Although treatment time seems long, it is actually a brief period, for example, 1½ minutes with the linear accelerator.
4 The radiotherapy staff will position the patient for treatment but will leave the room during actual treatment time. There is closed circuit TV or a viewing window and communication system for patient-staff interaction during actual treatment time.

5 The patient must maintain the position he or she is placed in and lie absolutely still during treatment.

6 After treatment the patient is *not* radioactive.

Initiation of Treatment and Discharge   Once treatment is initiated, the patient's feelings, concerns, and questions about the experience can be explored. This is also a good time to provide clarification and reinforcement of the previously discussed important aspects of treatment. Patient teaching with reference to side effects must also be accomplished and is discussed below. Discharge planning also should be initiated during the treatment phase. The patient does not usually remain in the hospital for the entire duration of the treatment period, hence will benefit optimally by early discharge planning. It is necessary to explore with the patient and family the nature of the home situation in order to determine if there are any apparent or anticipated problems in the patient's continuance in treatment. Some considerations may be as follows: How far is home from the treatment center? If it is a long distance, where will the patient stay? How will the patient get to and from the treatment center (bus, car, taxi)? Is this means of transportation feasible for the duration of the treatment? What is the family's financial status? Will a family member have to take time off from work? It must be impressed upon the patient and family that it is important for the patient to keep every treatment appointment.

Patient and family education must also occur before the patient's discharge. Each member of the family must be informed of the possible side effects, specific to the body area being treated. Assure them that there are symptomatic treatment for many of the side effects. They should be informed also of some general guidelines for care of the patient undergoing external radiotherapy. These guidelines include the following:

1 Activites must be scheduled to allow for adequate rest periods, especially after treatment. Rationale (R): There is an increase in cell-death waste products circulating in the blood; thus the patient experiences malaise. This situation is directly related to the dose and rate of delivery and to the volume and type of tissue treated.

2 Encourage or arrange for the patient to eat small feedings several times a day with an especially high nutritional content. It may not be best for the patient to eat immediately before or after treatment. R: Radiotherapy works best on well-nourished and oxygenated cells. Also, an increase in waste products in the blood may decrease the patient's appetite.

3 The patient should drink 2 to 4 qt of liquids per day. R: Cell death causes an increase of uric acid in the blood which is excreted from the body via the urinary system. The patient must be well hydrated so that crystallization of the uric acid is prevented.

4 The treated area should be kept dry. In addition, caution the patient not to wear clothing that is tight over the treatment area. R: to decrease the chance of skin breakdown and infection by preventing development of moist areas and by preventing constant irritation.

5 The treatment area should not be exposed to direct sunlight. Encourage the patient to wear hats, scarves, etc., if the area is on the head or neck. R: to protect the treated area from more radiation exposure.

6   Treatment area(s) must not be shaved. R: to decrease the chance of breaking skin surface and creating an open wound for infection.

7   Tepid or cold water should be used to wash the treated area. Abrasive soaps should not be used. If soap must be used, it should be one with a lanolin base and the area should be patted dry with a soft towel. It should not be rubbed or scrubbed. R: Use of abrasive soaps or rubbing and scrubbing leads to further drying and irritation of the skin and may lead to infection.

8   Skin markings should not be washed off. R: These markings delineate the treatment portal and are used by the radiotherapy staff. The delineation of these portals is very time-consuming.

9   A heating pad, hot water bottle, or hot compresses should not be placed on the treated area. R: Heat over the treated area serves as more irritation to the skin and may lead to infection.

10   Alcohol, creams, ointments, or deodorants should not be placed on the treatment areas. No metallic-based creams or ointments should be applied. The patient should confer with the radiotherapist before putting anything on treated area. R: These substances may further irritate the treatment area and lead to skin breakdown.

11   It is important that the patient not lie on the treated area for long periods of time. R: The vascular supply is compromised by pressure; thus the treatment area is more susceptible to skin breakdown and infection.

12   Adhesive tape should not be placed on treatment area. R: Placement and removal of tape may further irritate the treatment area and lead to skin breakdown and infection.

13   The patient should avoid people with colds or infections. R: With radiotherapy the patient's white blood cell count may be affected, and the patient is more susceptible to infections.

14   All discomforts or concerns must be reported to the radiotherapist. R: The side effects of radiotherapy can be treated symptomatically.

15   When the patient or family members have any doubts, the radiotherapist should be consulted. R: The radiotherapist is most aware of the patient's total treatment plan.

Possible Radiation Reactions   Reactions from radiotherapy can be systemic and/or local. Local reactions depend on the area of the body being irradiated and usually are associated with a disturbance of function of that body part (a side effect). Systemic reactions to radiotherapy are related to dose, volume of tissue treated, rate of dose delivery, and type of tissue. These side effects were discussed earlier in the chapter, under "Physiologic Effects of Radiotherapy" and "Effects on Normal Tissues."

Standard Care Plan   A standard care plan for patients receiving external radiotherapy (Figure 8-3) has been devised by the Queen's Medical Center Nursing Service. This standard care plan is initiated by the nurses when a patient is receiving external radiotherapy and serves to guide the care delivered to the

Figure 8-3 Standard care plan for external radiation therapy. (*Printed with permission from The Queen's Medical Center, State of Hawaii, 1975. Copyright © 1975 The Queen's Medical Center.*)

DISCHARGE
GOALS:
(See Expected
Outcomes
Below)
DATE: _____

USUAL PROBLEMS	EXPECTED OUTCOMES	DEADLINES	NURSING ORDERS
1 Anxiety and fear due to possible misunderstanding and/or lack of knowledge of radiation therapy	Verbalizes understanding and acceptance of treatment	(2 days after 1st treatment) √ qd	a Prior to initiation of therapy, assign knowledgeable R.N. or L.P.N. to discuss treatment plan with patient. Include the following information: 　1 Treatment is painless. 　2 Duration of daily treatment. 　3 Necessity of frequent lab work. b Arrange previsit to radiation department. If not possible describe room and equipment.
2 Potential skin changes due to cellular reaction to gamma rays	Demonstrates good skin care technique and verbalizes intent to continue technique after discharge	(Discharge) √ qd	a Prior to initiation of therapy, inform patient that changes may occur. —May vary from mild sunburn appearance to severe erythema.

USUAL PROBLEMS	EXPECTED OUTCOMES	DEADLINES	NURSING ORDERS
			b Prior to initiation of therapy, instruct patient:
			1 Do not remove special skin markings applied by doctor.
			2 Avoid strong soap, cream, or ointments on affected area. Check with physician before using any ointments.
			3 Do not use hot water bottle or hot compresses on area.
			4 Do not shave irradiated areas—beards may be shaved with electric razor q3d.
			5 Avoid pressure on area by not wearing tight-fitting or constricting clothing and by not lying on affected areas for long periods of time.
			6 Keep area dry—wear cotton clothing next to skin to absorb moisture.
			7 Avoid adhesive tape.
3 Potential lethargy due to increased metabolic rate	Carries out ADL with minimal fatigue (ADL = Activities of Daily Living)	(Discharge) √qd	**a** Plan daily care around time of radiation treatment.
			b Provide uninterrupted rest periods for 30 min after receiving treatment.

Figure 8-3 (*Continued*)

	USUAL PROBLEMS	EXPECTED OUTCOMES	DEADLINES	NURSING ORDERS
4	Potential nausea due to tissue breakdown which causes increased waste products circulating in the blood	Is free from nausea and tolerates diet	(Discharge) √qd	**a** Provide small feedings 4–5× a day. **b** Avoid meals 30 min before or after treatment. **c** Encourage patient to drink at least 2000 cc/24°. **d** Obtain antiemetic order from physician if necessary.
5	Potential side effects dependent on area being treated due to radiation treatment	Identifies possible side effects of radiation therapy which may occur after discharge Verbalizes intent to report effects to physician	(Discharge) √qd	**a** Day nurse to check with physician about possible side effects patient may expect, i.e., lung—pneumonitis; eye—conjunctivitis; GI tract—diarrhea. **b** Instruct patient regarding above. Use chemotherapy nurse, dietician, radiation therapist as consultants prn.
6	Potential inability to follow up as outpatient due to transportation problems	Identifies plan for transportation to hospital for treatments	(Discharge) √q day × 3d before discharge.	**a** Consult radiation therapist for best available appointment time. **b** Consult with patient and family member regarding availability of transportation to hospital. **c** Inform patient and/or family regarding availability of assistance with transportation if needed: • Cancer society • Social worker for taxi service for DSS patients

patient. When patient problems occur that are unique to the patient, an individual patient care plan is initiated by the nursing staff.

The nursing implications in the care of a patient receiving external radiotherapy are varied and numerous. The total assessment of the patient focuses on the following things:

1   The patient as an individual with unique needs but also as a member of a family system
2   The physical and nutritional status, activity level, and abilities of the patient
3   The treatment plan and the patient's comprehension of its many facets
4   The emotional status of the patient
5   The patient's inner resources, sources of support, and liabilities

The nurse must also initiate teaching of patient and family regarding actual and anticipated radiation reactions and what should be done when a reaction occurs. You are a direct care giver, liaison, counselor, and teacher for the patient receiving external radiotherapy.

Nursing Implications with Internal Radiotherapy

The nursing implications in the care of a patient receiving internal radiotherapy vary with the type of radiotherapy being used, e.g., systemic, interstitial, or intracavitary internal radiotherapy.

When working with patients who are receiving systemic internal radiotherapy, you must know which radioisotope is being used, what its half-life is, how is it administered, how is it excreted from the body, what precautions are needed, and what to do in case there is contamination. Systemic therapy can be given intraveneously, as with polycythemia vera and leukemia; by mouth, as with thyroid carcinoma; or into a body cavity, as in instillation into the pleural cavity via chest tubes for malignant pleural effusions. The radioactive isotopes are unsealed sources.

If the patient is to receive interstitial radiotherapy, the radioactive isotope is placed in a sealed container that is then inserted into the tumor. It is important that you know which radioisotope is being used, what its half-life is, what precautions are needed, and what is to be done should the source become dislodged, fall out, or be lost.

Intracavitary radiotherapy is commonly used in the treatment of caricinoma of the cervix. With this type of therapy, the radioactive isotope is in an applicator or sealed container. Usually radium is used. Radium has a half-life of 1600 years, which results in a fairly constant emission rate. Patients receiving this therapy usually have the applicators in place for 48 to 72 hours and therefore are isolated. The applicators used to deliver intracavitary radiotherapy for cervical carcinoma are of two basic types: one type contains the radium prior to insertion, and the other is loaded after insertion (after-loading type).

The after-loading applicator is placed in the patient in the operating room.

She is returned to her private room, and the applicator is then loaded with the radium. In caring for these patients, you must remember that during the time the applicator and radium are in the patient, she is radioactive. For this reason, each person having contact with her must observe the three cardinal rules of time, distance, and shielding.

Time, Distance and, Shielding   These are three cardinal rules for safety which personnel must observe when caring for patients with radioactive implants.

1   *Time:* From 10 to 20 to 30 minutes of contact, the amount of radiation received doubles and triples. Time is the one factor that is controllable: The faster you work, the lower the dose received. Hence, before entering the patient's room plan the care to be delivered, to increase your efficiency and decrease delay time. This is the key to reducing radiation exposure.

2   *Distance:* Radiation loses its intensity according to the inverse square law: Working twice as far from the radiation, one receives one-quarter the dose. (At 2 m one gets ¼ dose; at 4 m 1/16 dose; etc.) One should work as far from the source as is practical.

3   *Shielding:* Usually in caring for implant patients the nurse does not utilize any form of shielding, for example, a lead apron. No practical amount of shielding is effective for the very penetrating radiations from radium.

Initially you must explore with the patient her perception and understanding of what will be done in treatment and what it may mean to her. Usually the patient who receives an intrauterine radium implant is admitted to the hospital the evening before the insertion of the applicator. She may or may not have had previous external pelvic irradiation. Patient teaching at this time includes the following items:

1   Clarification of misunderstandings and/or misinformation regarding the procedure and purposes

2   Explanation of the routines that will be carried out the night before insertion, e.g., enemas, low-residue diet, etc.

3   Explanation of how and where the application/implant will be inserted

4   Explanation of routine care after insertion, i.e., daily care, isolation, precautions for staff and visitors, etc.

5   Reiteration of the precautions that family and staff will observe

You must remember that the patient will be radioactive for the period of time the radioactive isotope is in place, usually 48 to 72 hours. After the radioactive isotope is removed from the patient, she is no longer radioactive. She must be given explanations as to why she will be in isolation during the insertion period and why visitation times are limited. The patient must be allowed to ventilate her feelings and concerns at all times.

In delivering nursing care to an implant patient, you must be aware of safety precautions for yourself. Three basic questions that nurses should be aware of are as follows:

1 How much radiation can personnel receive? The National Council on Radiation Protection and Measurements recommends that one can receive 1250 mrem every 3 months to the whole body or 100 mrems per week.

2 How do we know how much radiation the personnel receive in caring for implant patients? Pocket dosimeters permit immediate determination of how much radiation has been received. To read the dosimeter, hold it up to the light and look through the eyepiece. The position of the indicating line is noted on the log sheet before the dosimeter is worn and the patient's room entered. After patient care is delivered, i.e., after exposure to radiation, the position of the line is again noted on the log sheet. If you then subtract the two readings, you obtain the dose in mrem received by the care giver.

3 How can a nurse reduce the amount of radiation received when caring for a patient? As previously discussed, the nurse must be aware of the three cardinal rules for safety: time, distance, and shielding. In the nursing care of the patient with an intracavitary cervical implant, shielding would be impractical in most hospitals. The principle of distance can be used at times but is impractical for physical care. Distance can be used when visiting or talking with the patient. The most important principle that the care giver has is that of time. The nurse should be organized and prepared for the type and amount of care that must be delivered and can control the amount of time spent with the patient.

Patient bed assignment and degree of isolation for patients receiving radioactive material is determined by the Radiation safety officer of the hospital. The patient has a "Radioactive Precautions" tag on the chart, on the room door, written on laboratory slips, etc. All personnel, whether nursing, house-keeping, laboratory, or other, may enter the patient's room and perform duties as usual unless they are pregnant, they think they are pregnant, or there are specific special instructions from the radiation officer. Family members and other visitors must also be instructed as to the safety precautions in effect.

You should check the position of the applicator approximately every 4 hours and should know the emergency procedures (steps to be followed) should the entire applicator or the radioactive source fall out. One important point should be emphasized: No one is to pick up the radioactive source with bare hands should it become dislodged. Long forceps should be used to pick it up, and it should be placed in the shielded transporter cart. If such an accident occurs, the radiation safety officer and other appropriate personnel should be notified immediately and visitors restricted. Should the entire applicator become dislodged, the patient should be removed from the bed, as she is no longer radioactive.

SUMMARY

Radiotherapy is an important and integral part of cancer management today. A nurse caring for such patients must be knowledgeable in the following areas:

1 Neoplastic diseases and their manifestations
2 Treatment modalities available for neoplastic diseases
3 Radiotherapy and its principles

4 The physiological effects of radiotherapy
5 The side effects with radiotherapy
6 The safety factors inherent in the care of the radiotherapy patients
7 Common patient and family concerns, fears, and reactions to radiotherapy

A nurse must also be aware of his or her own attitudes, fears, and anxieties in relation to cancer, radiotherapy, and the care of the radiotherapy patient and family. The nurse caring for the radiotherapy patient and family has various roles, including that of direct care giver, teacher, counselor, and liaison. Nursing in this particular area of oncology nursing is dynamic, challenging, and rewarding.

BIBLIOGRAPHY

Ackerman, L. V. and J. A. del Regato: *Cancer: Diagnosis, Treatment, and Prognosis,* St. Louis: C. V. Mosby, 1970.

Bloomer, William D. and Samuel Hellman: Normal Tissue Responses to Radiation Therapy, *New England Journal of Medicine,* 293:80–83 (July 10, 1975).

Bouchard, Rosemary and Norma Owens: *Nursing Care of the Cancer Patient,* St. Louis: C. V. Mosby, 1972.

Breeding, Mary Anne and Myron Wollin: Working Safely Around Implanted Radiation Sources, *Nursing '76,* 6:58–63 (May 1976).

Deeley, T. J. et al.: *A Guide to Radiotherapy Nursing,* London: E. and S. Livingstone, 1970.

Dolores, Thomas: The Nurse's Contribution in a Radiation Therapy Outpatient Department, *Nursing Clinics of North America,* 2(1)(March 1967).

Rubin, Philip (ed.): *Clinical Oncology for Medical Students and Physicians,* New York: American Cancer Society, 1974, pp. 66–89.

Walter, J.: *Cancer and Radiotherapy,* London: Churchill Livingstone, 1973.

Chapter 9

Nursing Management of the Oncology Patient in Pain

Linda Alexander and Jeanie Barry

Pain is a universal human experience and one of the most common phenomena with which oncology nurses must deal. It is a frequent accompaniment of cancer, yet no predictable relationship exists between the intensity of the painful stimulus and an individual's response to it. The integrity of a one's nervous system, one's personality, one's learned behavior in dealing with pain, one's cultural background, and one's psychological characteristics are just some of the factors that influence one's response to pain. Despite numerous research investigations of pain, much confusion exists about the pain experience. In order to define pain comprehensively it is necessary to encompass theories from a variety of disciplines, such as physiology, psychology, sociology, philosophy, and anthropology. Unfortunately the management of pain is often fragmented, with attention being given to just one isolated aspect rather than to the holistic actuality of the pain experience.

This chapter discusses the pain experience in a unified manner. Pain is viewed physiologically, intraspsychically, and interpersonally. In addition to this theoretical discussion, there is emphasis on the nursing assessment and management of the cancer patient in pain. Case studies are provided to illustrate important concepts involved in the holistic management of pain consequent to cancer.

STERNBACH'S MODEL

In an attempt to provide a more comprehensive holistic overview of pain, Sternbach's theoretical framework of pain has been utilized. Within this framework, Sternbach defines "pain" as a "total set of responses an individual makes to a stimulus which causes or is about to cause tissue damage. The responses may be described in *neurological, physiological, behavioral,* and *affective* terms."[1] An integrated description of the pain phenomena utilizing these terms provides the nurse with a more unified picture of human beings and their pain experience.

To facilitate clarity in the explanation of the various assumptions of Sternbach's theory, each aspect of the pain experience will be separately discussed. However, it must be emphasized that it is only through the integration of all four aspects that true understanding of the pain experience will be achieved.

Neurological Description of Pain

The "gateway control theory" is used here to explain the neurophysiological basis of pain. The distinctive concept of this theory is that pain impulses transmitted from peripheral receptors through the spinal cord to the brain can be modulated at various levels in the central nervous system. Small-diameter fibers of peripheral nerves transmit excitatory pain signals to the spinal cord. If unblocked, these impulses rapidly travel to transmission cells (T cells) and then ascend up the cord to the thalamus and cerebral cortex. It is thought that the *substantia gelatinosa,* which is also located within the spinal cord, is the site of the transmission-blocking action. These cells have the ability to close the gate to pain impulses entering the spinal cord and thus block their transmission to T cells and to higher centers (see Figure 9-1).

Several peripheral mechanisms can be activated to close the gate. Large-diameter nerves on the skin's surface can be stimulated by vibration, pressure, or rubbing. These inhibitory impulses act as negative charges to the incoming small-fiber excitatory impulses. The resultant balance between *inhibition-excitation* messages determines whether or not stimuli reach the transmission cells. If there is little large-fiber activity, the gate is open; then if small fibers are activated, pain will be felt. Large-fiber stimulation closes the gate, and pain is diminished. Of course, permanent closure of the gate would be disastrous, since the body would be deprived of an essential defense mechanism.

In addition to the blocking of peripheral afferent impulses, other pain-inhibiting mechanisms exist involving nerve fibers that descend from the brain stem, thalamus, and cortex. In fact, it is hypothesized that the whole brain is a "pain center."[2] Melzack and Wall propose that the cerebrum is responsible for pain perception and response and that the brain stem acts as a "central biasing mechanism" through its neural connections throughout the body.[3] Activation of this central control system triggers a descending blocking action that closes the gate to incoming pain signals. The central system is affected by factors such as attention, anxiety, anticipatory distress, suggestion, and memory of past experiences, all of which have tremendous impact on an individual's pain experience.

In summary, the gateway control theory provides a sound rationale for a beginning comprehension of the mechanism through which psychosocial and physical factors operate in the pain experience. It supports Sternbach's premise that pain is a complex perceptual experience that needs a holistic approach for definition and management.

Physiological Description of Pain

Any adequate stimulus, by definition, induces physical responses. If the stimulus is intense enough to be perceived by the individual as painful, a certain class of physiological responses, known as "stress responses," will occur. While much research has been conducted in evaluating the anterior pituitary–adrenal cortical response to prolonged pain,[3] these physiological changes are not readily discernible to the nurse. However, sympathetically induced alterations are easily assessed and will be described.

Sternbach has identified a number of parameters that should be considered

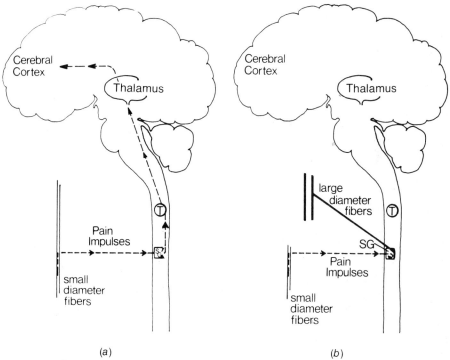

(a)   (b)

Figure 9-1   Diagram illustrating key concepts from the gateway control theory. SG stands for substantia gelatinosa; T stands for transmission cells. See text for complete explanation. (a) Open gate location. (b) Closed gate location.

by the nurse clinician in the assessment of the patient in pain. Numerous research projects have utilized these parameters in evaluating the success of nursing intervention aimed at relieving pain. The parameters include the following:

1 Increase in respiratory rate and depth
2 Pale, cold, clammy skin due to peripheral vasoconstriction
3 Increase in heart rate
4 Increase in both systolic and diastolic pressure
5 Decreased gastric motility, accompanied by reports of nausea[1]

Behavioral Description of Pain

Another way of conceptualizing a person's organismic response to pain is to consider observable behavior. "Observable behavior" may be defined as the individual's gross motor activity and verbal responses. Contained within this description are such concepts as perceptual styles of decision making (i.e., field-dependent versus field-independent, augmenters versus reducers); cognitive dissonance; personality factors such as extroversion, trait anxiety, and neuroticism; family factors; ethnicity; and aggression. A complete discussion of all the different influencing factors involved with each of these topics is beyond the scope of this chapter. However, to ensure continuity in Sternbach's theory of pain, a brief overview is provided. After analyzing a great number of studies, Sternbach organized overt pain behavior into four components:

Category 1: Pain tolerance   The duration of time or intensity at which a person is willing to endure a stimulus beyond the point where it begins to hurt is referred to as *"pain tolerance."* This tolerance is influenced by perceptual styles of judgment, personality factors, cognitive dissonance, amount of sensory input, and past experiences with pain.

Category 2: Pain expression   This term refers to an individual's style of responding to a painful stimulus and is closely linked to personality factors and ethnicity. For example, "exaggerated" expressions of pain may be found in individuals with extraverted personalities or Italian or Jewish cultural backgrounds.

Category 3: Complaints of pain   The readiness to present pain as a symptom is generally known as the *"complaint of pain."* Socioeconomic status, family factors (such as number of siblings, order of birth, and marital status), sex, personality factors, and ethnicity play important roles in determining an individual's willingness to report pain.

Category 4: Effects of pain   The pain experience frequently disrupts behavior. Learning ability, motor skills, and interpersonal communications are often impaired by the painful stimulation. Aggressive behavior is often caused by pain. In fact, environmental stimuli initially associated with pain can begin to elicit such aggression, even in the absence of pain.[1]

In summary, it can be stated that a person's pain tolerance, pain expression, pain reports, and behavioral manifestations of pain are influenced by a multitude of interrelated factors, all of which operate to determine overt pain behavior.

Affective Description of Pain

The affective, or emotional, responses elicited by painful stimuli may have early childhood associations of *pain with punishment*. Such childhood associations have two important components.

First, the threat of bodily harm by punishment may arouse a fantasy of the punitive parent. As a consequence, the patient not only has to deal with the potential harm signaled by the pain itself, but also must contend with the terrifying fantasy of an angry parent.

Second, the pain-as-punishment fantasy involves a childhood fear of abandonment. On a subconscious level, pain is seen not only as punishment that threatens permanent harm but also as lack of parental nurturance and love.

A prerequisite to the understanding of the development and elaboration of the affective part of the pain response is the recognition that an individual regards his or her body as an *object*. In psychoanalytic terms, "object" refers to a person or symbol invested with emotional significance. The body is, of course, an object invested with much feeling quite above the biological sense of survival. Insofar as the body is viewed as an object by the individual, the threat of damage arouses the affect *anxiety*. A common definition of "anxiety" is that it is an affective response to a real or imagined threat to self. Thus, pain that is a signal to the body about current or impending tissue damage evokes anxiety. There are innumerable factors in an experience with pain which can be perceived as threatening to the individual, for example, uncertainty about the pathological significance of pain, or a degree of certainty that the pain indicates advancement of the disease. No matter what the cause of the accompanying anxiety, there is ample empirical evidence for the assumption that increased anxiety is associated with increased pain. It would appear, then, that an investigation of various means of reducing anxiety is warranted for use by nurses who care for cancer patients who have pain.

There are many ways to alter anxiety, such as hypnotic and/or placebo interventions, relaxation therapies, biofeedback, tranquilizing drugs, and diversion techniques. In addition, interpersonal activity that assists the patient to understand his or her feelings and to structure the anxiety-producing event often reduces anxiety, strengthens the ego, and enhances the patient's coping capabilities.

INTERPERSONAL DIMENSIONS

Cancer and its related discomforts are different from many other kinds of illnesses and their concomitant pain. Cancer is a life-threatening disease. Its related discomforts are increased by fear, uncertainty, and anxiety. They are also increased by diminishing control of things around the patient, diminished competence, diminished productivity, and consequently diminished self-esteem. The "diminishing returns" of an illness-restricted, illness-preoccupied life make any discomfort or painful sensation less tolerable and acceptable than it might otherwise be. The biologic, intrapsychic, and intrapersonal dimensions of pain and illness have been discussed. The *interpersonal* aspects will now be explored.

A Conceptual Shift

Nursing training and experience tend to reinforce a somewhat simplistic view of cancer and of pain. Cancer is often viewed only as a condition of a patient and pain only as a characteristic of an individual. Health professionals learn to see illness as an attribute of a person: just as the person has red hair and freckles, nurses say the person has cancer or the person has pain, thus locating the illness within an individual and the pathology or problem within an organism. This simplistic but convenient *assumption* overlooks the fact that the illness and pain are also the subject matter of a communication between patient and nurse. That is, the cancer and pain are not simply located in the patient; they are also the basis for a human interaction or relationship. Shifting to this level of perception, the locus of the cancer and pain is seen to be *between* people rather than simply *in* people. This view is necessary for a responsible understanding of the treatment relationship.

The patient also relates to family members: spouses, parents, children, and siblings. The content or subject matter of much of their communication will be cancer and pain. On this more abstract level it can be seen that families and human relationships, not simply the patient, are afflicted with illness and pain. This is not an *easy* way of understanding pain, but it is an essential prerequisite to the holistic approach.

Pain Myths

The false assumption that pain and disease are solely the characteristics of patients leads to some *mythical ideas*. The patient who has a known lesion or pathology and yet reports no pain, or who has a known lesion but is sufficiently medicated to be pain-free and yet complains, presents a problem. If nurses confine their understanding to only neurological, physiological, and intrapsychic domains, the pain will be perplexing and the myth of *real pain* will arise.

The present state of the medical arts does not permit verification of the reality or nonreality of any subjective sensation. Yet, viewing pain as being within the patient, it becomes necessary to verify the *truth* of the patient's behavior and report. Thus terms such as "real" and "imaginary" pain are generated. These terms lead to the myths of "All pain is real." and "Even imaginary pain is real." These distinctions are clinically useless.

They result from our persistence in locating the pain *within* the patient while overlooking the fact that its locus, as it concerns the nurse, is in the nurse-patient relationship. Pain itself is a personal experience that is not *directly* communicable: one cannot feel another's pain. But it is possible to communicate about pain, and it is this communication *itself* that can be modified.

The myth of real pain is closely related to another myth, the *myth of medication.* Again, the persistent view that the neurological, physiological, and intrapsychic aspects are a sufficient definition of pain is responsible. When looking only at these loci, we think that surgical or chemical manipulations are sufficient to relieve or remove the pain. In fact, it is impossible to treat a *relationship* with an analgesic; it is impossible to surgically modify *communication*. Pain is the subject matter of a human interaction, and this level of reality is not controlled by medication.

Patients as well as health care professionals entertain these myths, which are derived from a partial or limited understanding of the relationship component.

Pain Communication

Once it is accepted that pain is a kind of communication, it is possible to look at pain from a communicational framework and to better understand it. As a result, a more productive alternative to the real/imaginary distinction as well as to the simplistic medication approach may be formulated.

All communication occurs between human beings on three levels. The first is *verbal,* the second is *relational,* and third is *situational.* Each level will be discussed in turn. Participants in communications use information on each of these levels to make sense of what is being expressed or shared.

The "verbal" level is the "I hurt" or "ouch" level. The patient expresses pain in sentences that describe it and locate it. But this information is not enough. It does not tell the nurse what to do or how to interpret the information. It does not relate the pain to the nurse. In order to make sense of the verbal level, it becomes necessary to use the nonverbal, or kinesthetic, level. *How* the patient tells the nurse "I hurt" is as important as the words used. Is the patient grimacing, sweating, clenching, and tensing muscles? Are there nonverbal signs of pain? If there are, the two levels are *congruent.* But is the patient smiling and laughing while saying "I hurt"? When the nonverbal message does not go along with the verbal message, they are *discrepant,* and the nurse may be confused about what exactly is being communicated. Because the nonverbal level interprets how the verbal statements are to be taken and how the nurse should respond, it may be called the "relational" level.

There is still another level, the "situational" level, which often receives much less attention than the other two. As a result, the nurse and patient may engage in incomplete or incorrect communications. The situational level contains still more information about the other two levels. The situation in which the communication occurs is always complex and rich. Part of the situation is the extent of illness itself, the patient's response to it, and the nurse's response to it. Another part is the patient's social system and support group, as well as the nurse's. Another situational variable is the place in which the communication occurs.

The situation is critical to communication. Someone may verbally say "I love you" and show affection by nonverbal expression (so far, congruent), but if the situation is such that the person is a stranger, something is discrepant. A patient may announce intense pain while clenching and sweating, but if there is no lesion, no organic pathology, as part of the situation, the nurse will find the communication discrepant. With cancer patients the situation may well include a lesion, but not always a lesion sufficiently damaging to explain the intense persistent verbal and relational expressions of pain.

A Communication Model   These three levels of information, the verbal, relational, and situational, can be arranged in a diagram or matrix. The major elements of each level of a pain dialogue can be analyzed, and a communication model can be constructed. On the verbal level, consider whether or not the patient's communication includes the report of pain (+) or does not include such a report (−). Then consider the relational level. As a nurse, the role is to treat the patient, to give expert care and skilled intervention. This is the nurse's ongoing contribution to the relationship. In this relationship, one must observe whether the patient responds positively, with relief of *symptoms* or nonverbal signs of pain (+), or negatively, continuing to show signs of pain and need for help (−). Finally, what is the medically verifiable situation of the patient? Is there a lesion or organic pathology that justifies the other two levels of information (+)? Or are the disease or iatrogenic problems resulting from treatment insufficient to explain these other two levels of communication (−)? See Table 9-1.

Every patient with pain can be identified on this matrix. The matrix clearly illustrates the level on which the discrepancy occurs. It permits an understanding of the relational aspects of pain. It forces the nurse away from assumptions and myths and into another dimension of possibility. It indicates where the nurse and/or the patient may be operating with *insufficient information*.

In considering each of the following clinical patient examples, refer to Table 9-1.

Clinical Examples of Pain Communication   Case 1 (+ + +) is an instance of congruent communication. There is a report of pain, a positive response to the nursing intervention, and a known lesion which is pain-producing. In case 1, the nurse is not inspired to look for more information on any level. Case 1 describes, for example, acute postoperative pain in the mastectomy patient. *Case 8* is the null case, an ideal state. Pain is not a reference in this case.

The remaining cases (2–7) are forms of discrepant communication. One descriptive instance of each is provided below. Each of these paradigms, or cases of discrepant communication, will be translated into directives for nursing plans and treatment.

Table 9-1   The Pain-Communication Matrix
(Presence = +   Absence = −)

Report of pain	+	+	+	+	−	−	−	−
Responses to care	+	+	−	−	−	+	−	−
Lesion	+	−	+	−	+	−	+	−
Case	1	2	3	4	5	6	7	8

Case 2 is not usually represented in cancer patients, since generally there is a known lesion or organic basis for the pain as part of the situation. However, sometimes, as in the case of Miss L., a 26-year-old Chinese-American, the site of a lesion adequately treated continued to be referred to as painful. Miss L. complained frequently to her doctor of pain at the site of a radiated neuroblastoma. The physician responded with a modest maintenance dose of analgesia, reassurance, and frequent examinations, but could not find any organic basis for the pain. Miss L. responded positively and with relief to the doctor's relational input and help, but the pain often recurred and did not go away. The patient felt, by association, that the pain indicated a recurrence of a malignancy. Her anxiety grew, and her verbal references to pain increased. The authors encountered her when the physician hospitalized her for tests and more thorough examination. The nursing input in this case is discussed in the next section.

Case 3, Ms. U., was a 48-year-old Creole woman with advanced intestinal cancer and obstruction. Her pattern of communication throughout her final hospitalization was "+ − +." She indicated in persistent verbal terms that she was in pain, she "clock-watched" and asked the nurse for pain medication on every encounter. Over a period of 2 weeks this patient had managed to elevate her medications to double the amount ordered by sheer persistence and demand. As her verbal content became more and more focused on her pain, the nursing staff became less and less interested in relating to her, knowing that every encounter would be a contest over medication—a *relational* contest.

The resultant interactional cycle and the corrective change in relationship indicated by this "+ − +" paradigm are discussed under "Nursing Intervention" below.

Case 4 (+ − −) is a more extreme variant of Case 2, but now the discrepancy occurs on another level of information. Mr. T. was a 64-year-old Caucasian with multiple medical problems, including alcoholism. His cancer was treated surgically, and his physicians did not feel that the residual lesion justified the extent of his complaints about neck pain. Nevertheless, he received narcotic medications for 2 weeks postoperatively, due in part to his extensive verbal reports about pain, delivered in a demanding and hostile fashion. He showed no relief or response to the help given him for pain. Socialization, support, and psychotherapy also failed to modify his demands.

Case 5 was a 45-year-old Japanese-American hospitalized with cancer of the cervix. She had received extensive radiotherapy with resultant painful scarring. Nevertheless, whenever asked how she was feeling, Mrs. Y. would answer, "I'm all right." or "I'm fine." She did not verbally report discomfort. However, her eyes were teary much of the time, her hands clenched, her neck tendons taut with tension. The secondary, relational message was, "I hurt, please help me." The situational level supported that she was suffering. Here the discrepancy is in the absence of verbal references to the pain. Mrs. Y.'s analgesics were ordered "prn," or as needed: as a result, she did not ask for, nor did she receive, any analgesic medication.

Case 6 is a bit odd or bizarre and may be encountered sometimes among psychiatric patients. It additionally describes an erroneous medication order or help given by the nurse but not solicited by the patient, which is not so rare an occurrence as it might seem.

Case 7 is represented by Mr. C., a 70-year-old Chinese-American with primary lung cancer (CA) and spinal metastases. Mr. C. was first encountered when he was admitted for possible depression. His symptoms were social withdrawal, almost total immobility, invalidism, anorexia, and weight loss. Pain was not apparent on the verbal level, and response to treatment was negative on the relational level. However, given his situation (metastatic CA), the presence of pain was probable. Mr. C.'s immobility and unwillingness to move his body were secondary, relational signs of pain. His age, the extensiveness of his illness, and his lack of motivation suggested a hopeless case.

NURSING INTERVENTION

Assessment of the Problem

Several pain cases have been described. The emphasis in this section is to consider what, specifically, the nurse can do. First, intervention requires a careful assessment and understanding of the problem. Systematic methodical interviewing of patient and family members is almost always sufficient to clarify the problem. Since most of the therapeutic work done with cancer patients occurs in some sort of institutional framework—hospital, clinic, physician's office, or at home by visiting nurse—an interview strategy is suggested which can realistically be implemented in these situations. In all the above situations, the nurse is in the best position to effectively assess *the total situation*.

The Interview Strategy

It has been suggested that pain be understood as the subject matter of a communication or relationship and that the nurse shift focus from the patient to the relationship between nurse and patient. Further observation by the nurse will include the patient-family communication about pain.

Two areas of communication should be explored:

1 *The patient's expectation of medical treatment:* Is the patient viewing his or her role as *passive* and anticipating that everything therapeutic will be done to or for him or her? Or does the patient expect to *control* what will happen? What are the nurse's related expectations? What are the family members'?

2 *The patient's beliefs about what the pain signifies:* Does the patient believe pain means tissue damage, progressive deterioration? Anxiety and fear are usually related to pain beliefs, and much of the patient's reference to pain may be in fact a search for information and reassurance. What are the nurse's related beliefs? What are the family members'?

The first area concerns the ways a patient will use pain to obtain help. Patients may use pain to elicit sympathy and support or to manipulate others to care for them. Pain may thus be used to serve broad relationship needs and expectations.

The second area concerns the ways a patient reacts to pain and interprets it. This area of communication is always best served by giving information.

It is not important what precise questions a nurse uses in the interview. It is important that the nurse develop a strategy, a purpose for the interview, and consistently apply it. The cases described above as instances of incongruent communication can now be considered, along with appropriate nursing interventions. (Cases 1 and 8, as previously stated, were not problematic.)

Case 2 (+ + −)   There are a number of important nursing considerations involved in this case. First of all, the *possibility* that the pain is secondary to an unknown organic lesion is always present, and an extensive physical examination is mandatory whenever a "−" occurs on the lesion level of information. The nurse can function as a patient advocate and assist the patient in obtaining thorough diagnostic care. Second, the nurse must assess the patient for extraorganic factors, such as anxiety-producing ideas, experiences, and expectations. Whenever discrepant pain messages are being received, it is essential that all health professionals look beyond the body.

In case 2, the patient made an equation, by association, that "pain-at-the-site-of-tumors = tumors." This was an erroneous equation that led the patient to be preoccupied with the pain and its possible implications. Later, scarring or radiation fibrosis was found as the organic bases for the pain *sensations*. But the nursing intervention, which corrected for the broader area of situational concerns, was to help the patient distinguish the tumor experience from the pain experience. With help, Miss L. was able to understand these as separate events and to react more objectively and with less anxiety to her pain.

Case 3 (+ − +)   This type of discrepant communication indicates a *non-response* to the help offered and leads to the question, "What is unsatisfactory about this help?" It may be that the analgesic is inadequate or that the patient is mistrustful of the health team. As a result, he or she may be using the presence or absence of pain as a means to assess progress of disease and does not want it modified. Another possibility is that an addiction problem has developed, and it is only through a steady flow of verbal pain messages that the patient will receive analgesia. Again it is essential for the nursing staff to look beyond the body for possible clues. In this case, clearly the relationship messages are at issue.

With Ms. U. the need for human relationship far exceeded those needs satisfied by analgesics. Ms. U. was dying, frightened, and alone in a private room. She was deprived socially and had no activities or diversions. She needed emotional and social support and comfort from some human relationship. The nurse was available to her to meet these needs, but the patient felt she could not demand that a nurse just sit and talk. Ms. U. felt that contact with this other human being required some medical and nursing basis, and so she tried to increase her encounters with the nurse by increasing her medication requests.

The nurse was able to correct the behavior. The previous cycle that consisted of *diminished responses* for contact was reversed through providing socialization unrelated to medication. The interpersonal, nonmedical relationship is in fact a nursing function; the patient's assumption was erroneous. Talk, visiting, and diversion were offered Ms. U. as often as medication, but separated from it. The socialization was therapeutic and corrective of the discrepant communication problem. This type of therapy is just as essential as analgesia and should be noted as a nursing order on the patient's treatment sheet.

Case 4 (+ − −)   The discrepancy in this case is on the verbal level. It is essential that the nursing staff precisely clarify the referents of the patient's communication. If the words are taken only literally, it would seem quite apparent that the patient is referring to his pain. But more investigation is indicated, since words are easily and voluntarily manipulated to say one thing and mean another. (Note that it is much harder to manipulate the other two levels of information.) Mr. T. was not looking for a one-to-one supportive relationship, since this was offered and did not modify his behavior. Restricting the view of the situation to "−" lesion was also uninformative. In fact, Mr. T. was addicted to narcotics. His verbal reference to pain was accurate to the extent that his tolerance to the analgesic was increasing and its efficacy was diminishing. If an addiction problem is present, the nursing staff must begin to keep a meticulous record of the time and dosage of all pain and tranquilizing drugs. Also, the precise verbal and relational messages that the patient sends at the time of administration must be noted.

The nurse *must not* limit assessment to a possible addiction problem. Sometimes a "+ − −" message alerts the health team to a wide range of needs: needs for attention and reassurance, for information, for secondary gains that can be attained only by claiming a disability or condition warranting certain treatments. What is important is that professionals not assume that the "+ − −" presentation relieves them from medical and nursing responsibility. It is a condition needing proper identification. Once this particular type of discrepant pain message has been identified, the nurse can function as the patient's advocate. Understanding this kind of discrepant communication is the prerequisite to planning for treatment or referral. Even malingering is a treatable condition.

Case 5 (− − +)   There are many reasons why a patient may adopt the role of martyr or "silent sufferer." Once recognizing the discrepancy in this communication, the nurse must begin to explore with the patient the reasons for the resistance to refer to pain. A few possible reasons may be as follows: a loss of self-esteem for appearing weak, a fear of demanding too much, or a religious belief that connects suffering with eternal rewards.

In Mrs. Y.'s case, there were expectations the nurses and doctors, all of whom were "experts," would *automatically* know of her pain and help her. Mrs. Y. had become increasingly anxious and hostile toward the staff since they did not respond as she felt they should.

It is obvious that prn medications are of little assistance in treating this type of patient. One of the first interventions with Mrs. Y. was to arrange for regularly scheduled medications. In addition, the nursing staff assisted this patient to become more assertive by encouraging her to verbalize her needs for analgesia and to feel comfortable about this new behavior.

Case 6 (− + −) Rarely encountered, case 6 does invite nurses to explore their own *projections* about cancer and about pain. Does the nurse sometimes offer help or relief to a patient for problems the nurse *assumes* are the case but which may not be operating?

Case 7 (− − +) When presented with this type of patient, often the staff reacts first by feeling hopeless, frustrated, and equally withdrawn. However, in Mr. C.'s case, some rather dramatic changes were instituted once the cause of the discrepant communication was identified.

The situational discrepancy was modified when the staff learned, by careful interviewing, that Mr. C. actively wanted to die. He was responding to this wish rather than to his cancer pathology alone, and he believed that any verbal reference to pain would result in more medication. He believed that more medication would prolong his life, and he did not want to live. He did not refer to his agony, nor would he take his analgesic. Thus he refused the help given and could not respond positively to it. This "stoicism" masked a misconception. The nurse took time to explain that analgesia would make him more comfortable but would not alter the course of his illness. His wish to die was not contested; his life of pain was. Mr. C. did finally accept analgesia, on a regular non-prn basis, and his communication during his last week of life was "+ + +," a congruent set of messages.

A very important misconception is implied in Mr. C.'s case study. Many patients, families, and health professionals believe that a diagnosis of terminal cancer equals unremitting pain. This often *is not* the case. What often is the case is that inadequate analgesia and unrecognized organic and extraorganic factors equal intractable pain. Nurses can do much to relieve the agony of cancer pain through assessment of the patient based on the pain-communication model and interventions directed toward removing the discrepancy.

Summary

Nursing has an important role in the management of the cancer patient with pain. In order to fulfill this role, the nurse requires a broad theoretical base for intervention and care planning. The theory and approach should reflect a comprehensive understanding of pain behavior in its broadest aspects. A conscious effort to avoid fragmenting a patient's pain experience should be made by all members of the health care team.

REFERENCES

1   R. Sternbach. *Pain: A Psychophysiological Analysis,* New York: Academic Press, 1968, p. 159.

2 R. Melzack and P. D. Wall. "Pain Mechanisms: A New Theory," *Science,* **150**:973, 1965.
3 D. Siegle. "The Gate Control Theory," *American Journal of Nursing,* **74**:500, March 1974.

BIBLIOGRAPHY

Bruegel, M. A. "Relationship of Preoperative Anxiety to Perception of Postoperative Pain," *Nursing Research,* **20**:26–31, January –February 1971.
Chambers, W. and Price, G. "Influence of Nurse upon Effects of Analgesics Administered," *Nursing Research,* **16**:228–233, Summer 1967.
Dudley, D., Masuda, M., and Marlin, C. J. "Psychophysiological Studies of Experimentally Induced Action Oriented Behavior," *Journal of Psychosomatic Research,* **9**:209–221, 1965.
Fordyce, W. "An Operant Conditioning Method for Managing Chronic Pain," *Postgraduate Medicine,* **53**:123–129, May 1973.
Jacox, Ada and Stewart, Mary. *Psychosocial Contingencies of the Pain Experience,* Iowa City: University of Iowa Press, 1973.
Johnson, Jean and Rice, Virginia. "Sensory and Distress Component of Pain: Implications for the Study of Clinical Pain," *Nursing Research,* **22**:203–209, May–June 1974.
Lacey, J. I., Baleman, D., and Van Lehn R. "Autonomic Response Specificity: An Experimental Study," *Psychosomatic Medicine,* **15**:8–21, 1953.
Lynn, R. and Eysenck, H. J. "Tolerance for Pain, Extraversion, and Neuroticism," *Perceptual and Motor Skills,* **12**:161–162, 1961.
McBride, M. A. "Nursing Approach, Pain and Relief: An Exploratory Experiment," *Nursing Research,* **16**:337–340, Fall 1967.
McCaffery, Margo. *Nursing Management of the Patient with Pain,* Philadelphia: Lippincott, 1972.
Melzack, R. and Casey, K. L. "Sensory, Motivational and Central Control Determinants of Pain: A New Conceptual Model," in Kenshalo, D. (ed.), *The Skin Senses,* Springfield, Ill.: Charles C. Thomas, 1968.
―――― and Chapman, C. "Psychologic Aspects of Pain," *Postgraduate Medicine,* **53**:69–75, May 1973.
―――― and Wall, P. D. "Pain Mechanisms: A New Theory," *Science,* **150**:971–979, 1965.
Moss, F. and Meyer, B. "The Effects of Nursing Interaction upon Pain Relief in Patients," *Nursing Research,* **15**:303–306, Fall 1966.
Schalling, D. and Levander, S. "Ratings of Anxiety-Proneness and Responses to Electrical Pain Stimulation, *Scandanavian Journal of Psychology,* **5**:1–9, 1964.
Seyle, Hans. *The Stress of Life,* New York: McGraw-Hill, 1956.
Siegle, D. "The Gate Control Theory," *American Journal of Nursing,* **74**:498–502, March 1974.
Sternbach, R. A. "A Comparative Analysis of Autonomic Responses in Startle," *Psychosomatic Medicine,* **22**:204–210, 1960.

Sternbach, Richard. *Pain: A Psychophysiological Analysis,* New York: Academic Press, 1968.

Szasz, T. S. *Pain and Pleasure,* New York: Basic Books, 1957.

————. "Language in Pain," in Arieti, S. *American Handbook of Psychiatry,* New York: Basic Books, 1960.

Zborowski, Mark. *People in Pain,* San Francisco: Jossey-Bass, 1969.

Chapter 10

Rehabilitation in Cancer: Concepts and Application

Doris Y. Ahana and Amy Takeuchi

Cancer patients are living longer! There are approximately 1,500,000 Americans living today who have been free of disease for at least 5 years after diagnosis and treatment. About 225,000, or one-third, of all Americans who get cancer this year will be alive at least 5 years after treatment.

The increase in the quantity of life, though measurable and dramatic, does not guarantee quality living to the cancer patient. Dr. Robbins, a renowned proponent of cancer rehabilitation, succinctly describes the importance of human values in the treatment of the cancer patient. He states:

> It doesn't matter how early cancer patients are diagnosed or how we treat them if efforts are not made to readjust them to society. I think we haven't done the job. That is the price that one must pay for cancer cure and control if, in fact, it has left an individual a recluse, non-productive, virtually an emotional cripple.[1]

Some cancer patients state that feelings of anger, fear, depression, and rejection are more difficult to cope with than the cancer itself. Rehabilitation addresses the human problems as well as the disease condition. Emphasis is placed upon the patient as a human being having hopes and fears.

Cancer rehabilitation is an attempt to provide quality survival for the cancer patient using the following criteria:

1   The general health and physical well being of the cancer patient enables him to resume personal living and work responsibilities.
2   The cancer patient is comfortable, and free of pain and distress from immobility.
3   The cancer patient is able to readapt to family and communal living.
4   The cancer patient does not deplete his or her financial resources.

Rehabilitation encompasses all phases of illness from the time the diagnosis is made to the curative, chronic, or terminal stage. It recognizes the cancer patient as a unique and holistic person who requires a continuum of care utilizing the skills of a multidisciplinary team.

Rehabilitation provides the cancer patient with hope for the future and the opportunity to live with the disease in a meaningful and productive way. To live with cancer, the patient must be assisted to adapt to the bio-psycho-social tasks of living. These tasks include maintaining and restoring relations with significant others, enhancing the potential for restoring and maintaining bodily functions, reshaping a personally valued and socially acceptable life-style after maximum recovery has been attained, minimizing the effects of changes in self-concept, and capitalizing on strengths. Every patient regardless of the increasing limitations imposed by the disease process and treatments is capable of self-growth.

The family or significant others must also "live with" the patient's illness and with the concomitant changes and problems that it brings. Helping the family through this difficult period of adjustment necessitates a rehabilitative focus. Rehabilitation offers the supporters of a patient—family, friends, relatives, neighbors—appropriate help, so that the strengths of these people are renewed and they can continue supporting the patient. Where cure and management are no longer the aims of therapy, the dignity of the person is still respected by enabling him or her to make choices and decisions about care.

In summary, the following concepts, illustrated in Figure 10-1, can be utilized in cancer rehabilitation:

1   The comprehensive needs of the patient are met by the utilization of a multidisciplinary team approach.
2   The continuum of care is a rehabilitative component in all phases of the patient's illness and all settings of the patient's interactions—hospital, home, and community.
3   Early and continuous involvement of the family and significant others is important to the patient's adaptive process.
4   Living with cancer requires the patient to engage in bio-psycho-social adaptive tasks.
5   Human problems and needs demand a holistic approach to the cancer patient and family.

Figure 10-1 Rehabilitation is. . .

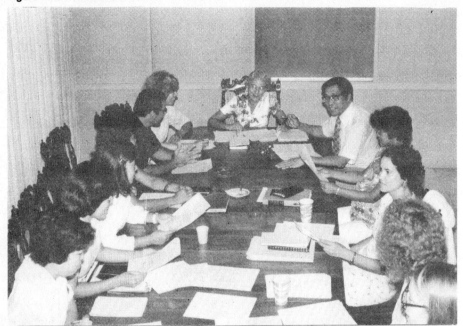

Meeting the holistic needs of the cancer patient through a multidisciplinary approach.

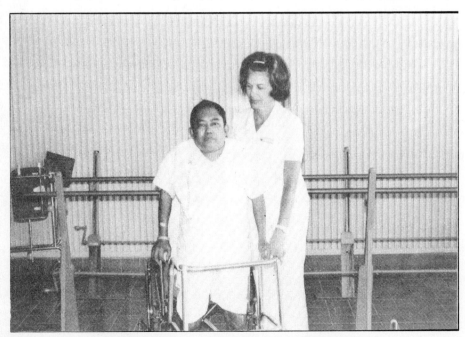

Physical therapist assisting the patient in achieving maximum dependence.

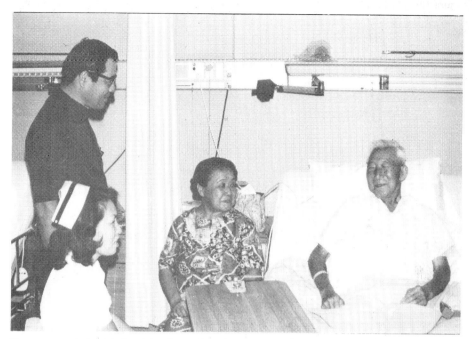

The nurse and chaplain involving the patient and his wife in establishing rehabilitation goals.

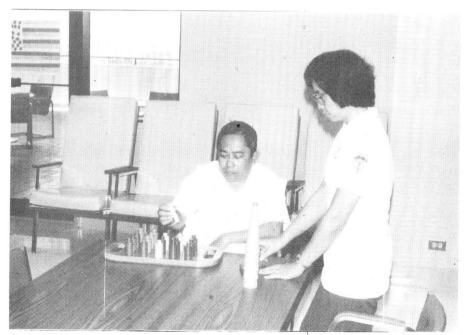

Occupational therapist assisting patient to regain control and independence.

6 Despite the cancer and its limitations, the patient has the potential for self-growth.

PROCESSES/COMPONENTS OF EFFECTIVE REHABILITATION

Rehabilitation: An Attitudinal Process

Successful rehabilitation begins with attitudes. The interaction of attitudes between the cancer patient, significant others, and health personnel creates a climate for rehabilitation.

Cancer has negative connotations for many people. The world "cancer" generates feelings of fear, shame, terror, hopelessness, and helplessness, as shown in the following statements made by patients and families:

> Cancer is a silent killer. It's worse than leprosy because you may look well on the outside but still have it hanging in there.

> Cancer is like an octopus whose legs are similar to the roots of cancer. You can't cure it until you can get at the roots.

> I don't want people to find out that I have cancer because they may be afraid to touch me.

> "Cancer" is a terrible word. Whoever thought of it should get rid of the word from the dictionary.

One's attitudes are largely influenced by one's experience with cancer. With the rising incidence of cancer, many people have become aware of it via families, relatives, and friends. People have a tendency to recall the negative aspects of such experiences and consequently may hold pessimistic views of the disease. They are seldom aware of the many kinds of cancer, each having a potential for control and some for cure.

When told the diagnosis of cancer, the patient and the family frequently are immobilized and unable to look beyond the emotional impact of the diagnosis. Perhaps no other chronic illness is equated with such strong feelings of imminent death as is cancer. At this point rehabilitation and cancer appear diametrically opposed. Changing this attitude of hopelessness to one of rehabilitation is the goal of health professionals and community organizations. Attitude change often depends upon who presents the information. The physician is seen as an expert by cancer patient and family, thereby exerting significant influence on the patient's willingness to participate in a program of rehabilitation. Volunteers of the Reach to Recovery and ostomy organizations are instrumental in changing the attitudes of patients. Because these volunteers have had cancer but lead normal and productive lives, they, more than any other professional group, lend credibility to the concept of rehabilitation.

Health professionals have attitudes toward cancer that are similar to the general public's attitudes. They rationalize and intellectualize that the cancer patient is unable to benefit from an aggressive program of rehabilitation. They have a "wait and see" attitude about providing rehabilitative services. Evidence of delay is noted in remarks such as: "How much does the patient know about the illness?" and "We can't get involved unless the patient really understands that he (she) has cancer."

The nurse is in a strategic position to inculcate a healthy and realistic attitude toward cancer rehabilitation. The nurse's interaction with the patient and family and ministrations of care convey the attitude of hope, responsiveness, and involvement in rehabilitating the patient.

Other care providers constitute the larger community of the patient and family. Their positive attitudes toward the cancer patient potentiate the rehabilitative process. Rehabilitative goals are facilitated in an environment free of stigma, in which the patient, the family, health professionals, and ancillary staff relate first as human beings.

Rehabilitation: An Integrative Process Based on Patient Needs

Health care today is increasingly complex, with multiple specialists responding to different aspects of patient care. Though desirable, specialization brings with it the inherent problems of fragmentation, conflict of goals between disciplines, and depersonalization. Rehabilitation services can be integrated if there is commitment to meeting the needs of the patient. Health professionals accept this premise in theory, but patient needs frequently are poorly articulated in practice.

In any health care delivery system, there are three types of behavior orientation in each profession; the organizationally oriented, the self-oriented, and the patient-oriented. Below, nurses are depicted in examples of this typology.

Nurse 1: Organizationally oriented nurse   Nurse 1 follows rules and regulations to avoid risks. She delays any form of rehabilitation until it is prescribed by the physician. Exercises and self-care activities are initiated after there is a physician's order. This nurse has difficulty exercising judgment, adhering to policy, procedure, and tradition. Families are asked to follow the visiting hour policies and are frequently viewed as an obstacle to the delivery of care to the patient. Nurse 1 appears task-centered and relates to the patients through nursing procedures and treatments. This nurse provides little time to sit and listen to the patients.

Nurse 2: Self-oriented nurse   Nurse 2 perceives the cancer patient as a stereotype with needs that are determined by the nurse's own values and goals. This nurse speaks for the cancer patient to the extent of deciding what rehabilitative interventions are necessary and which discipline should provide them. There is minimal participation and collaboration with the patient and other health professionals. For example, Nurse 2 aggressively seeks a physician's order for an ostomy club volunteer to see the patient. As an afterthought the patient is told of the planned visitation. It does not matter to Nurse 2 that the patient is refusing this visit because a friend with an ostomy is providing support and encouragement.

Nurse 3: Patient-oriented nurse   Nurse 3 perceives the cancer patient as an individual with unique problems and needs. Recognizing the impact of a crisis on the patient and family, this nurse provides time to listen and offer crisis counseling. Nurse 3 includes the patient and the family in the plan of care. This nurse views cancer rehabilitation as a team effort and collaborates with other health disciplines to deliver services the patient requires. Nurse 3 sees the patient as an active and responsible member of the team and as the unifying component in an integrated approach to rehabilitation.

Rehabilitation: A Creative Process

New insights and skills in cancer rehabilitation are emerging from the integration of a multitude of specialties. The complexity of each patient's problems requires the interaction of a multidisciplinary team. As each discipline discusses with the other disciplines alternative ways of helping the patient adapt to the cancer, creativity in interventions is enhanced.

Modification of conventional approaches to rehabilitation to meet the needs of the patient is an example of creativity. The following example illustrates the use of occupational therapy in replicating the patient's work role:

> Mr. M. is a 48-year-old patient who works for a construction firm as a foreman. He is admitted to the hospital for treatment of cancer in his liver. Intra-arterial infusion using 5-FU is planned.
>
> His wife describes the patient as a "workaholic" who enjoys helping his laborers beyond the duties of his job. He has become increasingly angry and frustrated with the prolonged confinement in the hospital.
>
> In the multidisciplinary planning conferences, the occupational therapist recommends that the patient be encouraged to pursue an activity of interest to him while on chemotherapy. Knowing that the patient is accustomed to helping and supervising his laborers, the nurse suggested that Mr. M. teach other patients fishnet making, a handicraft in which he excels.

The patient, as a participant in rehabilitation, should assist the health team in finding innovative solutions to his or her problem. Stryker defines rehabilitation as a creative process in which patients will ultimately create their own environment and ways of coping with it.[3] An example of patient creativity is described:

> Mr. W. is a 67-year-old patient who was formerly employed as a draftsman. He had a cystectomy with a urinary diversion for cancer of his bladder. The home care nurse was called in to assist the patient with the care of his ileo-conduit at home.
>
> The patient knew the procedure for changing his appliance but had difficulty in assembling its parts. The lack of strength in his arthritic hands prevented him from attaining complete independence. With the nurse's encouragement, he designed,

and had his son fashion, a tool that enabled him to assemble the appliance without assistance.

As can be seen from the example, the patient's inventiveness contributed to his own independence. Creativity is fostered in a familiar home environment in which adjustments must be made to normalize a patient's life-style.

STAGES OF CANCER: THEIR IMPLICATIONS FOR REHABILITATION

Cancer patients enter the hospital in varying stages of illness. With each admission and readmission, realistic appraisal of the nature and extent of the patient's illness, level of functioning and dependency, adaptive abilities, and family relationships needs to be made. As cancer progresses, short-term and long-term goals are redefined. As depicted in Figure 10-2, rehabilitation is an ongoing process regardless of the prognosis and/or declining levels of performance that may be apparent.

Early Stage of Cancer

In the early stage of cancer, the patient's illness is potentially curable. Usually no further treatment is required after the initial intervention. A large percentage of patients in this category have surgery as an initial mode of treatment.

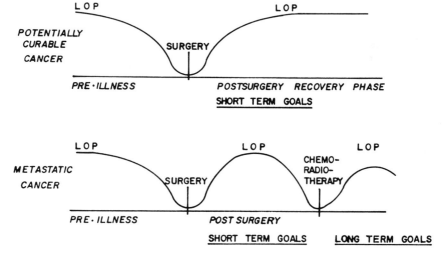

Figure 10-2 With potentially curable cancer, short-term goals are set which seek to reestablish levels of performance during the postsurgery phase. The patient with metastatic cancer requires both short- and long-term goals that may retain optimum levels of performance for a period of time. Over time, the level of performance gradually declines as the disease progresses.

The length of hospital stay of the cancer patient in the early stage is dependent upon the extensiveness of the surgery and the development of postoperative complications. Preoperative preparation influences the patient's postoperative course and necessitates the initiation of preventive rehabilitation prior to the patient's hospitalization. Patient and family participation in a preoperative class will mobilize their strengths so that they can deal effectively with the postoperative routine of care.

The concept of rehabilitation in the preoperative period is more viable while the patient is independent and not institutionalized. An outpatient program of preoperative teaching, including a multidisciplinary team, should focus on the immediate concerns of the patient and the family rather on than the professionals' concern of what *should* be taught in class. Such a program (1) facilitates earlier identification of the problems and services required and (2) stimulates the patient and the family to initiate actions to resolve their own problems prior to surgery.

Postoperatively, the appropriate disciplines must be available at the proper time to facilitate the patient's return to his or her former level of independence. Since timing is important to the success of rehabilitation, and since nurses are in direct contact with the patient 24 hours a day, they should develop guidelines that indicate the time to initiate specific actions or referrals. The mastectomy protocol* in Figure 10-3 *a* directs the nurse in anticipating common problems and implementing rehabilitative actions. The protocol also shows the time frame within which a particular discipline should be called. A nurse who has difficulty in carrying out or reinforcing actions or instructions can refer to an example shown in Figure 10-3 *b*.

Although surgical patients will rationalize that body image changes can be compromised for one's life, they still need to reintegrate their self-concept. Multidisciplinary interventions for the resolution of body image problems are described in Figure 10-4.

Most surgical patients are able to resume a preillness level of functioning after discharge. When they go home, they may require the services of the home care nurse or a public health nurse. Visits by professionals are usually necessary for a short period of time. Psychosocial and physical adjustments extend beyond hospitalization and agency follow-up. For example, sexual problems become a reality as the patient recovers physically and attempts to meet the spouse's needs. These problems usually will not be magnified during the patient's contact with the rehabilitation staff. The office nurse, significant others, family members, and friends are the people with whom the patient will have a continuing relationship. Therefore, efforts should be made to involve them in the rehabilitative process.

---

*A "protocol" consists of guidelines to help the nurse and consulting multidisciplines in solving common problems.

Chronic Stage of Cancer

Progression of cancer is anticipated in those patients who have evidence of metastasis. Controlled by current modalities of treatment—radiotherapy, chemotherapy, surgery, hormonal therapy, immunotherapy—chronic illnesses have periods of remission. The treatments, however, produce varying side effects that may be devastating to the patient. For example, the use of alkylating agents such as vincristine causes a form of myopathy in varying degrees of peripheral neuropathy. A program of range-of-motion exercises can prevent posttreatment deficits. Prevention and control of side effects are essential during the chronic phase of illness.

Repeated hospitalizations of the chronically ill cancer patient result in role changes, family disruption, marital stress, and financial difficulties. Adherence to restrictions and precautions over a long period is difficult for the patient on continuing therapy. Changes in life-style can be life-threatening, particularly among the young, as exemplified by the following patient:

A 16-year-old male with leukemia was admitted with cellulitis in his right leg, having sustained an abrasion falling off his motorcycle. Three months ago while hospitalized for chemotherapy, he had boils on his face and in the axilla.

The patient described himself as "carefree and wild" and typical of all his friends. His personal hygiene habits were poor. The ancillary staff informed the nurse that the patient was reluctant to bathe. According to his mother, the patient seldom took a bath at home, but she didn't know about his personal habits since he spent a large portion of his time at his friend's home.

Changes in the patient's life-style required the support of his peers as well as his family and health professionals. Each minor change was interpreted as a personal loss. His leukemia was viewed as a threat to his independence, particularly when restrictions were imposed by family and health professionals to protect him from infection and trauma. For patients to maintain control over their situation, they must be given an opportunity to make decisions and modify activities in a way that they can accept.

Chronically ill cancer patients can continue to be independent and to participate in many useful and social activities:

The wife of a cancer patient identified her husband's need to be useful to his family and allowed him to assume a simple household task. Both she and her daughter worked during the day. Prior to the patient's illness, he frequently assisted his wife with the preparation of "little side dishes." Since he enjoyed being in the kitchen, the tasks of shopping for groceries and starting the dinner for the family were given to the patient. Grocery shopping proved to be therapeutic for the patient because he visited his friends along the way. As the cancer progressed he still continued to buy the groceries, until only one item, such as a loaf of bread, was purchased each day.

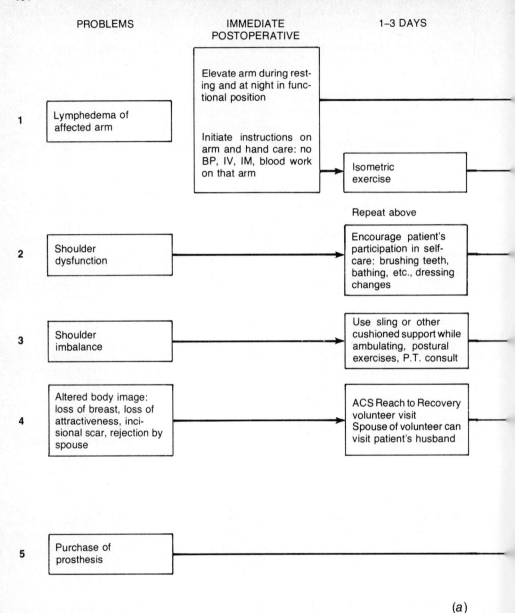

	PROBLEMS	IMMEDIATE POSTOPERATIVE	1–3 DAYS
1	Lymphedema of affected arm	Elevate arm during resting and at night in functional position Initiate instructions on arm and hand care: no BP, IV, IM, blood work on that arm	Isometric exercise
			Repeat above
2	Shoulder dysfunction		Encourage patient's participation in self-care: brushing teeth, bathing, etc., dressing changes
3	Shoulder imbalance		Use sling or other cushioned support while ambulating, postural exercises, P.T. consult
4	Altered body image: loss of breast, loss of attractiveness, incisional scar, rejection by spouse		ACS Reach to Recovery volunteer visit Spouse of volunteer can visit patient's husband
5	Purchase of prosthesis		

(a)

Figure 10-3 Mastectomy protocol—modified radical and radical. Proper exercises will help decrease stiffness, heaviness, and pain in shoulder or incision so the patient can (a) regain normal shoulder range of motion, (b) regain strength in shoulder and arm, and (c) relieve or prevent swelling of arm. Postoperative day 2: Isometric exercise of squeezing rolled gauze or ball, with patient frequently being given the instruction, "the more the better" or "the longer the better." (a) Protocol. (b) Example. (*Acknowledgment is made to St. Francis Hospital Cancer Rehabilitation Services Program in Honolulu, Hawaii, which was funded through the National Cancer Institute Contract No. NO1-CN-45118.*)

3–7 DAYS   POSTDISCHARGE—   GOALS
                                7+ DAYS

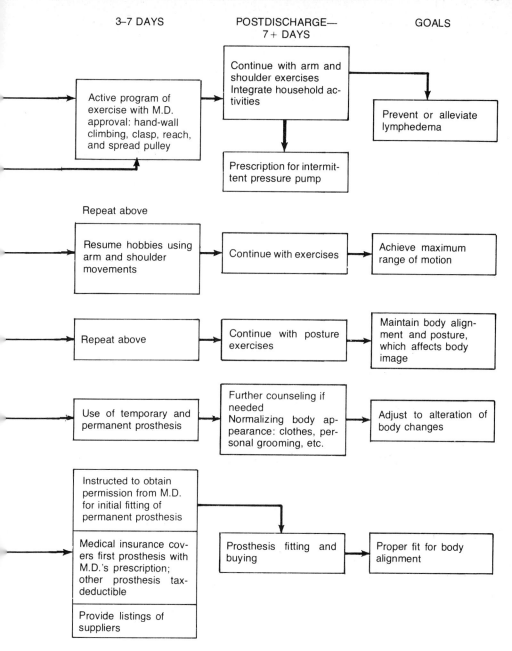

Active program of exercise with M.D. approval: hand-wall climbing, clasp, reach, and spread pulley

Continue with arm and shoulder exercises Integrate household activities

Prevent or alleviate lymphedema

Prescription for intermittent pressure pump

Repeat above

Resume hobbies using arm and shoulder movements

Continue with exercises

Achieve maximum range of motion

Repeat above

Continue with posture exercises

Maintain body alignment and posture, which affects body image

Use of temporary and permanent prosthesis

Further counseling if needed Normalizing body appearance: clothes, personal grooming, etc.

Adjust to alteration of body changes

Instructed to obtain permission from M.D. for initial fitting of permanent prosthesis

Medical insurance covers first prosthesis with M.D.'s prescription; other prosthesis tax-deductible

Provide listings of suppliers

Prosthesis fitting and buying

Proper fit for body alignment

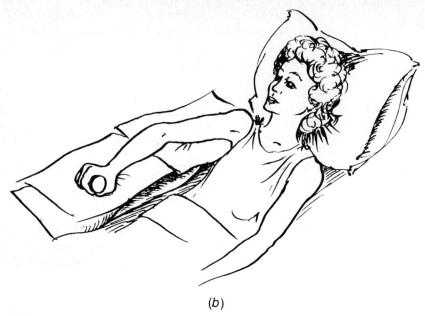

(b)

Figure 10-3 *(Continued)*

Family members can reinforce a sick person's role by seeing and treating the person as an invalid. Before long the patient responds in a similar manner, and a cycle is established making it difficult for everyone to change. Through a discharge planning conference with the multidisciplinary team members, the family has an opportunity to raise questions about the care and rehabilitation measures required.

Table 10-1 shows a multidisciplinary planning conference in which the following goals are facilitated:

1 Continuing care and rehabilitation
2 Allaying anxiety of family members
3 Ascertaining roles of family members and health professionals upon patient's discharge to home
4 Strengthening the supportive system in the family

The supportive role of the family has been identified as one of the criteria for determining the successful outcome of rehabilitation. Family members have the major responsibility in helping the patient return to the maximum level of independence and productivity. Health professionals should feel a moral obligation to guide the family through its difficult transition from seeing the patient as a sick person in the hospital to viewing him or her as a person with potential for remission and health after discharge.

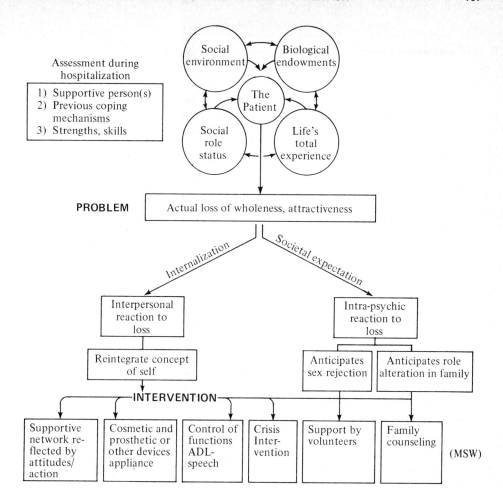

Assessment during
hospitalization

1) Supportive person(s)
2) Previous coping
   mechanisms
3) Strengths, skills

PROBLEM   Actual loss of wholeness, attractiveness

Internalization   Societal expectation

Interpersonal
reaction to
loss

Intra-psychic
reaction to
loss

Reintegrate concept
of self

Anticipates
sex rejection

Anticipates role
alteration in family

─INTERVENTION─

Supportive
network re-
flected by
attitudes/
action

Cosmetic and
prosthetic or
other devices
appliance

Control of
functions
ADL-
speech

Crisis
Inter-
vention

Support by
volunteers

Family
counseling

(MSW)

Figure 10-4 Postoperative change in body image. Changes in body image begin during hospitalization and are influenced by social and biological factors as well as by life experience and social status. With identification of the body image problem, appropriate interventions can be designed. (*Acknowledgment is made to St. Francis Hospital Cancer Rehabilitation Services Program in Honolulu, Hawaii, which was funded through the National Cancer Institute Contract No. NO1-CN-45118.*)

Advanced Stage of Cancer

At the stage of advanced cancer, the patient's response to treatment is poor. Symptoms due to the effects of the cancerous process become exceedingly difficult to palliate. Problems of debility, immobility, and pain contribute to the patient's feelings of hopelessness and the family's feelings of helplessness. Limitations in the patient's physical resources increase dependency on others. The elderly person with cancer often has other health problems that contribute to

Table 10-1 Multidisciplinary Discharge Planning Conference

Family members present

Husband
Son and his wife
Two daughters (another daugher unable to attend)

Health team members present

Attending physician
Chaplain
Nurse
Social worker
Occupational therapist
Physical therapist
Home care nurse liasison
Dietitian

Ms. S. W. is a 65-year-old housewife with a diagnosis of left temporal astrocytoma, grade III. She had a left temporal craniotomy with partial excision of the tumor. Her motor and sensory functions are within normal limits. However, she has a right homonymous hemianopsia. Ms. S. W. understands simple commands and is able to follow instructions. Her verbal communication is slow and repetitive.

  Prior to her illness, Ms. S. W. led an active and independent life. Her major hobbies included knitting, sewing, and other hand crafts.

Problem areas	Actions/recommendations by group
Bathing, dressing, feeding, and personal hygiene	1 Supervise patient but encourage her to do as much for herself as she can, at her own pace. 2 Obtain bath brush so she can wash her back. 3 Place chair in shower for bathing. 4 Encourage self-feeding. Patient needs sufficient time to complete her meals.
Mobility	1 Supervise ambulation with cane. 2 Wheelchair not recommended to encourage ambulation. 3 Armchair should be of appropriate height in order to facilitate standing. 4 Teach body mechanics to patient and family —sitting and standing.
Nutrition	1 Chop foods until her upper dentures are replaced. 2 Dietitian will review written instructions on high-protein diet with family.
Vision	1 Occupational therapist will evaluate visual and mental abilities through activities. 2 Visual deficits should not limit her participation in socialization and activities of daily living. 3 Articles should be placed on her left side.

Table 10-1 *(Continued)*

Problem areas	Actions/recommendations by group
Socialization for patient and husband	1 Continue occupational therapy on an outpatient basis. 2 Husband will continue with his usual socialization and activities (e.g., shopping, meeting with his friends) while patient is in occupational therapy.
Bladder care	1 Nurse will continue teaching bladder care to patient's husband. 2 Foley catheter will be changed by the home care nurse.
Spiritual needs	1 Patient's minister with United Church of Christ will maintain contact with the family.
Radiotherapy	1 Son will provide transportation for his mother's treatments. 2 Social worker will arrange for transportation through the American Cancer Society if son has difficulty in taking time off from his work. 3 Daughter will knit a cap for her mother if she loses her hair after radiotherapy. 4 Nurse will explain radiotherapy skin care to patient and family.
Chemotherapy	1 Nurse will review chemotherapy brochure with the family. 2 Physician will initiate chemotherapy with 1,3-BIS-(2 chloroethyl)-1-nitrosurea (abbreviated as BCNU).
Equipment at home	1 Home care nurse will do predischarge home evaluation to assess environmental situation. 2 Occupational and physical therapists recommended bed rail at night, toilet guard, shower bench, and extended nozzle for shower.

further physiological impairment. During this phase of illness, control of symptoms, prevention of secondary disability and complications, and provision of comfort are essential rehabilitation objectives.

The institution of comfort measures and the presence of health personnel to meet care needs communicate to the patient and the family that they have not been abandoned. Usually when a spouse has been ministering to the patient's care needs, there is an unintentional tendency on the part of the nurses to assume that the spouse does not need help or relief. The spouse or significant other is heavily taxed by the increasing care needs of the patient and the demands of other members of the family. If the patient chooses to die at home, the health professionals should assist the family in preparing for this event. Assisting the family through anticipatory grief enables them to deal effectively with the patient's dying.

Treating the patient as a human being until death reflects the ultimate philosophy of rehabilitation.

THE TEAM APPROACH IN CANCER REHABILITATION

There is a growing impetus toward the development and application of the team concept in the delivery of optimum rehabilitation services for cancer patients and their families. Cancer, like other chronic illnesses, requires the use of many disciplines to help patients to achieve maximum rehabilitation. Fragmentation of rehabilitative services can be prevented if certain professionals function as coordinators to integrate the team. (See Chapter 19 for an example of a nurse functioning in such a role.) Such persons must be able to perceive the medical, social, and behavioral aspects of care and must have the leadership skills necessary for facilitating teamwork.

The nurse clinical specialist with educational preparation and experience in cancer is a possible team coordinator in the hospital. Having a broad base of knowledge in the physical and behavioral sciences, the nurse clinical specialist is able to identify the needs of the cancer patient and family.

The medical social worker can function as co-coordinator, making the scope of assessment more inclusive by involving the family, community, and other support systems. Figure 10-5 demonstrates the roles envisioned for the nurse clinical specialist and the social worker on the health team.

In addition to the coordinators, there should be a formal group designated within the health care setting to respond to the needs of cancer patients and their families. The basic team consists of available disciplines, such as the primary physician, minister, physical therapist, occupational therapist, and nutritionist. The team approach does not, however, negate the importance of consulting team members such as the psychiatrist, dentist, speech therapist, and other resource persons in the community.

The establishment of a cancer rehabilitation team in a small community hospital can be a costly undertaking in terms of the personnel required to implement this concept. A more economical approach is to expand the rehabilitative knowledge and skills of staff nurses who are in direct contact with the patient. Many of the disciplines can be called upon as consultants.

Team Development

The evolution of a health team is a formidable task, particularly when people with diverse backgrounds and personalities come together to use their special skills, knowledge, and occupational languages in a joint undertaking. As a group, they need to formulate a philosophy of cancer rehabilitation, develop objectives, identify the roles and responsibilities of team members, and determine team

Referrals: Initiate contact with physician to obtain patient referral to cancer
rehabilitation program
Explain program and roles of disciplines
Program: Orient patients and families to program
Interpret services offered to patients and families

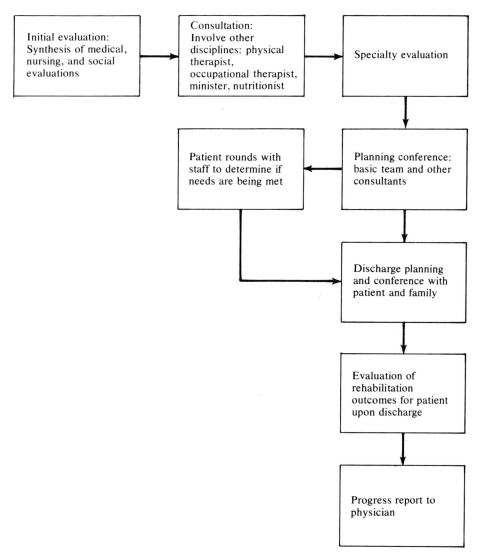

Figure 10-5   Role of coordinators in the health team. *(Acknowledgment is made to St. Francis Hospital Cancer Rehabilitation Services Program in Hololulu, Hawaii, which was funded through the National Cancer Institute Contract No. NO1-CN-45118.)*

procedures. To avoid the pitfalls of a poorly functioning team, health professionals must set aside time for joint planning.

A mutual understanding of the philosophy and objectives of cancer rehabilitation is necessary for efficient functioning of the team. Differing philosophies and orientations of professionals may create frustrations within and between individual team members. Statements of philosophy and objectives may sound academic, but these have profound influence on the professionals' expectations of patients and of each other.

Definition of the roles and responsibilities of team members allows each discipline to realistically look at the distribution of work in relation to the time the person has allowed for cancer rehabilitation. It is suggested that the health team determine and coordinate roles as each setting, each circumstance, personal qualifications, and time permit. For example, responsibility in crisis intervention is shared by the physician, minister, nurse, and social worker, as all may be qualified, but circumstances may dictate intervention by a specific team member.

In the acute hospital, one professional cannot expect to handle the crises of all the cancer patients. Team members should be encouraged to look at their unique as well as their shared functions. Roles will expand and overlap as each discipline is exposed to the expertise of the others.

Team procedures and policies should be developed prior to the implementation of the program. The following questions have to be dealt with by the team to elicit cooperation of its members: How are decisions made? What forms will be used by the group for collection of data? Systematic approaches to team communication facilitate coordination and continuity of rehabilitation and achievement of goals.

The viability of the team depends upon the interpersonal relationships of the health disciplines. Professionals, like their patients, are persons with needs for recognition, achievement, and security. A built-in system of support from one's own colleagues should be developed at the beginning of health team growth, since team members may not be supportive of each other as interdependent roles are established.

Early provision for an educational program in teamwork, cancer, and rehabilitation will maximize the productivity of health team members so that less time and energy will be expended over a period of time. Knowledge in those areas described does not ensure commitment to the team concept in cancer rehabilitation. It is in actual practice that the true test of teamwork is applied.

REHABILITATION IN THE GENERAL HOSPITAL

Every general hospital admitting cancer patients for diagnostic studies and treatment should have a program of early rehabilitation. Cancer rehabilitation must be placed in a proper time perspective if it is to minimize the physical, psychological, and social impact of a cancer diagnosis and treatment for the patient and family. The traditional view of rehabilitation presupposes a sequential time relationship, with rehabilitation occurring at the end of definitive therapy. This is an unfortunate assumption because rehabilitation can begin prior to the confirmation of diagnosis and treatment.

There are forces that influence rehabilitation in the hospital. Cancer care programs, oncology units, and the Professional Standards Review Organization all contribute to the efficacy of rehabilitation.

Cancer Care Programs

A progressive and aggressive program of cancer care consisting of a broad range of services for the patient—prevention, diagnosis, therapy, and follow-up— gives impetus to comprehensive care. Bringing to the patient the best available medical treatment is a fundamental aspect of comprehensive care. Innovative approaches to rehabilitation develop when knowledge of current concepts of cancer can be applied in clinical practice. Investigational data are exhaustive in the field of cancer. As a result, new rehabilitation concepts can be expected to develop when treatment modalities are combined.

Oncology Units

Where there is a distribution of cancer patients in all clinical areas of the general hospital, rehabilitation can be costly in terms of time and personnel. Placement of cancer patients on an oncology unit permits consolidation of the services of the multidisciplinary team. Intraprofessional and interprofessional communication are fostered when rehabilitation staff are accessible to one another. The nursing team and key members of the multidisciplinary staff are able to strengthen their rehabilitation concepts and skills through participation in joint patient rounds, patient planning conferences, and in-service programs.

The Professional Standards Review Organization

Today cancer patients in the hospital find themselves returning home or transferring to another long-term facility as soon as their acute care symptoms subside. This trend toward shorter confinement in an acute care setting is being influenced by the Professional Standards Review Organization (PSRO).

Utilization review programs in the hospital include three major areas: reviews of admission and length of stay, medical care evaluation, and discharge planning. The utilization review guidelines emphasize the viewpoint that the acute medical care needs of the patient are justification for hospitalization. The rehabilitation needs of the patient, particularly the psychosocial needs, are seldom viewed as justification for an extended hospital stay.

Plans for rehabilitation can be projected across time and implemented within the specific time period expected according to length-of-stay data available in every hospital. For example, the length of stay on a patient with an uncomplicated radical mastectomy may require approximately 9 days of hospitalization. Therefore, a short stay is anticipated for a patient having this type of operative procedure, and an early and coordinated plan to involve health disciplines and the Reach to Recovery volunteer is needed. In an effort to initiate teaching of the treatment during this short period of time, health professionals may overlook the feelings the patient has about coping with the diagnosis and altered body image as well as the physical discomforts of surgery.

The rehabilitation staff in each hospital must have an understanding of the role of the PSRO and the constraints that may be placed on meeting the total needs of the patient and family.

The Acute Hospital

In the hospital, routine tasks, diagnostic procedures, and treatment regimens may take precedence over activities directly related to helping the patient become self-sufficient and adapt to the illness. Factors that contribute to prevention of patient problems and initiation of rehabilitation efforts are frequently missed when the major emphasis is placed on meeting the acute needs of the patient. Consider the following example:

> A 56-year-old woman with cancer of the lung was admitted to the hospital. She had just finished taking a shower and decided to rest in bed because of shortness of breath. Upon entering the patient's room the nurse discovered her dyspneic and immediately started oxygen therapy. The patient was then told that someone would assist her with the bath the next morning.

Nursing actions to support this patient's need for independence were overlooked. Connecting a long tube to the oxygen source would have permitted the patient to use oxygen while showering. Energy-saving devices such as a shower bench would also have minimized the need for oxygen.

Health professionals, especially the nurse, tend to appear hurried and preoccupied due to continual distractions and interruptions. Schedules for therapy are made on the basis of the needs and convenience of health professionals rather than the patient's needs. What is important to the patient is overshadowed by the professionals' interest and specialty.

Recently, changes have occurred within general hospitals to promote a more holistic approach to cancer care. These changes include the following:

1 Primary-care concept of health delivery, in which the nurse assumes complete responsibility for the 24-hour per day care of the patient
2 Flexible visiting hours for families and visitors
3 Rooming in of significant others with the patient at night
4 Rearrangement of the work hours of disciplines so that they can meet the needs of the cancer patient and family
5 Sitting and talking as a treatment for cancer patients
6 Specific time set aside for counseling and cancer education
7 Modification of the physical setting to encourage maximum participation in activities of daily living; promotion of socialization; giving patients more control over their environment.

REHABILITATION AT HOME

Rehabilitation and recovery of the cancer patient continue in the home once the acute care and treatment of the disease are completed in the hospital. The rehabilitative focus in the home should be physical and psychological adaptation to cancer and integration of the patient into the community. In cases of chronic or terminal illness, the focus at home is on palliative care.

A smooth transition from hospital to home care and vice versa is ensured through communication between the multidisciplinary teams in both settings. This is accomplished by a written referral that includes notes from participating team members and also through telephone contacts.

Discharge planning, as previously mentioned, must be implemented prior to the patient's discharge to the home. A substandard living arrangement, lack of family support, and inaccessibility to centers of treatment could prove detrimental to effective rehabilitation. Appropriate plans must also be made when the patient is discharged from home care services or readmitted to the hospital. Should the patient require it, referrals for follow-up can be made to the physician's office nurse, state public health nurse, or private and community agencies specializing in long-term counseling therapy.

The Home Setting

Positive factors within the home which contribute toward the rehabilitation of the cancer patient include a familiar environment, cultural influences, situational control, and family support. The multidisciplinary team must evaluate the effectiveness of each area in order to determine the need for supportive services.

Familiar Environment   The feeling of security in one's home environment can greatly improve a patient's ability to cope with stress. Territoriality and idiosyncratic territorial structure can provide useful personality support. Familiar sounds, sights, and smells of home are equated with love and security. The patient who was confused and belligerent in the hospital often becomes stable at home. The colostomy patient can make the necessary adjustments in the physical layout of the bathroom and also can have the privacy required.

Adaptive changes can be made in the home to aid rehabilitation. Toilet guardrails, shower grabbars, and even the simple rearrangement of furniture can assist the patient toward independence.

Cultural Influences   Established modes of living can be resumed and cultural preferences can be observed once the patient is at home. The patient with anorexia in the hospital frequently has a better appetitite at home, where ethnic foods are prepared. The familiar language spoken at home also increases the patient's comfort.

Variations in ethnic values and traditions must be recognized by the multidisciplinary team in determining their approach toward initiating rehabilitative measures in the home. For example, a warm, hospitable Hawaiian family may reject an aggressive, direct approach and explanations that a Caucasion family frequently expects. The belief in medicinal qualities of certain foods and herbs among the Orientals must be respected by the nutritionist giving diet instructions in the home.

The patient is in his or her own element, and the visiting multidisciplinary team member, as the intruder or guest, must make necessary adaptations.

Situational Control   At home the patient does not have to conform to the rules and restrictions of the hospital setting. He or she participates in the plan of care and can even terminate service, although this is not common practice. Flexibility is the rule of thumb, with the patient awakening at the hour desired or irrigating the colostomy at a personally convenient time. The privacy of the home is also conducive for discussions between patient, family, and nurse.

Family Support   The family support system is a major factor in the care of the cancer patient at home. Only in the home setting can the patient maintain physical and emotional closeness to loved ones. However, the decision to care for the patient at home should be influenced by the presence of a viable family support system, willingness of family members, an understanding of what the illness entails, and a schedule that permits flexibility. Without these elements, comprehensive care at home will be difficult to provide.

Effective rehabilitation requires the cooperative efforts of all family members within the home. Primary and secondary care givers need to be identified and supported in their roles. In situations in which only one family member is rendering care, measures for providing relief must be investigated. This relief can be in the form of significant others such as close friends or such individuals as private duty nurses employed through an agency.

Demands and stresses on the family increase if the patient's condition deteriorates, so the multidisciplinary team should periodically assess and reevaluate the family's ability to cope with new problems as necessary.

Restorative Rehabilitation

The following case studies illustrate the rehabilitative focus in which the multidisciplinary team assists the cancer patient at home to resume activities and relationships within the family and the larger community. Limitations caused by the disease or definitive treatments given may necessitate a modified life-style but one that still may be productive and fulfilling.

Mrs. H. is a 43-year-old woman who works as a secretary for an automobile dealership. She developed a wound infection after a right radical mastectomy and also suffered a pathological fracture of her right humerus due to bone metastasis. The affected arm was immobilized in a sling to promote healing.

The patient was followed at home by the nurse, occupational therapist, and psychiatric social worker to meet the following rehabilitation objectives: to assist with wound care, to provide exercises to maintain upper-extremity function, to provide counseling, and to assist with financial support.

In the multidisciplinary conference, the team decided that the patient had the desire and potential to return to work despite a permanent right shoulder subluxation and decreased function. The occupational therapist (OT) therefore concentrated on providing tasks to prepare Mrs. H. to return to work, emphasizing the use of her left hand and arm. These tasks included typing and using a pencil to dial the telephone and flip pages.

Upon the patient's return to work on a part-time basis, the OT visited her office to assist Mrs. H. in adapting the physical environment to meet her needs and offered encouragement during a time of fear and uncertainty. Several visits were made to the patient's office by the OT and Mrs. H. was later able to resume full employment.

Another example of the teamwork involved is shown in the case below:

Mr. P. is a 65-year-old Portuguese male who had a radical prostatectomy done for carcinoma of the prostate. He was followed by the nurse on the team to assist with the care of a decubitus ulcer.

During the home visit the patient eagerly recounted his past sexual experiences and made coarse remarks to the nurse even in the presence of his wife. Recognizing that the psychological impact on a man faced with permanent impotency following a life-saving surgical procedure frequently necessitates professional counseling, the nurse referred the patient and his wife to the psychiatric social worker on the team.

The psychiatric social worker was able to initiate sexual counseling sessions at home with the couple and later to refer them to a sex counseling agency for long-term follow-up.

Palliative Rehabilitation

Death at Home   When the patient's condition is terminal, consideration should be given to the possibility of death occurring at home. Terminal patients not infrequently request to remain at home to die. The continued presence of loved ones within the familiar surroundings of one's own home is a source of comfort no institution can provide.

This desire to die at home can place a heavy burden on the family. The multidisciplinary team needs to assess the family's ability to cope and decide if death at home is realistic. If the dying patient is not reasonably comfortable or the situation is causing undue stress and disruption for the family, it probably will be necessary to hospitalize the patient.

Conflicts arise when the patient elects to remain at home but the family is unwilling to comply mainly out of fear. The home care nurse is faced with feelings of guilt, anxiety, and helplessness generated by both the patient and family members. The nurse may be asked by the family to intervene and encourage the patient to be hospitalized. When this situation occurs, the nurse, often in conjunction with the psychiatric social worker, will ask to have a family conference where concerns and fears can be aired. In many cases, informing family members of the physical signs and symptoms of impending death and reassuring them that the patient in a coma is free of pain are deciding factors in their compliance with the patient's request to die at home. The family is also concerned about the notification procedure to follow when death occurs. Despite attempts to assist family members in managing death at home, they may be unable to cope with the notification procedure. Occasionally, a compromise can be reached in which the patient is hospitalized when he or she goes into a coma.

OBSTACLES TO THE DELIVERY OF COMPREHENSIVE SERVICES

The provision of comprehensive care services from the patient's point of entry into a health care facility until discharge to the home is essential to effective rehabilitation. The philosophy that underlies this concept is widely accepted, but its implementation is often hindered. Role rivalry among disciplines, limitations of third-party payments for services, physician decision-making powers, and patients' misunderstanding or lack of acceptance of rehabilitation are obstacles to the attainment of comprehensive care.

Role Rivalry

The traditional roles of professionals are changing as more specialists are becoming involved in the delivery of comprehensive services. Role overlap is anticipated as professionals expand their functions, but its acceptance is fraught with problems. The need to maintain role identity inhibits the effective utilization of services.

Health professionals protect their roles to justify their existence in health care institutions. A more expedient and economic approach to comprehensive care cannot be accomplished by team members who have difficulty in sharing some aspects of their functions. As each professional renders direct service to the cancer patient, the professional's consultative and evaluative roles expand to a treatment focus, thus necessitating additional therapists. However, staff nurses explain that patients' problems are not always predictable, frequently occurring during evenings, nights, and weekends, when other professionals are not available to render services. Staff nurses are expected to initiate, implement, and follow through on rehabilitative functions of the team members. Role rivalry occurs among staff nurses and other disciplines particularly when roles are overlapping and appropriate disciplines are not credited for their work. As a result there is usually a subtle defensiveness among nurses and other disciplines to the detriment of patient rehabilitation.

The role of the professional is rigidly guarded in an individual who is threatened by another discipline's competence in an area the person feels is his or her "unique function." For example, there are many professionals who are psychosocially oriented and have varying degrees of skills in therapeutic counseling. The social worker, minister, and nurse are some of the disciplines that have overlapping functions in counseling. However, each person in a professional role must recognize his or her limitations and confer with others so patient needs are ultimately met. The inflexibility of any professional prevents that person from working toward the patient's successful rehabilitation.

Third-Party Payments

Present health insurance contracts differ in the type, amount, and extent of benefits to cancer patients. The private insurance system often encourages the use of inpatient services because outpatient services are usually not reimbursed under the standard policies. Medicare and Medicaid offer outpatient alternatives to most types of inpatient services. For example, in some private insurance plans, occupational therapy is nonreimbursable on an outpatient basis. However, Medicare covers the services of the occupational therapist when provided as part of home health services and the Medicaid program covers occupational therapy on an outpatient basis.

Psychosocial rehabilitative counseling is usually covered by insurance if given by a psychologist or psychiatrist. Yet most of the individual counseling for the cancer patient is conducted by either a psychiatric nurse specialist, social worker, or chaplain. These health professionals are seldom paid for their services because their credentials are not recognized by the health insurance contracts.

Physician Decision-Making Powers

In the present system of medical practice, the extent and nature of rehabilitation are controlled by the physician. The physician plays an important role in rehabilitation by selecting health professionals who will be helpful to the cancer patient. Aggressive rehabilitation is often delayed or not implemented because of the lack of a referral.

Physicians may be reluctant to refer patients to a cancer rehabilitation program when they do not understand the roles of health team members. Unless exposed to rehabilitative medicine during medical training and/or practice, they may not value the contributions made by a multidisciplinary approach. They will continue to have this difficulty unless team members, including the physician, establish an effective interdisciplinary communication system.

Another reason why physicians do not refer cancer patients to a cancer rehabilitation program can be stated as follows: "A physician may not know what his patient needs or he doesn't want to know . . . perhaps because of his own fears of cancer and all it implies . . . and his patients are being denied the ultimate in good rehabilitation."[4] Other factors identified by physicians themselves include a concern with the acute medical needs of the patient, the threat of rising malpractice expenses, and attempts to control rising medical costs.

Patients' Misunderstanding of Rehabilitation

The average lay person has minimal knowledge of the health professionals available to help in recovery from cancer. The physician is viewed as the primary person who can solve the patient's problems, while the nurse is seen as the one who assists the physician. Even after the roles of health team members have been explained, the patient may still focus on immediate tangible gains. For example, among Orientals, there is a willingness to pay if something is being physically done for the patient. "Actions speak louder than words," related one patient who was seen by a public health nurse.

> I had to do all the colostomy irrigation by myself. The nurse stood by and observed the procedure with suggestions as to where to place my irrigation bag. She asked if I had any problems with my diet. I don't think I need her help anymore.

In a similar fashion, physical therapy is easier to justify to the cancer patient than is the need for counseling services.

Rehabilitation interventions must also be reviewed carefully with the cancer patient and family so that the relevance of care is understood. For example, if radiotherapy is planned for 4 weeks after surgery, the cancer patient and significant other should know early that arrangements for transportation need to be made, and instructions on skin care and diet should be given prior to treatment. Without such preplanning, rehabilitative interventions may be viewed as irrelevant until a problem or complication occurs.

THE ROLE OF THE NURSE IN CANCER REHABILITATION

With increasing emphasis on the team approach in cancer rehabilitation and the emerging role of other health professionals, nurses must identify their role in relationship to others. Because nurses are "grass roots" professionals in close proximity to the patient, they need to critically examine their rehabilitative functions before relinquishing responsibilities in this area. Problems related to implementation of the rehabilitation program tend to arise regardless of the number of disciplines called upon to help the patient if the nurse lacks the commitment, leadership, knowledge, skills, and assistance from other personnel. Stating that others have the time to do the job is an unsufficient reason for passing nursing functions to others.

In the acute hospitals, nurses tend to call upon specialists when a patient has specific types of problems, often failing to realize that the nurses themselves play a significant role in exploring the reasons for the patient's problems. It becomes imperative, then, that they come to value their assessment of the patient and the person's present or potential care needs.

Professionally oriented practice promotes the concept of rehabilitation. Alfano[5] grouped behaviors that contribute to professionally oriented practice and compared it with behaviors that exemplify task-oriented practice. Some behaviors that relate to the rehabilitative aspects are listed on the next page.

Being present during the critical periods of the patient's hospitalization, the nurse is in the advantageous position of helping the patient and family. It is usually the nurse to whom the physician relates plans. A nurse who is aware of the patient's and family's needs can discuss with the physician the feasibility of specific interventions. In this way, needs are communicated and services initiated early.

Task-Oriented Nursing Practice	Professionally Oriented Nursing Practice
• Other therapists give their care to patients. The nurse acts as a scheduler and has little opportunity to incorporate off-floor activities into patient's activities for daily living or on-floor care.	• Other therapists act primarily as resources. They participate in direct care alongside the nurse in their distinctive area of practice. The nurse incorporates the therapist's suggestions in the care plan.
• The nurse acts as the surrogate of the M.D. and other disciplines.	• The nurse works collaboratively with the M.D. and other disciplines. The nurse acts as the surrogate of the patient.
• Major priorities of care include medications, treatment, and assistance to physicians.	• Major priorities of care focus upon the patient's feelings, concerns, and goals and on assisting the patient and family through medical therapy.
• The nurse interprets the M.D. and the M.D.'s orders to the patient.	• The nurse interprets the patient and the patient's concerns to the M.D. and helps the patient directly approach M.D. in discussing the plan of care.
• The quality of teaching is mostly explanation, orientation, fact giving.	• The quality of teaching emphasizes listening and reflecting what the the patient does and says.

Other functional areas of the nurse's practice include teaching, counseling, and discharge planning.

The Nurse as a Teacher

Rehabilitation of patients with any chronic illness begins with their understanding of the condition and its treatment. However, the cancer patient is usually not afforded the same educational opportunity as patients with other chronic illnesses. This often happens because of the "hang-ups" of health professionals toward the diagnosis of cancer. Fundamental to the successful rehabilitation of the cancer patient is participation in a program of education. A teaching program needs to meet the informational needs of the cancer patient and family. Such a program provides basic information about cancer and its treatment in an understandable and nonthreatening way. It dispels fears based on unfounded beliefs and myths while encouraging a realistic approach to the patient's illness.

As the largest group of professionals on the health team, nurses have an important role in helping patients understand their illness. In order for patients to achieve this goal, nurses must first relate to the patients' feelings about their diagnosis before any teaching is initiated. The disclosure of a cancer diagnosis has an emotional impact on patients which directly influences their readiness to learn. Response to the following patient questions must be considered on two levels: the feeling level and the informational level: "Will I give my cancer to my family? I didn't expect cancer to strike my family twice. My brother died of cancer in his liver and, now me. Is cancer hereditary?"

By first acknowledging the patient's fear of transmitting cancer and then giving information about the subject, the nurse can minimize the patient's anxieties and help him or her learn about the condition. The nurse with an understanding of the facts about cancer and a sensitivity to the emotional needs of patients is able to offer patients relevant information at the appropriate time.

Instructions about treatment side effects must be a shared function of the physician and the nurse. Chemotherapy and radiotherapy nurses who work collaboratively with physicians should reflect confidence and competence when teaching about the undesirable effects of therapy. However, a staff nurse usually reinforces and interprets to the patient what the physician has taught the patient. Some physicians may object to the nurse's instructions on chemotherapy and radiotherapy because of the patient's vulnerability to suggestions of potential side effects. Therefore, it is imperative that the nurse develop a cooperative plan with physicians which delegates specific areas of instructions to the nurse.

Another area of teaching that the nurse emphasizes is the patient's participation in care. The nurse monitors self-care activities while working with patients and ancillary staff. The nurse is more involved than ancillary staff in teaching patients and families procedures of self-care. For example, an initial colostomy irrigation should be taught by the nurse so astute observations of the patient's emotional response, physical strengths, and limitations can be evaluated and followed up. The nurse can call upon the enterostomal therapist to assist if specific areas of management require this person's expertise. The nurse can ascertain at what point the family should be brought in. By utilizing teaching skills, the nurse can prevent fostering of dependent behaviors that are difficult to reverse when the patient is discharged from the hospital.

Coordination of Teaching   Integration of instructions from the different therapies (occupational therapy, physical therapy, respiratory therapy, nutritional therapy, etc.) into the patient's activities and plan of care is an aspect of the nurse's teaching function. The nurse collaborates with other disciplines in formulating a comprehensive teaching plan. This plan is shared with the ancillary staff so similar learned behaviors and goals are stressed in their care of patients. Problems contributing to discrepancy of behaviors in therapy and on the clinical unit need to be identified and resolved. These problems usually occur because of the following reasons:

1 Lack of staff's awareness of the goals of different disciplines
2 Lack of communication between the nurse and other disciplines
3 Inconsistent information given to the patient by the nurse and other disciplines

4 Deficiency of the ancillary staff in implementing rehabilitative interventions

Instructions to patients may also be contradicted in actual practice, as reflected in the following example:

> A mastectomy patient is given initial instructions on hand and arm care. She is told to avoid having venipuncture in her arm on the same side as the mastectomy. A sign is posted at the head of the patient's bed. Since the intravenous infusion is being administered in the unaffected arm, the laboratory technician withdraws blood from the affected arm. The patient tells the technician that she has been advised not to have blood drawn from her affected arm. In reply, the technician explains that blood test results will be inaccurate if blood is taken from the side with the intravenous therapy.

Communication with other departments is essential for mutual resolution of problems in teaching.

Teaching is a distinct component of rehabilitation nursing. As an initiator, coordinator, implementor, and evaluator of teaching, the nurse has a key leadership function in patient and family education.

The Nurse in Counseling

The psychosocial impact of cancer on the patient and family necessitates the existence of nurse counselors. As a primary deliverer of care, the nurse should initiate short-term patient and family counseling. When the nature of the problems becomes too complex and intense, other disciplines may be called upon to assist the nurse. The nurse must, therefore, be aware of personal limitations in therapeutic counseling. (Refer to Chapter 12, "The Nurse as Counselor," for an in-depth discussion of the role.)

It has been difficult for nurses to assume the counselor role due to the traditional emphasis on performance skills in nursing curriculums. With the present shift toward psychosocial skills in the educational arena, with particular reference to interviewing and crisis intervention, however, nurses are now more prepared to assist the patient and family in achieving the goals of psychosocial rehabilitation.

Within the hospital, the nurse must develop unique methods of providing an atmosphere for counseling. An uninterrupted private time for counseling must be scheduled just as are other treatments in the hospital. Consistency of staff assignments facilitates and maintains a relationship between the nurse and the patient, thus enabling opportunities for effective, continual counseling.

Often the home is more conducive to counseling than is the hospital. When away from the busy atmosphere of the hospital, with minimal staff to relate with and privacy restored, the patient and family are relaxed and inclined to speak openly.

Counseling is an important rehabilitative armamentarium of the nurse, but is seldom a rewarded function in the hospital. It should be afforded the same recognition as other task-oriented treatments in cancer care. The role of the nurse in counseling must be viewed as normal. Conveying to the patient the nurse's availability and willingness to engage in a helping relationship through counseling is a major contribution of the nurse in cancer rehabilitation.

The Nurse in Discharge Planning

Through assessment of the comprehensive needs of the cancer patient, the nurse can anticipate problem areas that will influence discharge planning. The nurse consults with other health team members for an accurate and complete assessment of the patient's functional abilities, adaptive capacities, financial resources, nutritional requirements, living and transportation accomodations, and family support systems.

The discharge flow chart in Figure 10-6 shows the basic situational questions that the nurse can use as a guide in identifying potential problems as well as identifying disciplines that can assist in resolving those problems. In addition, the flow chart provides guidance as to where the patient can be cared for upon discharge—home, skilled nursing facility, intermediate-care facility (ICF), or care home.

The nurse's primary role in discharge planning is to ensure continuity of rehabilitative services for the cancer patient and family after discharge from the hospital. The nurse initiates discharge plans and teaches self-care with the patient and family as early as possible. Through early discharge planning, the nurse can assist the patient to gain independence and a sense of responsibility for care in a gradual and progressive way.

For those patients with multiple, complex problems requiring inputs from various disciplines, the nurse must attempt to arrange a discharge planning conference involving the physician and the whole family. In the acute hospital, the nurse may not be able to get all family members to attend the discharge planning conference. However, the person primarily responsible for the care of the patient must be identified and encouraged to participate in this conference.

The nurse, with the help of other health professionals, can prepare the patient to make a smooth transition from hospital to home or long-term facility (see Figure 10-7).

SUMMARY

As increasing numbers of patients survive cancer, equal importance must be given to the quality and the quantity of their life. Living with cancer is the primary thrust of rehabilitation, regardless of the increasing limitations imposed upon the patient by the illness and treatment. Rehabilitation concepts emphasize the preservation of human values through exploration of the cancer patient's attitudes, feelings, fears, and hopes and through reorganization of the person's potential for growth and adaptation.

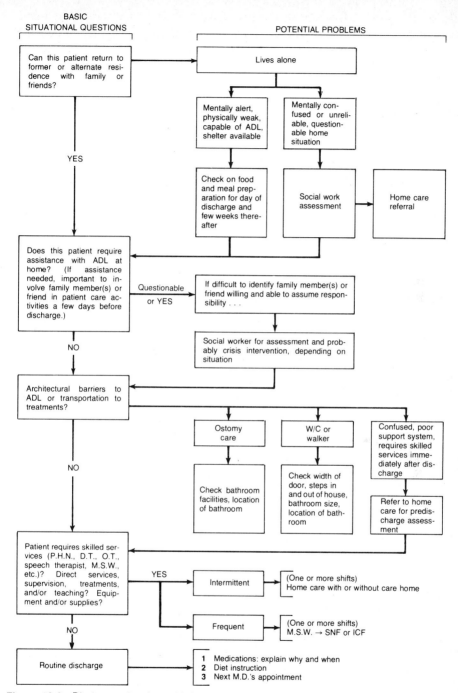

Figure 10-6 Discharge planning guidelines. (*Acknowledgment is made to St. Francis Hospital Cancer Rehabilitation Services Program in Honolulu, Hawaii, which was funded through the National Cancer Institute Contract No. NO1-CN-45118.*)

Nurse in hospital: counseling patient.

Home care nurse; teaching the patient.

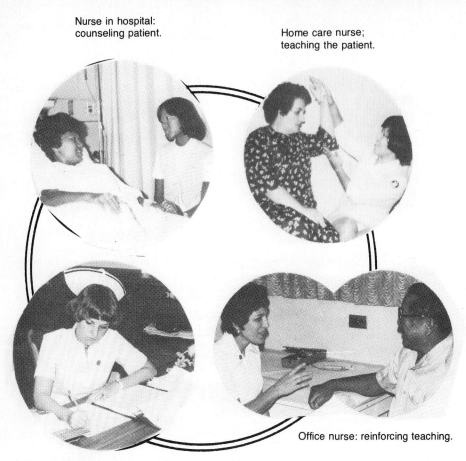

Office nurse: reinforcing teaching.

Nurse in skilled nursing facility: writing a discharge summary.

Figure 10-7 Continuity of rehabilitation functions.

Rehabilitation also means ensuring comprehensive, continuous care for the cancer patient. The patient's problems and needs are of paramount importance. As an active participant and consumer of professional services, the patient's decisions in rehabilitation must be of immediate concern to the health team.

The complexity and diversity of the cancer patient's needs require a coordinated multidisciplinary team approach. There must be a commitment by the health team, along with family and significant others, to helping, guiding, and supporting the patient during the various stages of the illness. This team approach can enhance innovative thinking and action in rehabilitation.

The delivery of rehabilitative services may be difficult because of role rivalry among disciplines, limitations of third-party payments for services, decision-making powers of the physician, and patient misunderstanding or lack of acceptance of rehabilitation. Environmental forces within the hospital may also impede the process of rehabilitation.

The nurse, who represents the largest group of professionals on the health team, has a significant contribution to make to the rehabilitative process, by virtue of the roles of teacher, counselor, and discharge planner. The nurse must reexamine and define the roles in relationship to others on the health care team. Today, with the advent of the team approach to health care, the nurse will find other disciplines as supportive allies in cancer rehabilitation.

REFERENCES

1 "Higher Cancer 'Cure' Rates Create Human Problem—Rehabilitation," *Journal of the American Medical Association,* 1972, **222**(4), 418–419.
2 R. Hardy and J. Cull: *Counseling and Rehabilitating the Cancer Patient.* Springfield, Ill.: Charles C. Thomas, 1975, pp. 26–27.
3 R. P. Stryker: *Rehabilitative Aspects of Acute and Chronic Nursing Care.* Philadelphia: W. B. Saunders, 1972, p. 9.
4 "Helping Your Patient Stage a Comeback from Cancer," *Medical Opinion,* 1975, **4**(8), 17.
5 G. Alfano: "Healing or Caretaking—Which Will It Be?" *Nursing Clinics of North America,* 1971, **6**(2), 275–276, 279.

BIBLIOGRAPHY

Alfano, G.: "Healing or Caretaking—Which Will It Be?" *Nursing Clinics of North America,* 1971, **6**(2), 273–280.
Barckley, V.: "Caring for the Cancer Patient at Home," *Journal of Practical Nursing,* 1974, **24**(10), 24–27.
"Cancer Patients' Organization Helps Them Deal with Problems of Living," *Journal of the American Medical Association,* 1976, **235**(19), 2065–2067ff.
Coelho, G. V., et al.: *Coping and Adaptation.* New York: Basic Books, 1974.
Cox, B.: "The Fine Art of Educating the Patient," *Medical Opinion,* 1975, **4**(8), 31–35.
Gentry, J. T.: "A More Rational Approach to Health Care Delivery," *Hospital Progress,* 1973, **54**(8), 94–103.
Hardy, R., and Cull, J.: *Counseling and Rehabilitating the Cancer Patient.* Springfield, Ill.: Charles C. Thomas, 1975.
"Helping Your Patient Stage a Comeback from Cancer," *Medical Opinion,* 1975, **4**(8), 12–21.
"Higher Cancer 'Cure' Rates Create Human Problem—Rehabilitation," *Journal of the American Medical Association,* 1972, **222**(4), 418–419.
Izsak, F. C., et al.: "Comprehensive Rehabilitation of the Patient with Cancer: Five-Year Experience of a Home-Care Unit," *Journal of Chronic Disease,* 1973, **26**, 363–374.
Kane, R.: *Interprofessional Teamwork,* Manpower Monograph Eight. Syracuse, N.Y.: Syracuse University School of Social Work, 1975.
Krusen, F., et al. (eds.): *Handbook of Physical Medicine and Rehabilitation,* 2d ed. Philadelphia: W. B. Saunders, 1971.

Madelon, G., et al.: "The Comprehensive Health Team: A Conceptual Model," *Journal of Nursing Administration,* 1971, **1**(2), 9–13.

Newhard, H.: "The Nation's Health: Some Issues," *Annals of the American Academy of Political and Social Science,* 1972, **1**.

1976 Cancer Facts and Figures. New York: American Cancer Society, 1975.

Peitchines, J.: "Therapeutic Effectiveness of Counseling by Nursing Personnel," *Nursing Research,* 1972, **21**(2), 138–147.

Rinear, E. E.: "Helping the Survivors of Expected Death," *Nursing '75,* 1975, **5**(3), 60–65.

Schoffer, P.: "The Utilization Review Coordinator," *Nursing '76,* 1976, **6**(2), 95–97.

Sheldon, A., et al.: "An Integrated Family Oriented Cancer Care Program: The Report of a Pilot Project in the Socio-emotional Management of Chronic Illness," 1970, **22**, 743–755.

Stryker, R. P.: *Rehabilitative Aspects of Acute and Chronic Nursing Care.* Philadelphia: W. B. Saunders, 1972.

Part Three

Psychosocial Implications of Oncology Nursing

Chapter II

The Psychological Aspects of Cancer

Graceann Ehlke

The psychological effects of cancer are totally encompassing. Dealt with in this paper will be the psychological effects of cancer on the patient, the family, and society as a whole. Specifically, the chapter will focus on the feelings that the patient, the family, and society have about cancer.

The patient with cancer may experience a wide gamut of feelings from the very negative to the very positive. Because any illness tends to constitute a crisis for the individual, how the person feels about having cancer may be influenced by the person's response to crisis. It may also be influenced by the response of those around the person to crisis.

Perhaps the most frequent feeling a patient with cancer has, at some point, is that of fear. Three fears that will be discussed here are fear of death, fear of the unknown, and fear of altered body image.

FEAR OF DEATH

Fear of death is very real in Western society. It arises for a multitude of reasons. The first reason is Western society's *life* orientation. Life or living, in Western society, takes place while people are in young or middle adulthood. One example of this attitude is the heavy emphasis placed on sports in Western society. The individuals who are the stars in sports are in either young or middle adulthood.

A second reason why fear of death arises is that the health profession, until very recently, focused on curing the individual. Inability to cure an individual was equated with failure for the profession. Generally speaking, health professionals have not dealt with personal feelings of hopelessness and failure.

A third reason why fear of death is strong in Western society is that in recent years death has usually taken place in the sterile environment of the hospital. It has been taken out of the family and society settings. Death is not a normally seen experience for the average person in Western society. In societies in which death routinely occurs in the home, the dying process is generally less frightening.

FEAR OF THE UNKNOWN

The second fear that is commonly experienced by oncology patients is fear of the unknown. To face the unknown is to have no direction. Most people formulate life goals, but when they are told that they have cancer, many times those goals are abruptly ended or changed. They are suddenly faced with the fact that they do not know what is going to happen to them or if they can handle whatever occurs. This reaction is partly due to the fact that individuals have rarely faced the imminence of their death. Death is a taboo topic.[1] Consider the number of individuals who put off having a will made until they are middle-aged or even older. Why this hesitation? Part of the answer lies in the fact that having a will drawn is an admission that one will die someday. Discussions of death are many times limited to issues such as "the social consequences of capital punishment or euthanasia."[2] Because the dying process is not generally discussed and because dying persons are removed from society, the dying process is an area most people know little about. Cancer often is equated with death; thus fear of the unknown is often encountered in oncology patients.

FEAR OF ALTERED BODY IMAGE

Fear of altered body image is also expressed by cancer patients. Alteration of one's image results in a feeling of loss. This feeling of loss may be totally unexpected by the health professionals caring for the cancer patient. For example, numerous individuals have had colostomies only to grieve for the removed colon. They were able to adjust to the actual colostomy, which health professionals often consider to be the greatest hurdle, but were unable to resolve the loss of the missing colon until a much later date. An individual who had large breasts had often received many compliments about her cleavage. Her greatest difficulty was in understanding that with the sternal split surgery she was to undergo, the cleavage would never be the same. This loss seemed to be a larger problem for this individual than the threat of possible death.

These, then, are the most common fears experienced by cancer patients: fear of death, fear of the unknown, and fear of altered body image. Each of these fears will be dealt with further when we look at ways to assist the patient who encounters these fears.

DEPRESSION

Depression is another feeling that cancer patients frequently have for a variety of reasons. The overall reason for depression is a feeling of loss. As discussed in relation to altered body image, this feeling may be due to the loss of a body part or a change in how one feels about one's body. The loss may be more concrete. It may be the loss of a job or home. The loss may be that of a role that may or may not be related to the individual's occupation.

LONELINESS

Loneliness is also a common feeling for the cancer patient. All people experience loneliness at least once and probably several times in their lives. Loneliness may have both positive and negative components. Any experience that is unique will cause loneliness in an individual. One example of such an experience is that of falling in love: No one can really share what the individual who has fallen in love is experiencing. Individuals not in the love experience cannot grasp the feeling that the two individuals involved evoke for each other. Thus the individual involved is really alone or isolated with his or her feelings. Loneliness is a widespread feeling today in our society. Many authors believe that this situation is due to the fact that we have lost much of the community life in which people used to be involved.[3]

Loneliness may initially bring on feelings of desolation, despair, and terror for the cancer patient. However, many individuals have described being able to go beyond these initial feelings and have been able to gain deeper insight into themselves. The experience of loneliness has left these individuals with a greater "now" orientation in which they are able to focus with greater intensity on the present. This experience may prove to be highly satisfying.

DEPENDENCY

Cancer patients also may experience feelings of dependency. Many times these feelings are thrust on them by societial expectations. To begin with, the individual may not feel particularly sick upon entering the hospital. Perhaps the individual initially comes in for diagnostic tests. However, shortly after admission to the hospital, the person is made to feel that she or he is ill. One cancer patient attributes the development of dependency to rapid loss of identity after entering the hospital setting. Loss of identity occurs through a series of steps.

First, the patient is given a wristband that identifies name, doctor, insurance company, and number within the company. Second, the individual is taken to a room after answering the necessary questions in the admission office and is put into a patient gown. She or he looks like everyone else. Slowly but surely, the rights of the individual—those things that make the person unique—are taken away. The individual must conform to hospital regime. To do this, the individual must depend on the hospital for certain basic needs. The individual can no longer go to the refrigerator for a bite to eat and must ask the hospital staff to order the food. Dependency feelings may be either negative or positive and will be discussed in more detail later.

RESPONSIBILITY

Along with dependency feelings experienced by patients, there may be those feelings having to do with responsibility. Ted Rosenthal has very accurately recorded experience with these feelings.[4] Prior to being ill, the individual has many roles to play in society. These might include that of father, president of a corporation, husband, son, treasurer in a social organization, and peer in a professional organization. Suddenly the individual is placed in a hospital and diagnosed as sick. In the sick role all responsibilities and obligations are taken away. The person no longer lives from meeting to meeting or on a tight work schedule. All duties are taken away, and the individual is suddenly allowed to experience whatever she or he wishes to experience. A negative response consists of fear at the loss of the normal routine. A positive response will allow the person to feel very free. It can be like starting all over. The person can be whomever or whatever she or he wants to be.

SATISFACTION IN LIFE

Another positive feeling experienced by cancer patients is one of satisfaction in living. Because these people often become very now-oriented, they develop acute awareness of their surroundings. This awareness becomes very exciting and new to them. Many cancer patients have said that they feel they are the lucky ones because, once told they had cancer, they really began to live. Life can become very satisfying to the cancer patient.

These are the feelings most often experienced by cancer patients at one time or another during the course of the illness. Many of the feelings discussed here are intertwined and related to other feelings as well. It is important for the nurse to identify the feelings expressed both verbally and nonverbally. However, it is vitally important that the nurse go one step further and be able to assist the patient in dealing with both positive and negative feelings. The remainder of this section will deal with the nursing care related to the psychological reactions of the cancer patient.

NURSING INTERVENTIONS

Fear of Death

Fear of death is represented by patients who say, "You can't let me die." or "I don't think I am going to wake up from the anesthesia." or "I think it is bad this time." How should the nurse respond to these patients? How can the nurse help? With the first patient the nurse should promise to help the patient as much as possible (that is, if the nurse really means it). A nurse should never promise a patient something that is not meant or something that is impossible. After acknowledging the patient's plea for help, the nurse should ask why the patient thinks she or he is going to die. Often the patient's problem or frustration is not the total experience of dying but some smaller aspect of the process, such as pain or nausea. If the patient responds that death is anticipated because of pain, then at that point the nurse needs to talk with the patient about the pain. What does pain mean to the individual patient? The nurse needs to find out about the pain medication the patient is receiving. Is it effective? For how long does it help? At this point the nurse should have some information with which to proceed with support that will be meaningful for this particular patient at this point in time.

With the second patient the nurse needs to find out why the patient does not think she or he will wake up from the anesthesia. Is it something that was said to the patient by another person? Was it something that the patient overheard the staff say? Or was it a nonverbal message that the patient received from someone? With the background information received from the patient, the nurse should be able to proceed with effective intervention, e.g., providing information on the action of the anesthesia or the operative sequence that will be followed.

In the case of the patient who says, "I think it is bad this time." the nurse might consider the example of the patient readmitted to the hospital. While previously there had been no indications of metastasis, the patient now is emaciated and has lost 20 lb since last seen. The nurse might start the conversation with this patient by asking why she or he thinks it is bad this time. The patient might answer, "Well, look at me. You can see that I have lost all of this weight." The nurse might then reply: "I have noticed the weight loss. Why do you think you have lost the weight?" It is important to find out what the patient thinks is happening. Perhaps the patient thinks that the weight has been lost due to nausea from chemotherapy rather than realizing that the cancer has metastasized. Whatever the patient's response, the nurse should focus on the specific statements made by the person. If nausea is the patient's focus, then work should be done with the patient to try to alleviate this frustration. If the patient says that the cancer has spread, then the nurse needs to work with this, perhaps by asking if this idea is frightening. If the answer is yes, the nurse might then ask what is most frightening at this time. Whatever the patient's response, the nurse needs to make every attempt to act on the problem. Otherwise the patient feels frustrated.

Fear of the Unknown

Fear of the unknown is very difficult to deal with for both the patient and the nurse. The frustrations associated with not knowing what is happening can place the patient in a constant crisis situation. The nurse can best help by providing some structure to the situation. The patient needs help in thinking through what she or he should do. This fear can occur in the patient who is undergoing diagnostic tests or in the patient who is undergoing treatment and is very unsure of the potential results. For those who fear the unknown, intervention must focus on the here and now. Not tomorrow or next week or next month, but right now—today.

Fear of Pain

Many people fear pain. When a patient tells of this fear, the first thing the nurse might do is ask the patient to describe what the pain will be like. Next the nurse might ask about the patient's past experience with pain. The nurse should also find out what was done or not done when the patient was in pain. Other things that need to be considered include the patient's sex, ethnic background, and what the person is afraid will happen because of pain. Many things pain will cause in terms of behavior are of concern to the patient. Some of these are loss of control and loss of sleep. Further in-depth information on the nursing care of a patient who fears pain is discussed in Chapter 9.

Fear of Changes in Body Image

Fear of body image alteration is a topic that encompasses the entire person. In dealing with people who may have this fear, it is extremely important to assess how they feel about the part of the body that is being altered. For example, for a person who feels that her hair is one of her greatest attributes, the loss of the hair may be devastating; but the individual whose hair has not been one of her greatest attributes may not feel alopecia to be as great a problem.

There are three groups of people who seem to need more help with the fear of body image alteration than others do. These groups are children, adolescents, and women.

Children   Children need stability. They cannot deal with abstracts. If their fear becomes a reality, nursing support needs to be very concrete. They need to know how long the medications will continue to cause the effects they are experiencing. One very good way of dealing with this problem is to have children mark off the days as they go by. For example, if a child is to be on a medication for 3 weeks, the child can be shown the days on a calendar and can then mark them off day by day.

Adolescents   Teen-agers are already at a point in life where they are having to make adjustments to a changing body. Having to adjust to the additional changes produced by the treatment for cancer may be almost impossible in teen-agers' eyes. They will need a great deal of support. Many times teen-agers will need to feel that they have some independence. If, for example, a teen-ager has gained weight because of steroid therapy, the teen-ager may wish to be on a diet. The nurse can help the patient accomplish this although dieting will not alter the moon-shaped contour of the patient's face. The nurse can make sure that the patient is adequately nourished, encourage the patient to drink diet beverages rather than Coke, and eliminate potato chips or other fatty snacks. Many times actions such as these will help patients to feel better about what is happening to them, for the actions help give patients some control over their lives.

All teen-agers have a need for identity and acceptance. Teen-agers with cancer may tend to shy away from friends by not keeping in contact with them by telephone or by refusing to allow their friends to visit them in the hospital. Teen-agers need peer support and acceptance to maintain their self-image. Thus, the nurse needs to watch for indications that a teen-ager is decreasing the peer support system and attempt to prevent this from happening. It is important to allow patients to make some decisions about what happens to them. Active participation in decision making allows teen-agers to feel good about themselves, which builds ego strength. As a result the patients may feel less apprehensive about their acceptance by others.

Women   Women in general have more difficulty with the fear or threat of a changed body image than men seem to have. This situation may be due to a societal emphasis on feminine beauty. An alteration of the body, such as a hysterectomy, may be a threat to a women's fundamental concept of femininity.

Depression

In dealing with a patient who is depressed as a result of a loss, it is important for the nurse to keep in mind that the person will probably display grieving behavior. Granger Westberg discusses 10 stages in the grief process.[5] The nurse should realize that time limits may be placed on some of the stages of grief. This does not mean that exceeding these limits of time is pathologic. It merely indicates that a patient who exceeds the suggested time limits may need some other type of help and/or support. The 10 stages that Westberg has identified are as follows:

   1   State of shock
   2   Expression of emotion
   3   Depression and loneliness
   4   Physical symptoms of distress
   5   Panic
   6   Sense of guilt
   7   Hostility and resentment
   8   Inability to return to usual activities
   9   Hope
  10   Affirmation of reality[6]

Loneliness

Loneliness has both positive and negative aspects. For the person who is unhappy about loneliness, the nurse needs to communicate interest in that person. The person needs to know that she or he is a worthwhile human being. The nurse needs to communicate with the patient so that the person feels comfortable in expressing feelings. Doing this will help the patient not to feel completely isolated in this experience. Remember, the nurse cannot go through the experience with the patient but can be the patient's ally.

Dependency

Dependency feelings can also have both positive and negative connotations. For those individuals who need additional attention, dependency can initiate receipt of the needed attention. With dependency, the nurse needs to first assess his or her own values with regard to dependency. What does this word mean to the nurse? Does the word "dependency" create positive or negative feelings? The nurse needs to realize that negative attitudes toward dependency may be communicated to the patient, thereby making the situation more difficult or frustrating for the patient.

The nurse also needs to assess how the patient feels about being dependent. If the patient does not like feeling dependent, the nurse can assist the person to feel more like an individual. The patient can gain some feeling of identity by wearing her or his own night clothes. If possible, the patient should be allowed to bring some personal effects into the hospital. A nursing history helps to identify the patient's usual patterns of activity as well as likes and dislikes. This information can then be utilized as much as possible within hospital constraints.

The patient will have a feeling of more control and more independence if consulted about care and allowed to make decisions about it. For example, the nurse might say, "Would you like me to help you with your colostomy irrigation now, or would it be better if I came back in half an hour?"

Positive Responses

As far as the positive experiences that the patient may have, the nurse needs to be happy for the patient. The nurse should not permit personal attitudes to deny the patient the joy of feeling free and should not disbelieve that this is the way the patient feels. The nurse needs to support the patient in these feelings while allowing room for them to change.

NURSING CARE OF THE FAMILY

Many of the psychological effects the cancer patient experiences also occur within the family. Before these effects are discussed, "family" must be defined. For the purpose of simplicity, the family discussed herein will refer to the mother, the father, and their children. Other members of the family will be referred to as the "extended family."

One of the most important things to consider when looking at the family are the roles that each member plays. What kinds of rewards do family members get from each other? Who provides the financial support for the family? Who provides the emotional support? Usually the financial support is provided primarily by the father figure. However, in recent years a great number of women have joined the workforce and have been contributing to the financial support of the family. Frequently the mother is the individual who provides a major portion of the emotional support for the family as well as the social education of the children. If the father or mother becomes ill, there are some major gaps in roles that must be filled. Thus, depending on what roles are to be filled, the ability of the family or others to fill the roles may be one indication of how well the family is able to deal with the crisis.

If family members feel too burdened with the additional roles they are having to fill or in finding replacements for the absent family member, they may react with anger. The nurse should not react negatively to the anger, but must remember that it is important for the family to be able to express feelings. The nurse should support the family members by acknowledging the feelings, giving sanction to express them, and conveying understanding of why they might be angry. If the family members are not allowed to express their anger, they may internalize the feelings and experience guilt or self-condemnation.

Another important factor to assess with the family of the patient is the gratifications that various family members normally received from the ill person. For example, there are numerous family members who receive various and sundry gratifications from a child. Perhaps the child is being given all those things that the parent would have liked when he or she was a child. The child may be the one who verbally communicates love for the family members. He or she may be an important member of the workforce, assisting with the financial support or housework. Perhaps the child assists with the education of other siblings.

Suddenly the child is ill. He or she can no longer provide the gratifications to family members that were previously provided. This loss must be dealt with in the family unit.

Family members may display any or all of the defense mechanisms normally seen with any individual in stress. These include isolation of affect, sublimation, repression, displacement, projection, or introjection. The nurse should assist the family members in the same way she or he would assist the patient who is under stress.

There have been a number of studies done which deal with the effects of serious illness on various family members. If the illness results in death, the children may respond to the illness and death in a number of ways, depending on the age of the child.

If the child is below the age of 5, death is often not equated with finality but with sleep, and as a result, the child may have an easier time dealing with this portion of the crisis than do children older than 5.

If the child is between the ages of 5 and 9, death is often personified as an evil being. In working with families who have children in this age range, the nurse needs to explain to the rest of the family what the child might experience. This is the age of ghosts and demons. It would be this child who might have nightmares. It might be wise to suggest to the families that they keep a night-light on in the room of children of this age range.

After the age of 9, the child is able to understand that death is permanent. The child of 9 and above, then, should be dealt with as would an adult in terms of the loss that this death may create.

Another important concept to consider when looking at the effect of cancer on the family is the communication pattern within the family unit. For example, the author once cared for a patient who did all of the verbal communication within the family. None of the children communicated with the father. If something was needed that the father controlled, the children would communicate through the mother. Then the mother became ill. Communication within this family unit was severely impaired. New communication patterns needed to be established. The nurse should be aware of what the communication channels are within the family so as to be of assistance in the development of alternate communication patterns while the family member is ill.

Communication between the patient and family may be severely hindered. Patients communicate different things during different phases of their illness. In her article, "The Patient with Cancer—His Changing Pattern of Communication,"[7] Ruth Abrams states that the type of communication a patient exhibits with people can be divided into three stages. These are (1) the initial stage, (2) the advancing stage, and (3) the terminal stage. It is the advancing stage of the disease that presents the greatest communication problems for all people, including the family. At this point the patient knows that treatment thus far has been unsuccessful and that further treatment will have to be tried in the hope of cure or remission. When the family possesses this information, a very stressful period is created during which direct communication frequently does not take place. The nurse needs to be aware of and sensitive to the excessive stress that the patient and family might be experiencing at this time.

EMOTIONAL REACTIONS OF THE FAMILY
Grief

Considering the emotions that affect the family of a cancer patient, one of the most frequently displayed emotions is that of grief. This grief may be due to real losses, such as the grief that a husband may experience when his wife has a mastectomy or hysterectomy. Family members may also experience a type of anticipatory grief. The family members may grieve over the future death of the patient while the person is still alive. Nurses need to be aware of this possibility so they do not think of, or treat, unkindly the family member who seems to have resolved the loss and no longer exhibits an active interest in the patient's welfare.

Protection

Another common feeling seen with the families of cancer patients is that of the need to protect the patient or others from what is happening to the patient. The most common manifestation of this is seen in the family that does not want the patient told of his or her diagnosis. This may or may not be the correct avenue to take with the individual. The author supports the position that better communication lines, as well as better support, are provided to both the patient and the family if all individuals concerned know all of the facts.

Another common manifestation of the protection need is seen when healthy young siblings are involved. The mother and father may feel that it would be best to protect the other children from knowing what is happening with the sick child. This protection can cause difficulties for the other children, for they are excluded from what is causing the disturbance in the family and so may feel personal guilt. As a result, they may feel they are being punished for something they have done. It may take years to repair the damage that can occur to the siblings of the sick child.

Families in Western society have become isolated units that function independently. The immediate and the extended family are no longer under the same roof. Because of this situation, the isolated family unit must assume total responsibility for family functioning. In times of crisis, other people are needed to assist in the normal responsibilities of the family, but they are not always available. Thus "because of the very nature of the modern family, the resources it possesses to cope with the impact of illness are relatively weak."[8]

The family members may also experience all the same feelings experienced by the patient. Both the patient and the family may greatly fear abandonment. The fear of abandonment will be lessened if two conditions are met for the family and patient. First, the patient and family must be offered some hope. Second, the patient and family want the individual delivering the news (i.e., the physician and/or nurse) to "stick it out with them."

If the patient is seriously ill for a long time, the family life changes. Other family members assume the roles that were previously assumed by the patient. The patient in many cases is no longer a member of the family, which fosters and reinforces feelings of abandonment in the patient. Nursing staff needs to recognize that this change may be happening within a family unit. Counseling of family members needs to be done to encourage the family to continue having the patient participate in decision making within the family unit.

Care of the cancer patient in the past has been just that—care of the cancer patient. The family has not been included in the nurse's plan of care. All too often the patient may become increasingly sick and die, and the nurse's primary contact with the family has been to present the family with the patient's belongings.

The author's personal experience, along with support from the literature, strongly indicates that this limited approach is inadequate. A higher annual death rate has been found among widows and widowers than that occurring among married people of the same age.[9] The increased mortality rate was not limited to spouses, but included other relatives as well. In another study, bereaved relatives were compared with a control group that included people who had not had a recent family death over a 6-year period of time. Over that time period it was found that bereaved relatives had a higher mortality rate than did people who had not had a recent family death.[10]

Why is this higher death rate seen in bereaved relatives in comparison with individuals who have not encountered death of a close family member? What, if anything, can nursing do to assist in the decrease of the mortality of bereaved relatives?

Perhaps one reason for the increase in mortality of the bereaved is that the individuals have for one reason or another not completed their grief process. For example, men are not encouraged to express emotion—particularly that associated with crying. If they have not had this emotional release, they may experience further depression. It has been shown that widowers in their twenties and early thirties exhibit a higher incidence of suicide than do other age groups of widowers. This is a time when the concept of manhood predominates. Perhaps some of these deaths could have been prevented if individuals within the patient's support system had been comfortable with encouraging the individual to express emotion.

Another aspect of the care of family members might include follow-up treatment. Rather than saying goodbye to the family and never seeing them again unless they enter the hospital as patients, perhaps the care of the family should include checkups following the death of the family member. These "checkups" would be used to see how the family is functioning. Are individuals within the family structure having difficulty adjusting to new roles and responsibilities? What about the children? What is happening to them in school and in their other activities? What support is the family receiving from the extended family and friends? The care of the family of a cancer patient is as important as the care of the patient.

Who is able to provide the support to the patient and the family? Who is able to assist with the communication between the patient, the family, and the health professionals? Society needs to provide this care for sick people and their families. As a consequence, it is important to evaluate what effect cancer has on society.

CANCER AND SOCIETY

The first area needing consideration is how society defines life and death. Life in Western society is centered around the young adult. Life represents being active, both physically and mentally. It means being independent and able to function alone.

Death, conversely, means the end of all these things. Western society says that the person who is dying may be dependent and may not be active either physically and/or mentally. No one wants to give away the things that life has to offer. Society has put very little value on things associated with dying. Religion has attempted to place value on dying by saying that individuals will have eternal life and that there will be no more suffering in the life after death. Until recently, little more than hope was attributed to these words. There was little factual proof in the religious doctrines. However, in recent times work has been done with individuals who have experienced "life after death" or as Raymond Moody and

Elisabeth Kübler-Ross describe it, "out-of-body experiences."[11,12] Perhaps in time society will not be so afraid of death and death will have more positive values attached to it. But for the present time, death has more negative attributes than positive ones for members of Western society in general.

Cancer has long been equated with death. Generally speaking, it is a disease that is feared. Society fears this disease for all of the same reasons that the patient and the family fear the disease. What effect then does this have on the patient and/or the family?

Society needs as much help as the individuals involved with cancer to gain an understanding of the disease and how it is viewed by society as a whole. Society must assess how it feels about death. Once attitudes and feelings about cancer and death are identified, society needs to express to the involved individuals its feelings—that society feels uncomfortable and it, too, fears cancer and/or death. Society should also be able to identify the origins of these fears. If this could be done by members of society, the actions of society might not be misinterpreted. Because this is seldom done, the patient often interprets society's reactions as abandonment, dislike of the patient, a desire to isolate the patient, or fear that the patient will be a burden. These attitudes bring about further anxiety for the patient, and the patient's responses further complicate the situation, which often becomes a knotted web.

Nurses, too, often are a part of society and display the same reactions that society does rather than becoming knowledgeable patient or family advocates. Both the medical and the nursing professions are cure-oriented, just as society is life-oriented.

According to Glaser and Strauss,[13] nurses may experience three types of loss when a patient dies. These losses are represented by feelings that nurses, as members of society and as individuals, have to deal with. Nurses' reactions, along with those of other members of society are interpreted by patients through their own feelings at the moment.

The first loss nurses may feel is a personal loss. This may result because many times patients who have been hosptialized repeatedly become friends of the health team. A patient may also be the same age as a nurse or a member of the nurse's family. This situation results in a degree of personal identification with the patient by the nurse.

The second loss a nurse may experience is work loss, or a feeling that one's best efforts have been in vain. Many nurses, including the author, feel that they have caused or contributed to the death of the patient when they first experience a death in their professional capacity. Many times nurses invest so much of themselves in an effort to help the patient live that the person's death is a real loss, not only of the patient who is now beyond the nurses' abilities to help, but also of the investment of themselves. These losses are not always easy to understand.

The third loss a nurse may experience is a social loss. "In our society we value people, more or less, on the basis of various social characteristics; for example, age, skin color, ethnicity, education, occupation, family status, social class, beauty, 'personality,' talent, and accomplishments.''[12] Age is one of the factors valued most. For example, if a young person dies, this death is usually considered a greater loss than the death of someone who has lived a long time. If a person is ''old'' when death comes, society tends to feel that this individual has lived a full life, whereas society feels that someone young has not had a chance to live. What society fails to put value on is quality rather than quantity. It appears that the loss of a criminal who has committed murder is not as great a loss, for the nurse or for society, as is the death of a president of university. Although nurses have been singled out in their losses, the other health professionals and all of society place this same value on social loss.

SUMMARY

The cancer patient, the patient's family, and all of society have a wide variety of feelings associated with cancer. Some of them, such as those discussed in this chapter, can be generalized. Others are very individual and may not be experienced by everyone. It must be remembered that seldom do all people experience every one of the generalized feelings either.

Important considerations in dealing with people's feelings are to assess the feelings and to communicate with the individual in an attempt to understand why the person feels as he or she does. It is extremely important to communicate honestly with other people, whether they be the patient, the family, or the rest of society. They must know the nurse's feelings and concerns for them.

With this type of a base, the patient, the family, and the rest of society can support each other. In addition, with provision of this kind of support, the difficult feelings of the cancer patient may be diminished or eliminated. In that way the patient, family, and significant others will not have to go through the cancer experience alone and alienated.

REFERENCES

1 Herman Feifel. ''Death.'' In Norman L. Barberow, *Taboo Topics*. New York: Atherton. 1973. pp. 8–21.
2 Barney G. Glaser and Anselm L. Strauss. *Awareness of Dying*. Chicago: Aldine. 1965. p. 3.
3 Clark E. Moustakes. *Loneliness*. Englewood Cliffs, N.J.: Prentice-Hall. 1961. p. 25.
4 Ted Rosenthal. *How Could I Not Be Among You?* New York: George Braziller. 1973.
5 Granger E. Westberg. *Good Grief*. Philadelphia: Fortress. 1962.
6 Ibid.
7 Ruth D. Abrams. ''The Patient with Cancer—His Changing Pattern of Communication.'' *New England Journal of Medicine*. 274:6. 1966. pp. 317–322.
8 Ruth F. Craven and Benita H. Sharp. ''The Effects of Illness on Family Functions.'' *Nursing Forum*. XI:2. 1972. p. 211.

9   Bernard Schoenberg et al. (eds.). *Psychosocial Aspects of Terminal Care*. New York: Columbia University Press. 1972. p. 211.
10 Ibid., p. 213.
11 Raymond A. Moody, Jr. *Life after Life*. Atlanta: Mockingbird Books. 1975.
12 Elisabeth Kübler-Ross. "Foreword," in ibid., pp. 7-8.
13 Barney G. Glaser and Anselm L. Strauss. "The Social Loss of Dying Patients." *American Journal of Nursing*. 64:June 1964. p. 119.

BIBLIOGRAPHY

Abrams, Ruth D. "The Patient with Cancer—His Changing Pattern of Communication." *New England Journal of Medicine*. 274:6. 1966, 317–322.

Agee, James. *A Death in the Family*. New York: Grosset and Dunlap. 1957.

Albright, David. *It's Not Easy Knowing*. Oregon: Creative Christian Communicators. 1974.

Alsop, Stewart. *Stay of Execution*. Philadelphia: Lippincott. 1973.

Celine, Louis-Ferdinand. *Death on the Installment Plan*. New York: New Directions. 1952.

Choron, Jacques. *Death and Western Thought*. New York: Macmillan. 1963.

Craven, Ruth F. and Benita H. Sharp. "The Effects of Illness on Family Functions." *Nursing Forum*. XI:2. 1972, 186–193.

The Dying Patient: A Nursing Perspective. New York: The American Journal of Nursing Company. 1972.

Epstein, Charlotte. *Nursing the Dying Patient*. Virginia: Reston. 1975.

Feifel, Herman. "Death." In Norman L. Farberow, *Taboo Topics*. New York: Atherton. 1963.

Glaser, Barney G. and Anselm L. Strauss. *Awareness of Dying*. Chicago: Aldine. 1965.

———. "The Social Loss of Dying Patients." *American Journal of Nursing*. 64:June 1964, 119–121.

King, Stanley H. *Perceptions of Illness and Medical Practice*. New York: Russell Sage Foundation. 1962.

Knutson, Andie L. *The Individual, Society, and Health Behavior*. New York: Russell Sage Foundation. 1965.

Kübler-Ross, Elisabeth. *Death, the Final Stage of Growth*. Englewood Cliffs, N.J.: Prentice-Hall. 1975.

———. *On Death and Dying*. New York: Macmillan. 1969.

———. *Questions and Answers on Death and Dying*. New York: Collier Books. 1974.

Mines, Samuel. *The Conquest of Pain*. New York: Grosset and Dunlap. 1974.

Moody, Raymond A., Jr. *Life after Life*. Atlanta: Mockingbird Books. 1975.

Moustakes, Clark E. *Loneliness*. Englewood Cliffs: N.J.: Prentice-Hall. 1961.

Nye, F. Ivan and Felix M. Berardo. *The Family: Its Structure and Interaction*. New York: Macmillan. 1973.

Parad, Howard J. (ed.). *Crisis Intervention: Selected Readings*. New York: Family Service Association of America. 1965.

Quint, Jeanne C. *The Nurse and the Dying Patient*. New York: Macmillan. 1967.

Rosenthal, Ted. *How Could I Not Be among You?* New York: George Braziller. 1973.

Schoenberg, Bernard, et al. (eds.). *Psychosocial Aspects of Terminal Care*. New York: Columbia University Press. 1972.

Scott, Frances G. and Ruth M. Brewer (eds.). *Confrontations of Death*. Oregon: Oregon State University. 1971.

Solzhenitsyn, Alexander. *The Cancer Ward*. New York: Bantam. 1968.

Westberg, Granger E. *Good Grief*. Philadelphia: Fortress. 1962.

Williams, Robert H. (ed.). *To Live and Die: When, Why, and How*. New York: Springer-Verlag. 1973.

Zborowski, Mark. *People in Pain*. San Francisco: Jossey-Bass. 1969.

Chapter 12

Counseling the Oncology Patient

Pamela K. Burkhalter

Nurses caring for oncology patients fulfill many roles. They become sources of emotional support, administer complex treatments, make sophisticated assessments of patient needs, act as patient advocates, and serve as an information and advice resource to patient and family. Within this wide array of nursing activities, each with a different level of responsibility and skill requirement, lies a central unifying role—that of counselor. How, when, and where nursing intervention takes place can be largely determined by the extent to which counseling has become an integral part of the nurse's role.

Oncology patients tend to have a history of highly stressful life experiences as compared with persons who do not have cancer. The diagnosis and treatment of cancer creates an additional source of intensely stressful experiences that may be of long duration. Thus, the oncology patient is faced with development of coping strategies that must contend with prior as well as present and future stresses. In seeking to assist the patient with cancer to cope with existing and potential stressors, the nurse will find it beneficial to consider how the counseling role can facilitate achievement of nursing goals. For those nurses who have not taken a position on whether or not to formalize the counseling role for themselves, this chapter will provide a basis from which such a decision can be made. Nurses who currently use a counseling approach to patient interaction situations will obtain information on application of counseling techniques to the oncology patient–nurse relationship.

NATURE OF COUNSELING

Definition of Counseling

In the context of the nurse-patient relationship, "counseling" can be defined as a *process* in which an interpersonal *relationship* is established between the nurse and a patient/family which is characterized by meaningful *interaction* and *involvement*. The definition is not restricted to nursing; it applies to other counseling situations involving a helper and recipient of assistance.

Counseling involves more than conversation, listening, reflecting, or any of the other techniques used during any particular interaction. The sum of all the components of counseling does not equal the whole. The counseling process consists not only of skills, but also of an entire feeling tone and sense of commitment on the part of the counselor to achieve identified goals.

Counseling as a Process

Over the course of a counseling relationship, the patient gradually experiences change(s) that ultimately result(s) in attainment of a specified goal or outcome. This transition from one state of being to another is called a "process." Counseling, then, is a process in which the nurse facilitates the patient's psychological, emotional, or physiological development and growth. The parameters of the counseling process are defined by the skills of the counselor, environmental influences, and the patient's ability to respond to the interactions that take place.

Characteristics of Counseling

Counseling versus Psychotherapy   One of the more common questions raised by those who seek understanding of the counselor role is, What is the difference between counseling and psychotherapy? These two major interpersonal assistance modalities often are taken to (1) mean the same thing, (2) do the same thing, or (3) be equally effective in helping others. Although trained mental health professionals may use theories or techniques that are derived from the body of knowledge called "counseling" or "psychotherapy," there *are* differences between the two. Nurses who are interested in developing an increased ability to meet the needs of oncology patients should not be deterred from doing so by the overt similarities between counseling and psychotherapy. The motivated nurse *can* acquire the ability to offer counseling services to the patient without undertaking the role of psychotherapist.

The primary differences between counseling and psychotherapy lie in the nature of the patient-helper relationship and the problems addressed. Psychotherapy focuses on

1   Identifying intrapsychic dynamics

2 Changing personality structure or overt behavior to enhance life functioning

3 Relatively severe emotional or psychological problems, e.g., neurosis, psychosis

The therapeutic process attempts to resolve underlying intrapsychic conflict such that the patient can reduce expenditures for nonproductive behavior patterns.

Counseling also emphasizes behavior change that allows the patient to achieve a more satisfying and meaningful life. The counselor, however (unless specifically trained to do so), does not ordinarily work with persons who have deep-seated or disabling emotional problems. In cases in which the patient or client begins to evidence severe emotional impairment, the counselor will usually refer the person to a psychotherapist or acute psychiatric facility.

Goals of Counseling   The counselor may seek to aid or assist the oncology patient to

1 Identify problem areas that are having an adverse impact on functioning
2 Resolve identified problems
3 Mobilize resources prior to problem resolution
4 Make plans or devise coping strategies
5 Reduce conflicts that impede effectiveness
6 Adjust to nonmodifiable stressors both internal and external in origin
7 Effect needed behavior change
8 Enhance feelings of effectiveness and satisfaction with living

While some oncology patients need comprehensive counseling services that aim at achieving all of the stated goals, others require a more limited emphasis. It must be remembered that oncology patients often experience a multitude of stressing events over the course of diagnosis and treatment. At the same time, many people tend not to actively request assistance in dealing with all the problems they may have. When the counselor overtly offers the patient help while using the outlined goals as guideposts to potential patient problem area identification, it is very likely that the person will then be able to acknowledge a general or specific need. It is important, then, for the counselor to be clear as to the goals identified.

Need for Counseling   Nurses caring for oncology patients may have questions related to identifying the need for counseling; e.g.: When does nursing intervention need to shift its emphasis from general supportive measures to counseling? What does the nurse look for in terms of patient behavior? In answering these questions, each nurse will base the decision of counseling versus no counseling on different sets of variables; i.e., each patient, as a unique being, will evidence needs in a slightly different manner, and each nurse, as a unique being, will perceive different patient needs.

In general, the oncology patient needs counseling services when attitudes or behavior are affecting relationships with others in an ineffective manner. The patient who argues with family or nursing personnel over every detail of care is displaying behavior that may be detrimental to the survival or quality of established relationships. Similarly, the patient with negative attitudes or uncooperative behavior with reference to treatment requirements may experience a reduced level of optimal responding to interventions. Here the patient's entire course of treatment and recovery may be jeopardized. Clearly, counseling (or, in some cases, psychotherapy) is indicated.

When the nurse is concerned about a patient's emotional welfare and stability but feels more specific information is necessary to verify problem existence, initiation of counseling is appropriate. In this situation, the goal of counseling is to identify specific problem areas, assess the level of need for intervention, and where applicable, engage the patient in a counseling interaction or series of interactions.

Frequently nurses working with oncology patients will identify patient or family behaviors that reduce the quality of life experienced by the care recipient. If the nurse believes that behavior change can be fostered which will enhance the patient's quality of life or overall recovery, counseling is indicated.

Knowing when and under what circumstances to initiate counseling services depends on a number of factors. The nurse must possess a degree of assessment ability and knowledge of human behavior that will permit awareness of patient need for assistance. Of equal importance is the ability to fulfill the counselor role comfortably and competently. In order to do this, the nurse needs to have a solid base of knowledge of the counseling process.

THE COUNSELING PROCESS

A counseling relationship has three phases. Each phase is subject to numerous influences that may facilitate, neutralize, or block the interaction that takes place in counseling sessions. The physical setting and extent of privacy may affect the subjects discussed as well as the intimacy and rapport that can be established during each phase. In order to engineer a high probability of meeting counseling goals, then, the nurse needs to construct the interaction milieu in such a way that external influences will be minimized.

The theoretical model upon which counseling is based will determine how the process unfolds. Counselors who base intervention on a behavioral model, for example, will use a problem-solving approach in which behavioral change can be engineered. A gestalt approach, however, will emphasize a more intrapsychic process as the vehicle for change. Regardless of the model used, the process of counseling occurs in the three phases to be discussed below.

A crucial variable in the counseling process is *time*. Not all counseling relationships last for weeks or months. In some cases, the entire three-phase sequence occurs in one or two sessions. In addition, while the phases are discussed separately, it is important for the nurse to realize that they can overlap considerably, as depicted in Figure 12-1. For instance, the initiation phase may be extremely short to the extent that the nurse is able to rapidly move into the work phase. As a consequence, the nurse's original plan for a session devoted to initiating the counseling relationship is replaced by progress to the intervention phase. The more flexibility that is possible, the greater the likelihood of a smooth transition from phase to phase.

Initiation Phase

At the beginning of counseling, the nurse focuses on (1) establishing a therapeutic relationship and (2) gathering information on the areas of conflict. The major tool used in this phase is the interview. Nurses learn interviewing skills as part of their basic nursing education. These skills and abilities are finely honed as the nurse interacts with different patients over time. As a consequence, only a brief review of interviewing concepts will be included here.

Interviewing seeks to gain an understanding of the patient through the verbal information gathered as well as through the observation of behavior evidenced by the patient. The nurse carefully plans and identifies the goal or purpose for the interview *prior* to initiating it. By so doing, it is possible to reduce tangential episodes that may occur with the anxious or stressed patient. However, the nurse need not rigidly adhere to this goal if the nature of the dialogue unearths significant problem areas. The goal merely serves as a useful guide for the skilled interviewer.

After introductions are made (where necessary), the nurse should specify the reason for the encounter. For example, "Ms. E., I've noticed over the past 2 days that you've become very quiet and sad. I'd like to find out if you have concerns about something that we might discuss." The clear indication that the nurse is interested and will not leave in a few minutes encourages the patient to respond to further queries. In general, it is extremely important for the nurse counselor to specifically state the *time* parameters of each encounter e.g., "Mr. J., it would be helpful to understand what you may be experiencing at this point in your course of chemotherapy. I would like to spend the next 20 minutes talking with you about this experience." Of course, there will be many occasions where a time limit will be completely irrelevant and will be abandoned because of the intensity of the interaction taking place. However, the patient who agrees to a certain counseling session length knows that for the period of time specified, he or she will receive the nurse's undivided attention and concern.

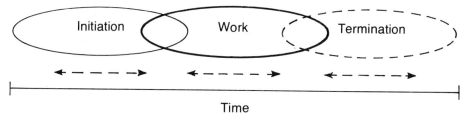

Time

Figure 12-1

The sequence in which information is obtained can vary greatly depending on the style of interviewing developed by the nurse. Often it is helpful to begin by asking nonthreatening, descriptive questions that permit the patient to become accustomed to the interview situation. After the nurse learns of the patient's living location, employment history, or family configuration, it is then possible to focus on suspected, anticipated, or potential problem areas. Because all patients do not respond in the same fashion, some will initiate the interview by asking for help, e.g., "I'm so depressed today. I don't know what's wrong with me." This is clearly an opening that the nurse can immediately explore.

As the nurse moves into discussion of the problem area, it is important to gather information on the antecedent events, feelings, and behaviors related to the patient's immediate concern. This information will assist in determining the patient's available coping strategies and sources of support. Questions designed to elicit a description of the current behavior and emotional experience constitute a second step of the problem discussion. A third area of information emphasizes understanding of the consequences of the patient's behavior and emotional responses. These three information areas can be addressed in different sequences than the one presented here. To facilitate the information-gathering process, the nurse will want to use combinations of open-ended and closed-ended questions and statements. Briefly, the "open-ended" question tends to require a descriptive response while the "closed-ended" question requires a yes-no reply. The former is more successful in eliciting larger amounts of information, whereas the latter can be responded to with only a "yes" or a "no"—no elaboration is implied.

Throughout the interview, the nurse observes how the patient responds to the overall situation. Valuable clues are obtained by noticing such things as increased anxiety when a particular topic is mentioned or discussed or silence following a particular inquiry. The pattern of eye contact with the nurse, body position during the interview, appearance, and general body movement and posture provide further information on the patient's comfort or discomfort during the exchange.

In some cases, it is necessary to conduct several interviews to gain an understanding of the patient's problem or concerns. At other times, the initial contact will include sufficient information collection and will then progress to intervention. The skill of the nurse counselor in identifying patient problems can determine the rapidity with which counseling moves from the initiation to the work phase.

Work Phase

The second phase may also be referred to as the "intervention" or "progress" phase of counseling. Work is composed of the theoretical model used by the counselor to guide the process and the specific techniques or skills used to implement the process. Most counselors adhere to a particular model of counseling that serves as a foundation or point of departure for the use of portions of other theoretical models. The nurse also may seek a model that best fits his or her particular style of relating to others. It is not compulsory to do so—many nurse counselors will be extremely effective and competent while using a variety of theoretical models. In the following sections, descriptions of several of the major theoretical approaches to counseling will be discussed. The specific skills and techniques used by counselors will then be presented.

Adlerian Individual Counseling   Within the context of Adlerian theory, human behavior is viewed as an attempt to achieve status in society. Dysfunctional behavior arises in response to feelings of inferiority and represents an attempt to deal with the feelings. An individual is not considered to be a victim of unconscious forces. On the contrary, the person is viewed as being capable of exercising appropriate control over behavior. To this end, the counselor focuses on promoting the patient's recognition of his or her true behavior and the development of ability to effect necessary change.

Client-centered Counseling   As formulated by Carl Rogers, the client-centered approach to counseling is based on a belief that each individual has the capacity to understand his or her behavior and possesses the ability to assume responsibility for behavior change. The purpose of counseling is to create an atmosphere in which the patient can freely express and explore feelings without fear or embarrassment. Because the patient feels no need for defensiveness, it is possible for the person to (1) achieve insight, (2) make better adjustments, and (3) attain self-actualization. Growth is achieved as the person gains insight and enhances self-confidence.

Behavioral Counseling   An emphasis on change of one's overt behavior or cognitions (thoughts) characterizes the behavioral theory of counseling. Developed primarily from the major learning theories (e.g., reinforcement and classical and operant conditioning), the behavioral approach to counseling is based on careful behavioral observation, assessment, and analysis. Interventions are designed which manipulate environmental or intrapersonal cue stimuli while fostering the development of alternative responses. Dysfunctional behaviors are considered to represent learned patterns of responding and, as such, are amenable to replacement with new, more adaptive patterns of behavior. The counselor facilitates and engineers the necessary behavior changes through the counseling process.

Rational-Emotive Counseling   Known as "rational-emotive therapy" (RET), this method of counseling was developed by Albert Ellis in the 1950s. It views human beings as both uniquely rational and irrational. Emotional dysfunction arises as a result of irrational or illogical thinking. The counselor seeks to promote the patient's ability to think logically about himself or herself instead of attributing negative qualities to the self. Over the course of counseling, the patient becomes able to recognize illogical thought patterns via the unmasking of such behavior by the counselor. Within the context of consistent confrontation, the counselor uses advice, explanation, direction, and teaching as methods to facilitate the development of more logical and efficient thinking about the self.

Gestalt Counseling   A holistic approach to the nature of human beings and their relationship with the environment is the basis of gestalt therapy. Each person is viewed as being equal to more than the sum of his or her parts—i.e., a unique whole operating within the context of present reality. The whole acquires meaning only within the context of the person's environment. Awareness of self and of present reality is emphasized in gestalt counseling. The counseling process seeks to actively reshape the individual's sensory capacities through encounter with the counselor. The goal is to develop awareness of feelings and to develop the ability to self-discover how one feels. As this capacity is developed, the person becomes better able to alter dysfunctional behavior patterns or methods of expression. Gestalt counselors use questioning, confrontation, telling, or instruction to restore the client to his or her gestalt (unified whole).

These five examples of theoretical formulations are representative of current counseling approaches. Each results in varying degrees of behavior change and addresses patient problems from different perspectives. Other theories not discussed include logotherapy, existential, developmental, and growth counseling. The nurse counselor may find that a particular theory is more appealing or appropriate to personal styles of interaction than another is. In any event, the nurse counselor needs to consider which model will best suit individual need and be compatible with the counseling needs of the setting and patient population. Ideally, the nurse who wishes to actively pursue development of the counseling role will initiate an organized plan of study to gain a solid understanding of a selected approach or number of approaches. Academic and practicum course work in counseling is one avenue to attain this knowledge. Self-study and continuing-education offerings provide acceptable alternative means of acquiring counseling abilities and knowledge. The brief summaries presented will hopefully act as stimulation for more in-depth study and consideration of the multitude of counseling strategies available.

Communication

Counseling could not exist without communication. Although this is an obvious statement of reality, the significance of communication can easily be overlooked in the rush to help the needy patient. Communication acts as the vehicle or channel through which purposeful and effective counseling takes place. According to Gilmore, "It is not possible to *not* communicate with your clients. It is indeed possible to communicate poorly or ineffectively with your clients, but not communicating at all is *not* an option."[1] Whether communication is clear or garbled, effective or ineffective, it occurs in every counseling interaction. Through communication at verbal and nonverbal levels, a process of creating meaning between nurse and patient evolves. All counseling theories rely on communication to accomplish identifed goals.

The basic communication sequence is illustrated in Figure 12-2. In the sequence, the patient or nurse verbally or nonverbally puts a message into the communication channel which is received by the nurse or patient. Although the originator of the message introduces it into the channel, which consists of each person's sensory organs, it may or may not be accurately perceived by the recipient.

The communication channel is subject to the influence of *noise*—stimuli, events, objects, or emotions that alter the quality of the message received. Noise may consist of such things as anxiety, fear, pain, treatments, or style of coping. The values, attitudes, expectations, and experiences of nurse and patient can also create noise in the communication channel. One's self-concept and sense of worthiness can impinge on and alter the message received in the counseling process. Each participant in counseling therefore contributes to the quality of the communication that takes place.

Two aspects of the communication process deserve special emphasis: congruence and silence.

Congruence   To the extent that the content of a message coincides with the behavior expressed, communication is said to be "congruent," or matching. Major problems in counseling can arise when nurse or patient perceives one meaning from a verbal message and another conflicting message from the behavioral message. Attention to one aspect of the overall message without attention to the other portion creates an incongruent message. Of equal importance is *failure* to attend to or be aware of both levels of communication. When this situation occurs, an escalating spiral of misunderstanding and confusion develops. The following interaction illustrates this problem.

Nurse: Good morning, Mr. Richards. I understand that you start chemotherapy today. How do you feel about it?

Patient: Just fine. (Smiling, shift in body position.)

Nurse: That's good. You know it won't hurt too much when the drug is injected. It'll be similar to having blood drawn.

Patient: Well, you know me. I've never been afraid of needles. Let's get on with it. (Looking away, voice tone higher, fingering wedding band.)

Nurse: How did you sleep last night? We had some noise in the hall when the elevator broke down.

Patient: Oh, just fine. No problem. Slept right through it. (Turning on TV, smiles quickly.)

Nurse: Well, I'll see you about 11 A.M. when the chemotherapy is administered.

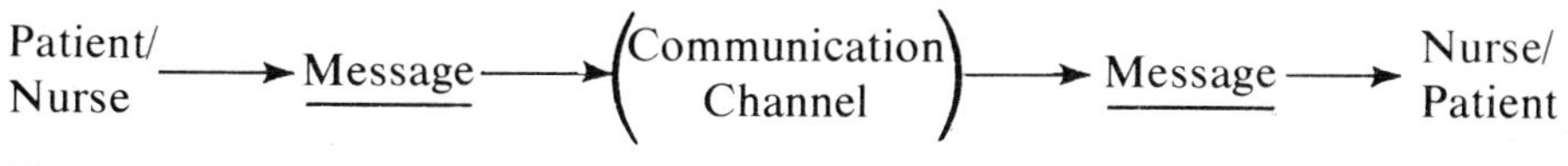

Patient/Nurse ⟶ Message ⟶ (Communication Channel) ⟶ Message ⟶ Nurse/Patient

Figure 12-2

Here the patient's verbal message of "everything's fine, O.K. with me" was incongruent with the behavioral cues of anxiety and apprehension. At the outset, perception of this discrepancy would have led the nurse to identify and deal with *both* levels of the message with something like this:

> Mr. Richards, I noticed that when I mentioned your chemotherapy you looked a little nervous. Many people do have questions and concerns about this form of treatment before it begins. What kinds of things are on your mind at this point?

This statement acknowledges the patient's verbal and nonverbal message.

Attention to both levels of the communication process reduces the tendency to misunderstand what is conveyed. Realization that one cannot ignore or be unaware of the complete message placed in the communication channel creates a situation in which the nurse can be truly responsive to the patient. With this in mind, counseling can progress in such a way that the patient and the nurse achieve identified goals.

Silence   Most counselors are able to respond to the verbal or highly verbal patient in such a way that progress is achieved during counseling sessions. However, many nurses and other counselors find it difficult to understand and be comfortable with periods of silence during a session. When the patient becomes nonverbal at some point during the interaction, the nurse needs to consider the possible meaning of the behavior:

1   The patient may be uncomfortable with the topic.
2   The end of a particular train of thought may have been reached.
3   The patient may have stopped or interrupted ongoing thought processes.
4   The silence may be necessary to formulate thoughts, comments, and questions.
5   The silence may indicate a need for "rescue" by the counselor.

These alternative explanations should not be assumed to be responsible for the silence without first being *validated*. A statement such as "You've become very quiet since we began talking about. . . . Are you uncomfortable talking about this?" allows the nurse to verify whether or not the patient is concerned about the nature of the topic. The nurse seeks to identify the reason for the silence and at the same time gains valuable information on the patient's tolerance for silence, anxiety, or ability to look at uncomfortable discussion topics. Silence need not be viewed as a negatively valenced part of counseling. In some cases, it allows both counselor and patient to relax, reflect, and consider future interaction directions.

Communication can be facilitated or impeded by the techniques used during counseling. The next section of this chapter describes many of the specific techniques the nurse may use in counseling the oncology patient.

Counseling Techniques

Implementation of a theoretical approach occurs through the techniques used by the counselor. Most counselors use a variety of techniques to actualize the counseling process, although some counselors confine the use of techniques to a limited few. In this writer's opinion, the nurse who assumes the counseling role can make use of an extremely wide range of techniques to assist the oncology patient to achieve quality living. The very context in which nurse counseling takes place, coupled with the severity of the illness and its treatment, may preclude rigid adherence to a particular counseling theory. In many cases, the nurse has minimal control over the complex variables that influence the oncology patient's behavior. For this reason, the emphasis here will be on counseling techniques that are directly applicable to the patient care situation. The techniques described are designed for use in all phases of the counseling process but tend to be used more frequently and intensely during the work phase of counseling.

Listening   As a primary counseling technique, listening consists of more than hearing through the auditory channel. It more accurately involves a total perceptiveness to not only *what* is said, but also *how* it is said. The nurse who can effectively listen to the patient remains silent much of the time while gaining a full understanding of the patient's problem or concern.

Summarizing   In order to gain a complete and accurate understanding of the patient's message, the nurse counselor will periodically summarize the content and feeling expressed. Part of summarizing consists of tying up the threads of thought discussed into a coherent bundle that clearly states the nature of the material covered. Because interactions may cover a wide variety of topics, an occasional summary by the nurse can help the patient gain insight into the extent of problems experienced. At the same time, the counselor may find the summary quite useful in identifying progress toward goal attainment. A summary statement might be something like the following: "Over the past several minutes we've discussed your feelings about employment, the radiation therapy you will start to receive, and your desire to take a vacation. Each of these topics involved your concern over whether you can continue to be physically active. Perhaps we can discuss this feeling and how it influences you."

Clarifying   At different times during a counseling session, the nurse will find it useful and indeed essential to seek clarification as to the patient's message. The nurse can make statements such as "I don't think I quite understand what you mean. Please tell me a little more about. . . ." Here the counselor wishes to be sure that a clear unconfused message is received.

Reflecting   Often the patient can begin to understand a problem as the counselor reflects the content and feeling expressed. Reflecting consists of restating in different words the message that has been conveyed. It also lets the patient know the degree of understanding the nurse has of the patient's unique problem or experience. A reflective comment could be something like "You really were hurt when your husband said that." or "You feel angry. . . ." or "It sounds like you resent having to return to the hospital for further treatment." The counselor may use the patient's words or substitute different terms when reflecting a feeling or thought. It is important for the nurse to avoid sounding like a "broken record" that repeatedly restates what the patient has said. This technique is useful to the extent that it assists the patient to increase understanding of concerns. When used excessively, the patient may cease participation in meaningful interaction.

Leading   Counseling progresses in response to leading by the counselor. The technique of leading consists of anticipating the direction of the dialogue and actively encouraging the patient to continue talking. Comments such as "Tell me more about that experience," or "What were you thinking when that happened?" are illustrative of indirect leading that helps the patient start to talk and also places some responsibility on the patient for continuation of the interaction. Direct leading consists of more specific items of information. Open-ended questions often directly lead the patient into discussion of specific areas of concern; e.g., "Try to describe the sensation you had when. . . ."

Informing   An essential technique in the counselor's repertoire is informing. Counselors frequently become significant sources of information for patients. In oncology nursing, the patient may have a tremendous need for information—often requiring several presentations of the same material over an extended period of time. As a counselor, the nurse is in a position to provide accurate and clear information in an understandable manner while at the same time assessing the patient's capacity to receive information.

Supporting   The counseling relationship is in essence a supportive one. The patient is free to be, feel, and think without being judged by the counselor. Giving support consists of acknowledging the patient's feeling state and allowing him or her to experience a reduction in aloneness with the problem. The counselor is able to reduce patient stress by supporting the patient's need to seek help. Nurses give support through care-giving activities, touch, and a genuine sense of concern for the patient's welfare. Statements like "This must be a very difficult time for you and your family." or "I'll stay with you until you feel more at ease with the infusion equipment." represent a desire on the part of the nurse to assist the patient to cope with a problem. Actions such as moving closer to the patient, touching a shoulder or arm, or sitting when talking with the patient each convey a supportive action—i.e., the nurse is not repelled by the disfigurement of surgery or the odor of the wound. Support giving is a vital element of the counseling relationship.

Problem Solving   The techniques presented above can be applied to the problem-solving aspects of counseling. In this technique, the nurse counselor assists the patient to (1) describe a problem area, (2) determine its significance, (3) identify alternatives for change or action, (4) gather information and consider the implications of each alternative, (5) decide on a course of action, and (6) implement selected choices. Teaching problem-solving strategies is a major purpose of counseling. The oncology patient may require particular assistance in problem solving when faced with the numerous unknowns of cancer treatment and recovery. Problem solving may range from developing emotional coping strategies, to seeking ways to mobilize resources, to devising ways to handle financial problems. Within this technique, the nurse can consider referral to other helpers when specific problem-solving tasks are beyond the realm of nursing.

Decision Making   Patient problems may involve a need or desire to make a decision paired with an inability or unwillingness to do so. In these cases, the nurse uses the problem-solving sequence outlined above and emphasizes the decision-making step. Here the counselor devotes attention to the patient's hesitancy, anxiety, or fear associated with a decision-making episode. By carefully identifying the emotions aroused in relation to the issue, the counselor can help the patient gain an understanding of the feelings experienced. With this understanding, the patient may be more open and accepting of attempts to consider available options. Exploration of the potential alternatives before making a decision allows the patient to gain a sense of control over events that influence his or her comfort and quality of living. In oncology nursing, patient participation in crucial decision-making processes can be greatly facilitated and promoted when the nurse counselor (1) assists the patient in developing decision-making capacities and (2) supports the patient in doing so.

Behavior Modification   Counseling may be initiated by nurse or patient with the expressed goal of modifying dysfunctional or unsatisfying behavior. Through the counseling process, the nurse may assist the patient in achieving understanding of his or her behavior as a means of promoting behavior alteration in the future. The theoretical background of the counselor will determine the methods used to bring about behavior change. The nurse may involve family, friends, or nursing personnel in the implementation of a behavior-change plan. When the problem involves an intrapsychic difficulty, the counselor may focus exclusively on stimulating patient understanding and insight as the primary method preceding alteration of emotional coping styles. In seeking to modify patient behavior, the nurse must be knowledgeable and competent in the theory used: The responsibility for changing another's behavior is awesome. It cannot be undertaken without careful consideration of the nature of the problem as well as the nurse's skill in introducing behavior change.

Summary of Techniques   These counseling techniques are representative of approaches applicable to oncology patients as well as other patient groups. Because the purpose of this chapter did not include a comprehensive teaching program in counseling techniques, the methods included here are merely representative of the multitude of available strategies. The nurse counselor will want to seek in-depth information on each of the techniques discussed in addition to those not covered, e.g., confronting, reviewing, interpreting.

Termination Phase

In a formal sense, the termination phase of counseling occurs when the reason for initiating the relationship has been resolved. In reality, however, termination begins with the first phase of the counseling process. The nurse counselor and the patient establish an agreement or contract at the outset which identifies the parameters of the counseling sequence. During the work phase, when the patient begins to progress in goal attainment, the prospect of eventual conclusion of the counseling relationship nears. The techniques discussed above continue to be used in this ending phase as the nurse summarizes counseling outcomes. Length of termination may be short or can occur over several sessions. How it is implemented is largely determined by the patient's emotional state of being and the amount of work that has been completed.

Part of the overall gestalt of the counseling relationship is the aspect of dependency. During the process, the patient experiences dependence on the counselor which allows the person to seek help. A need for help implies a reduced ability to manage a particular problem and creates a degree of dependence on the helper. The oncology patient who enters a counseling relationship is allowed to experience dependence with the understanding that as goals are achieved, dependence will gradually give way to independence. A basic, underlying premise of the majority of counseling relationships consists of facilitation of the patient's ability and capacity to control and/or modify his or her behavior. The counselor acts as the catalyst to this process. It is at the time of termination that the patient is assisted to realize the progress made and the ability gained to resume independent functioning.

Some patients resist termination of the counseling relationship and wish to continue it indefinitely. While certain cases may indeed warrant an indefinite continuation of dependence on the counselor or continued work on newly identified problems, the general purpose of counseling is to promote the patient's ability to function independently of the counselor. Be careful. This does *not* imply that the patient will be abandoned. The nurse counselor who has thoroughly assessed the patient's needs, strengths, and limitations will plan for continued support through patient resources, i.e., family, staff members, friends, clergy, etc. Thus, the catalytic role of the counselor is maintained, and the patient learns to make use of other available resources.

Termination has a very practical benefit for the nurse counselor. In working with oncology patients and their families, the counselor experiences varying degrees of stress and emotionally intense feelings. Some patients require more in-depth involvement than others do; some patients are terminally ill and need extensive counseling and support. Nurses who work with many oncology patients cannot continue to be effective when counseling relationships are never terminated. As a consequence, periodic review of goal attainment and stability of the patient need to be conducted as one means of retaining an awareness of priorities. When the *nurse's* need to continue the relationship exceeds the need of the patient, it is time to terminate. Frequent self-appraisal by the nurse will assist in identifying when termination is necessary, meaningful, and appropriate for patient and counselor.

QUALITIES OF THE NURSE COUNSELOR

Assuming the counselor role involves more than acquiring knowledge of and proficiency in the use of counseling theories and techniques. The manner in which these components are used and the extent to which they are effective in the counseling process are determined by the *qualities* of the counselor. As the nurse explores the counselor role, he or she will recognize that most training programs in counseling expend considerable energy and time in developing the qualitative components of the new counselor. Without attention to this aspect of the counseling dynamic, the probability of meeting with success in a helping relationship is significantly reduced.

In addition to having a *desire* to become an effective counselor, the nurse will want to consider the qualities discussed in the next pages in terms of the following questions:

1 Do I possess some of these qualities now?
2 Do I have the desire to develop these qualities?
3 What are my feelings about expending energy to acquire these qualities?
4 Are there role models that can serve as guides for the development of these qualities?
5 If I do not possess all these qualities, how effective can I be as a counselor?

By focusing on these introspective questions and the self-evaluation that they stimulate, the nurse will become sensitive to personal strengths and areas for development as a counselor. The qualities discussed below are not meant to be representative of all the qualities a counselor can or should possess. This discussion seeks to create an awareness of the basic qualities each counselor should possess in varying degrees of intensity. Of importance is the fact that qualities are not static personality components; they change, develop, and sharpen with experience.

Acceptance

The quality of acceptance involves the *feelings* of the counselor for the patient. "Acceptance" can be defined as the counselor's recognition and appreciation of the patient's uniqueness and individuality. It includes an acknowledgment of the patient's right to express behavior in many different ways. The nurse counselor who is accepting of a patient need not also condone inappropriate behavior. Acceptance should not be construed as a passive blandness—a kind of indiscriminate open-door policy. The patient must feel accepted as he or she is—and that includes behaviors or problems that may be changed during a counseling relationship. To acquire or develop one's ability to be accepting, the nurse needs to carefully examine personal attitudes, values, and expectations held about the patient, the illness, and its treatment. Only when one is truly aware of inner reactions to others can one begin to accept the uniqueness of others.

In the counseling relationship, the nurse's acceptance of the patient allows the person to experience a nonthreatening environment, one in which the person can *be* without fear of disapproval or judgment. The counselor continues to accept the patient while helping to foster a recognition of a need for change or development of effective coping strategies. By being truly accepting, the nurse's regard for the oncology patient necessitates attention to ways that will maintain or reestablish a climate of quality living. Acceptance should not imply a willingness to go along with or support dysfunctional feelings or behavior patterns.

Acceptance is conveyed by the counselor's facial expression, posture, and body position. The nurse who sits near the patient with arms crossed is communicating a less accepting attitude than the nurse who sits near the patient with hands folded in the lap or resting on chair arms. These seemingly fine nuances of nonverbal communication can be quite significant to the oncology patient struggling to reach out for assistance. The nurse should become aware of personal facial expressions and body posture as well. A relaxed facial expression, eye contact, and a slight forward leaning of the posture when seated convey a message of interest and acceptance to the patient. Quiet listening to patient verbalization without injecting judgmental or value remarks about the content also tells that the patient is accepted. When the content is indicative of inappropriate behavior or dysfunctional thought patterns, the nurse counselor can continue to accept the patient and acknowledge the content. For example:

> Mr. Peterson, it sounds like you're very angry with your wife for refusing to visit you. As you've been describing your feelings, you used words that reveal a deep sense of hurt. With the way you feel now, I can see how hard it can be to maintain loving feelings toward her.

Here the nurse counselor summarized the nature of the patient's comments, identified the feeling tone expressed, and told the patient he was still accepted by the nurse. In other cases, the nurse's active listening to the patient coupled with an occasional nod of the head or "I'm with you" comment tells the patient that the content is not creating rejection.

A nonjudgmental attitude characterizes acceptance. Openness to the patient and willingness to establish a counseling relationship are equally important. As the counselor communicates an open willingness to assist the oncology patient, a risk is created. The risk involves the chance that as the nurse invests emotionally in helping the patient, the nurse also may experience emotional hurt and loss. With oncology patients, the risk can be quite high. At different times during counseling, the patient may express anger, frustration, and dislike of the counselor while seeking to cope with the disease that may eventually take the patient's life. The accepting counselor tries not to personalize these expressions, but often will experience emotional pain when the relationship is intense.

Attentiveness

In the counseling relationship, the patient has the opportunity to experience the counselor's attentiveness to him or her as a unique human being. The nurse develops an ability to attend to and perceive the patient's feelings and behaviors without hidden agendas (those unspoken goals or purposes for an interaction). To facilitate attentiveness, the nurse constructs the atmosphere of counseling sessions in such a way that optimal privacy, quietness, and freedom from distractions occur. Within this context, the nurse *can* attend to the patient's concerns and how they are expressed. Acquiring the ability to turn off or turn down one's internal dialogue, or random thoughts that interfere with attending, can be accomplished as the nurse counselor becomes self-aware and understands the requirements of counseling. To be an effective counselor requires the sensitivity to realize when personal problems or pressures are interfering with meaningful attending behavior. One must never forget, "The counselor needs to have a counselor too!"

Attentiveness as a quality involves physical, intellectual, and emotional perceptions. The nurse actively listens to the content and feeling levels of the patient's verbalizations and uses counseling techniques to clarify, summarize, or reflect the messages communicated. The patient has a sense and feeling of confidence that the nurse's attention is undivided. In itself, attentiveness may have a high therapeutic value to patients who feel dehumanized by hospitalization, diagnostic tests, complicated treatments, and hurried care givers.

Understanding

To understand the patient the nurse needs to accurately and clearly receive the message conveyed. The major focus of counseling techniques is to facilitate understanding of the patient's needs, concerns, problems, and behavior. Understanding can take place with a counselor who is open, accepting, and attentive. Acceptance creates the situation in which the patient can be expressive. Attentiveness allows the nurse to hear, see, and experience the expressions. Understanding is the outcome.

Progress in the counseling relationship depends on the counselor's understanding attitude toward the patient. The oncology patient may desperately need to have behavior and feelings understood:

> I've just been to x-ray. Then the lab people came to draw more blood. They drew some this morning. When my tray came they forgot the coffee, and this medicine I get makes me sick to my stomach.

This patient needs to know that the counselor *understands* how she feels—perhaps overstressed, annoyed, angry, or confused. Statements of "You've really been busy this morning." or "That won't happen this afternoon." negate the message conveyed. Comments such as "With all this activity, I imagine you might be feeling. . . ." more accurately indicate that the nurse understands the patient's experience.

In counseling the dying oncology patient, understanding is crucial. The patient often wants someone to *listen, hear,* and *understand* what is communicated, not offer false reassurance that "Things will be better tomorrow." or "You shouldn't worry about that now." Understanding is a two-way street. Just as the nurse seeks to be understanding, so does the patient. In a counseling relationship with the dying patient, the nurse may want the patient to understand how his or her situation impacts on others:

> When you said how sad you were last night, I really felt sadness too. Perhaps if we talk about how each of us feels, we can learn to deal with these feelings better.

The nurse's understanding of the patient is clearly stated as the nurse reveals personal feelings. Sharing feelings often promotes understanding. In the counselor role, the nurse *can* share personal feelings and continue to facilitate goal achievement.

Empathy and Warmth

Developing the ability to see and understand the patient's world as the patient sees it is termed "empathy." It consists of understanding the patient's problem, concern, or emotions from that person's unique internal frame of reference. The counselor tries to think *with* the patient, not about or for the patient. By trying to put oneself "in the patient's shoes" and examining the problem or situation from that perspective, the nurse can then lead counseling efforts in a direction that will address the patient's concerns.

Conveying empathy often is viewed as one of the intangibles of the counselor's qualities. It involves a feeling of warmth for the patient, a sense of caring for and regard for the patient's welfare, a desire to offer support and assistance during a troubled time. Empathy includes cognitive and emotional components. The counselor attends to and seeks understanding of the patient through overt behavioral observation and interviewing skills. With this information, the nurse attempts to translate the "data" into an empathic frame of reference. For example,

> *Nurse inner monologue:* This woman is nervous . . . hands trembling, fidgeting, paleness. . . . She says the mastectomy surgery was successful. . . . She has one grown son; her husband is retired. She works part time. What is she feeling now . . . fearful of rejection or job loss due to hospitalization? What does her world look like right now?

As the counselor goes through this process, he or she becomes clear about what the patient's perceptions are. The nurse can also consider, "What would *I* feel, think, or do if I were this patient?"

As used by Carl Rogers, empathy is a mainstay of counseling. It should not, however, be relegated to one theoretical formulation. Empathy is an appropriate counselor quality for all counseling situations.

Honesty

Along with empathy, attentiveness, and other counselor qualities is honesty. The counselor must be honest with the patient during the counseling process. As the counselor presents an honest and genuinely sincere attitude, the patient is able to experience security and trust in the nurse. Being honest involves a willingness to openly communicate with the patient and answer questions forthrightly. Of course, technical queries about prognosis or validity of treatments, for instance, fall within the physician's realm of responsibility. The counselor needs to be honest with the patient when such topics arise; e.g., "I think I understand your concern and feelings about the outcome of chemotherapy, and I would answer that question if I could. But that specific information must come from your physician. I'll contact her and ask that she discuss this with you."

In addition, when the nurse counselor simply does not know the answer to a question or does not know how to respond to the patient's statement, this should be acknowledged. This does not absolve the nurse from responsibility to find an answer for the patient; i.e., a referral can be made, the patient and counselor can explore how the answer might be obtained—an exercise in problem solving which may be therapeutic in its own right. When the nurse experiences hesitancy or uncertainty about how to respond, a statement similar to "I don't know how to respond to what you just said. Could you explain further?" stimulate the patient to enlarge on an important point or concern.

Honesty within the counseling relationship must operate within the boundaries of realism. The patient may not be able to cope with confrontive honesty when under physical or emotional stress. In these cases, the nurse counselor must be sensitive to and aware of how honest communication is conducted. At times, information needs to be given in limited doses so as not to exceed the patient's stress tolerance. Oncology patients may have many concerns and a continuing need for information and support. Yet this need may not be adequately balanced with the capacity to integrate, comprehend, and respond to all the input possible. Part of the counselor's role, then, is to ensure that the patient is able to accept input without becoming overwhelmed.

SUMMARY AND EXAMPLES

The qualities, techniques, and theories presented assume relevance within a context of *commitment*. The nurse counselor needs to experience a sense of commitment to assisting the oncology patient achieve or retain a quality of living regardless of treatment outcomes or probabilities. Attainment of counseling goals takes on meaning and significance as this overall purpose is kept in mind. Again, the nurse wishing to assume the counselor role as part of daily nursing activities or as a singular role must devote considerable energy to studying and developing the qualities and knowledge necessary to actualize this desire.

In the following closing sections of this chapter, several examples of nurse counseling with oncology patients are presented. These case examples represent possible ways the nurse can implement the counselor role. As you consider each case, evaluate the approaches used and devise alternative interventions. In this way, you can gain understanding of the factors that each nurse counselor must consider during the counseling process.

Case 1: Mrs. T.

Mrs. T. is a 67-year-old female with metastatic carcinoma of the bowel. She is divorced and has one daughter who lives a long distance from her. Over the past few days, Mrs. T. verbalized, in a random fashion, that she does not want to "be treated" anymore. The nurse counselor visited the patient with the goal of finding out what concerned her. During the first interview, Mrs. T. began to talk about her pain, disease, and desire to die in a dignified manner. She was rational but depressed as she speaks. As the nurse continued to listen to the patient, she began to understand the patient's concern. Mrs. T. wanted to be allowed to die without being subjected to vigorous treatment. The counselor reflected and summarized in this message: "Mrs. T., I hear you expressing a desire to be allowed to die peacefully. You don't want more surgery or tube feeding or other forms of treatment. Is this how you feel?"

The patient responded: "Yes. I'm so glad you understand . . . (crying). What can I do?" Next the nurse focused on discussing why the patient wanted to control her manner of death. Over the course of two sessions, the counselor learned that Mrs. T. had led a full life, one that she was proud of. She had retired recently and felt that financial pressures were too severe. Of greater significance was her pain. She did not want to continue to experience the pain any longer that she had to. Her physician had explained her prognosis clearly in a supportive manner. Basically, she expressed a firm desire to continue to control her life.

As the patient gained an understanding of her inner feelings, she began to feel more relaxed. She discussed her desire with the physician, who agreed not to operate again. The patient was greatly relieved and made plans for a visit from her daughter and the management of personal affairs. The two counseling sessions took place within a week's time.

This case illustrates the counselor's role in (1) facilitating the patient's decision-making process, (2) supporting the patient's right to make such a decision, and (3) assisting the patient in becoming clear about the decision.

Case 2: Mr. P.

Mr. P. is a 37-year-old married father of three school-age children. He is diagnosed as having esophageal carcinoma for which a course of radiation therapy is planned. Upon learning of the diagnosis, Mr. P. became depressed and withdrawn. The nurse counselor was asked to assess the patient's emotional needs and initiate counseling if necessary. During the initial meeting, Mr. P. expressed surprise at his diagnosis. He was angry, and stated that he had to take a leave of absence from his job. As the nurse listened and asked questions, he began to undersand Mr. P.'s position. He was a successful owner of a small business who took pride in managing his affairs and caring for his family. He was active athletically with his children and enjoyed a rigorous outdoor life. Now he would be unable to continue with these activities because of the physician's orders; i.e., with too much stressful activity, esophageal bleeding might reoccur.

The counselor discussed his observations with the patient and acknowledged the patient's right to feel depressed at this time. At the end of the session, the counselor asked Mr. P. if he would like to continue to meet for further discussions. The patient stated that while he felt relieved to have talked about his problem, he did not want to continue the meetings. However, he wanted his wife to meet with the counselor so she could express her feelings.

In this case, the initiation, work, and termination phases of the counseling process occurred in one session. The patient made it clear that he did not wish to enter a counseling relationship *at this time*. The counselor noted this stipulation and decided to follow up in 2 weeks.

Case 3: Mrs. K.

Mrs. K. was a 53-year-old married woman with two grown children. She had metastatic breast carcinoma with metastasis to the liver. The nurse caring for Mrs. K. developed a counseling relationship with the patient and family during the patient's final hospitalization. The counselor spent time talking with the patient directed at ventilation of feelings, fears about dying, and hopes for recovery. Over the course of counseling, the patient became accepting of her terminal prognosis and decided that she wanted to die "without any heroics."

Concurrent with patient counseling, the nurse initiated and carried on counseling with the patient's husband and eldest daughter. These meetings were directed at helping these people express feelings of anger, frustration, and confusion over what was happening with the patient. Joint and one-to-one sessions were arranged. As time passed, the husband and daughter were able to accept the patient's wishes and support her desire to die peacefully. Before they reached this point, however, they experienced periods of guilt and anxiety about how they were reacting to the patient.

The counselor allowed the family members to *feel* as they did without applying a judgment to what was expressed. Within this atmosphere, the family gained an understanding that they were not "abnormal"; they could love the patient and still react to her wishes in their own way. As the family gained self-understanding and the patient also did, they were able to communicate their feelings to each other. At the time of the patient's death, patient and family had become accepting of the loss. Counseling with this family took place over a 4-month period.

Because this counseling relationship involved three people and was quite intense, the nurse counselor found it necessary to periodically share her feelings with a peer and seek support to continue the relationship.

These examples represent three possible forms of the counseling relationship: a short single-meeting example, two sessions over a week's time, and an extended counseling encounter. Each oncology patient will require a different amount of time to work through problems. As a dynamic nursing role, the counseling role offers the nurse a unique opportunity to provide quality, comprehensive, and intimate patient care.

REFERENCE

1 Susan K. Gilmore. *The Counselor-in-Training*. Englewood Cliffs, N.J.: Prentice-Hall, 1973, p. 230.

BIBLIOGRAPHY

Avila, Donald L., Coombs, Arthur W., and William W. Purkey (eds.): *The Helping Relationship Sourcebook,* Allyn and Bacon, Boston, 1971.

Belkin, Gary S. (ed.): *Foundations of Counseling*. Kendall/Hunt, Dubuque, Iowa, 1974.

Brammer, Lawrence M.: *The Helping Relationship: Process and Skills*. Prentice-Hall, Englewood Cliffs, N.J., 1973.

Coombs, Arthur W., Avila, Donald L., and William W. Purkey: *Helping Relationships: Basic Concepts for the Helping Professions*. Allyn and Bacon, Boston, 1972.

Downing, Lester N.: *Counseling Theories and Techniques: Summarized and Critiqued*. Nelson-Hall, Chicago, 1975.

Gilmore, Susan K.: *The Counselor-in-Training*. Prentice-Hall, Englewood Cliffs, N.J., 1973.

Loesch, Larry C., and Nancy A. Loesch: "What Do You Say after You Say Mm-hmm?" *American Journal of Nursing,* **75**(5): 807–809, 1975.

Manfredi, Claire: "The Nursing Supervisor as Counselor," *Supervisor Nurse,* **5**:19–22, April 1974.

Seeger, Patricia A.: "A Framework for Family Therapy," *JPN and Mental Health Services,* **14**:23–27, July 1976.

Shanken, Williard, and Phyllis Shanken: "How to Be a Helping Person," *JPN and Mental Health Services,* **14**:24–28, February 1976.

Smith, W. R., and H. Sebastian: "Emotional History and Pathogenesis of Cancer," *Journal of Clinical Psychology,* **32**(4): 863-866, 1976.

Tubbs, Stewart L., and Sylvia Moss: *Human Communication: An Interpersonal Perspective*. Random House, New York, 1974.

Chapter 13

Sexuality and the Cancer Patient*

Pamela K. Burkhalter

Cancer management is based upon a holistic view of each patient afflicted with the disease. Within this all-encompassing framework, care givers seek to identify patient needs, assess the intensity of the needs, and design interventions that will fulfill the needs. Nurses, caring for the whole person are aware of the patient's need for pleasurable sensations and meaningful relationship with significant others. In spite of this overt recognition, the sexuality of the cancer patient is seldom viewed as a crucial aspect of overall assessment. In addition, intervention energies tend to be primarily focused on facilitating physical and emotional recovery and rehabilitation. The sexual needs of the person often are ignored, avoided, or remain unperceived by the health professional.

In viewing the cancer patient as a generator of multifaceted needs and problems, as well as assets and strengths, the nurse *must* become aware of the sexuality of each individual cared for. The purpose of this chapter, then, is to (1) discuss selected components of human sexuality, (2) describe the impact of nurse attitudes on sexuality as they relate to cancer management, (3) explore the role of the nurse in facilitating sexual need fulfillment of the cancer patient.

---

*The author wishes to thank and acknowledge the assistance of Ms. Pamela Reid Russell in the preparation of parts of this chapter.

COMPONENTS OF HUMAN SEXUALITY

Human sexuality is not a separate, distinct aspect of being. It is an integral part of one's values, beliefs, personality, interaction pattern, and modes of self-expression. Humans are sexual beings who seek to express the components of their sexuality in many ways.

Development of Sexuality

The basis of human sexuality is *sensual behavior*. From birth, the human experiences the environment via the senses, receiving multiple stimulations from touch, smell, sound, taste, and visual inputs. While these sources of stimulation are at first generally perceived, they become differentiated over time, repetition, and cognitive development. One of the first differentiations made by the infant is that of internal versus external sensory input. The infant discovers that other persons specifically the parents, are necessary for the occurrence of certain sensations. Over time, the infant also learns to behave in ways that increase or decrease the occurrence of pleasurable sensations. This early learning represents the model for later sexual behavior.

With cognitive development, the experience of sensation takes on meaning. Sensations become associated with the contexts in which they occur and the response of significant others. Sensations become linked with emotional response and a cognitive understanding of their source in addition to physical experience. Pleasurable sensations take on relative value(s), and the child learns to control them to meet his or her unique needs. Because other persons become sources for pleasurable sensory input, sexual behavior acquires a social as well as intra- and interpersonal meaning.

In the formation of identity, the sexual value is the first to be defined. A child learns of being a boy or a girl before identifying with a religion, culture, social system, or ethnic group. Later personality develops within the assigned sociosexual context. The child learns about permissible and prohibited sexual behaviors for the socially defined gender role. Understanding of concepts such as masculinity, femininity, propriety, and social acceptance or rejection of behavior is quickly acquired.

In order for the experience of sexual pleasure to survive social conditioning, the child learns to be increasingly selective with the manner in which sexual behaviors are shared with others. This selectivity allows for the formation of special relationships that are unique in that sexual experimentation, discussion, and emotions are shared exclusively with a special person or persons. Best friends and first lovers are crucial to childhood and adolescent development of sexuality. These experiences represent opportunities to share intimate thoughts, feelings, and behaviors.

The ability to share intimacy is the major developmental task of young adulthood. Uniqueness and selectivity characterize adult intimate relationships and become the basis for mate selection, bonding, and the creation of the family unit. For the adult, sexuality is recognized as more than the experience of pleasure and becomes the most valued expression of communication and communion between persons.

The growth and development of each person's sexuality continues throughout adulthood into old age. With passage of time, the human establishes patterns of sexual expression that coincide with personal and societal mores and expectations. When the individual's mode of expressing sexuality comes into conflict with society's values, confrontation occurs which may result in social punishment, ostracism, or a revision of social expectations.

Social Expectations of Sexuality

Sociocultural values, beliefs, and expectations regarding sexual identity and expression are prescribed by each society. Certain sexual behaviors, e.g., rape or incest, are clearly proscribed in Western culture, while others, e.g., masturbation, homosexuality, or transexualism, have recently become more tolerated or openly accepted by large segments of the population. With relaxation of sexual prohibitions and development of effective birth control technology, expression of one's need for intimate sexual contact has become more feasible for many who would otherwise resist such behavior.

Values   Although societal values appear to be more liberal with reference to the interpersonal expression of human sexuality, many conflicting belief systems receive continued support. Young adults or adolescents who experiment sexually are subject to punishment from parents or society depending on the behavior exhibited. For example, while homosexuality is no longer considered a "mental illness" by most health professionals, adolescents who have experiences with homosexual-like behavior typically feel guilt and embarrassment that may be exacerbated if the encounter is discovered by adults or peers. Yet experimentation with sensual and pleasurable sensations between same-sex partners is a relatively normal part of development.

Variation in the means of expressing sexuality is influenced by many factors. The social "double standard" continues to support male sexual expression before marriage as normal, anticipated, and appropriate. Similar sanction has only recently been partially granted to females. This more enlightened viewpoint can be attributed in large part to the women's liberation movement and a general trend, beginning in the 1960s, to acknowledge the female's right to free sexual expression. The persistence of the double standard, unfortunately, continues to foster development of barriers to sexual behavior in the primary sanctioned intimate relationship—marriage. A female who has learned not to openly express sexual needs and preferences often is expected to acquire this ability spontaneously after the marriage ceremony. Under these circumstances, many newly married couples experience a potentially traumatic encounter when sexual freedom is bestowed upon them. Many adjustments are needed. While some couples are successful in discovering and facilitating one another's sexuality, many others remain unsatisfied with the manner and quality of sexual expression that evolves.

Culture   Cultural mores and values also influence the development and ultimate expression of one's sense of sexuality. In male-dominant cultures, the "machismo" aspect of manliness, control, and female submissiveness dictates a more passive female role consisting of childbearing and child-rearing responsibilities. Premarital and extramarital sexual behavior is prohibited and condemned as an insult to the male's virility and masculinity. Where the culture supports a more equally expressive role, the female also can develop and seek meaningful modes of sexual expression and satisfaction. Many of the traditionally conservative prohibitions against sexual expressiveness came about in response to environmental need, e.g., assurance of "purity" of descendants and control of family size. Unfortunately, although the need for (as well as the dubious historical usefulness) of such practices no longer exists, many persons continue to subscribe to these belief systems.

Western cultures are in the process of acknowledging and accepting the diversity with which sexuality may be expressed. With this recognition has come the realization that old belief systems, which rigidly established sex roles, can no longer continue to dominate. As women continue to enter previously male-dominated professions and occupations, adjustments in what and how behavior is expressive of sexuality will come into question. The question of what is "femaleness" or "maleness" and how these qualities *can* or *may* be expressed must be addressed by society as a whole. The consequence of seeking the answer will be change: change in how the culture views the roles of male and female, change in what will be acceptable behavior in general, and change in how sexuality is expressed.

Appearance   Outward appearance, consisting of manner of dress, hair style, body build, posture, and carriage, constitutes an important part of one's sexuality. In Western cultures, great emphasis is placed on physical attractiveness and a youthful, healthy appearance. Those who do not possess the idealized characteristics often expend considerable energy in trying to acquire the ideal "look" modeled in the media. One's appearance reflects one's self-image and how one wishes to be perceived by others. When the sexual aspect of one's self-concept is rejected or disapproved of by others, one is faced with a fundamental conflict or dilemma: Should one revise one's identity so that it coincides with the societal norm, or should one develop a more personalized, comfortable identity regardless of the expectations of others?

The significance of appearance as an outward manifestation of social acceptance and belongingness is increased when the person becomes ill. Loss of health tends to be reflected in physical changes that alter the exterior that is presented to the environment. As a consequence, the appearance component of sexuality is subject to the threat of potential rejection when a chronic illness such as cancer strikes.

Myths of Sexuality

Anxiety, fear, and frustration about sexual behavior and sexuality in general have fostered the development of numerous sexual myths. These legendary beliefs serve to perpetuate false conceptions of what is normal, healthy, and meaningful sexual expression.

Masturbation "People who masturbate can expect to experience dire consequences such as growing hair or warts on the palms or going blind or crazy." In fact, masturbation is a normal part of early maturation and may continue to play a significant role in adult sexual behavior. No harm comes to the sexual organs as a result of masturbation. Each person may learn to masturbate following self-exploration of the body's erotic zones or may acquire knowledge of the pleasurable sensations possible with a partner.

Orgasm "In order for the female to reach orgasm, intercourse must occur." Significant numbers of women experience orgasm with manual stimulation of the clitoral region without intercourse. Other women find it more pleasurable and stimulating to reach orgasm during intercourse. Each woman may differ in the manner in which she seeks to experience this intensely pleasurable feeling.

Normality "Sexual behavior is only normal when. . . ." Defining what is appropriate and normal sexual behavior between people has become extremely difficult over the past several years. In general, normal sexual behavior consists of that which occurs between the consenting persons. This does not include the legally proscribed behaviors that violate societal sanction, e.g., pedophilia or rape.

Age "Old people have no sex drive." As do all other body systems, the sexual system ages. Yet interpersonal sexual behavior continues to be expressed by persons well into the eighth and ninth decades of life. While frequency and intensity may change with aging, the meaning and desire for intimacy does not evaporate at a particular age.

Lovemaking "Intercourse is the goal of lovemaking." Love, affection, and caring for another can be expressed in a multitude of ways. Lovemaking between two persons need not culminate in sexual intercourse in order to have meaning. Other forms of genital or body stimulation, e.g., cunnilingus, fellatio, or body caressing, can be equally if not more stimulating for many people.

Homosexuality "Sexual behavior between like-sex persons is abnormal and indicates severe mental impairment." As perhaps the most damaging myth about the expression of human sexuality, homosexuality seems to represent the epitome of sexual dysfunction to many people. This false belief tends to be perpetuated in spite of the fact that homosexuality is no longer considered to be abnormal by many health professionals and large segments of the population. Homosexuality between consenting adults merely represents one way of actualizing one's sexual identity.

Arousal   "Males become aroused faster than females do." Both males and females experience sexual arousal within approximately 15 seconds of stimulation, as indicated by penile tumescence and vaginal lubrication. Therefore, physical arousal is rapid whereas psychological arousal may require longer periods of time for both partners.

The myths discussed here are representative of currently adhered to societal misconceptions about human sexuality. By no means does this discussion imply that all people believe these and other myths. However, enough people continue to subscribe to mythical beliefs that they maintain a level of credibility. Until such time that society as a whole becomes less rigid with regard to acceptable sexual expression, these myths and a multitude of others will remain a component of sexuality in Western culture.

Expression of Sexuality

The range of appropriate sexual expression is enormous: It is limited only by each person's belief system, values, and physical health. As a joyful expression of interpersonal intimacy, sexuality can be reflected in touch, smell, hearing, taste, and visual sensations and stimulations. Hugging, caressing, fondling, cuddling, kissing, or hand holding are clear expressions of sexuality between two persons sharing an emotional bond. As stated above, sexuality is not confined to sexual intercourse between a male and a female who happen to be married. Many people choose to receive sexual pleasure via the five senses without a desire for intercourse, while others find coitus to be essential to a sense of fulfillment and enjoyment.

Sexuality also is expressed and experienced as one takes pride in caring for oneself and creating a pleasing appearance to loved ones. The feedback of approval and pleasure that is received tends to reinforce the desire to be "pretty," "handsome," "cute," or "neat." While quality of physical appearance may not constitute a major source of sexuality for many people, from a philosophical point of view it remains an essential component of sexuality in a broader context. Thus, persons who experience trauma, surgery, or other treatments for disease very often also may experience a loss of sexual identity or, at a minimum, an alteration of how sexuality will be expressed in the future.

Human sexuality is composed of many things all of which contribute to a holistic view of each person. How sexuality is developed and what society expects of the sexual being represent the basis of human sexual behavior. Myths and beliefs about what sexual behavior *should* be, *can* be, and *must* be influence one's expressions of sexual need fulfillment. Nurses are subject to the influence of each of these components of sexuality. Their attitudes, in turn, influence the care received by the cancer patient.

NURSE ATTITUDES TOWARD SEXUALITY

Attitudes evolve and are shaped by education, experience, and sociocultural influences. In nursing, education on human sexuality has been largely excluded from the curriculums that prepare nurses to care for patients. Related content on the reproductive cycles and systems is taught from a physiological and anatomical viewpoint without attention to the qualitive, emotional, and inter- and intrapersonal aspects of sexuality. As a result, nurses who have negative attitudes toward sexuality, sex roles, and sexual expression are not exposed to information that might alter these attitudes to a more neutral or accepting stance. When these nurses encounter sexually expressive behavior in patients, the behavior is likely to be labeled "deviate," "inappropriate," "perverse," or "problematic." Further assessment of the potential *meaning* of the behavior is overlooked. In contrast, nurses who have studied the many components of human sexuality have a higher probability of interpreting patient sexual behavior in a more comprehending manner. In these cases, the nurse considers what need the behavior may represent and how the need can be considered in overall care planning

Self-Awareness

One means of recognizing and acquiring a more accepting attitude toward sexuality involves the development of self-awareness of the nurse's own sexuality. Because prejudicial attitudes and strong feelings can prevent or interfere with receipt of information on sexuality, it becomes *essential* that the nurse find ways to be nonjudgmental when presented with such content. A nurse's negative, rigid, or naïve attitudes and feelings toward sexuality may be reflected in several ways in the patient care context:

    1 The nurse may reject the patient's expression of sexuality, overtly indicating disapproval or rejection of the need conveyed.

    2 The nurse may not *see* or be *aware* of the message communicated by the patient's behavior.

    3 The nurse may overreact to the patient's behavior by being overly solicitious or probing in the information-seeking interview following an "incident" of sexual expression.

In each instance, the *nurse's* values and attitudes result in some degree of mislabeling or misperception of what the patient may be conveying. Anxiety about one's own sexuality clearly interferes with and impedes communication about sexual concerns or needs of patients. Many opportunities to identify and resolve sexual concerns of patients can be missed when the nurse *and/or* the patient experience anxiety in anticipation of such discussion.

    To become more aware of personal attitudes and feelings about sexuality in general and as it relates to one's self-image, the nurse may find it helpful to ask questions such as "How do I feel about masturbation, homosexuality, heterosexuality, orgasm, etc?" "How open am I to the discussion of sexual concerns with patients?" "What verbal and nonverbal messages do I convey about *my* sexuality?" In answering these questions as they relate to inner feelings, the nurse can become aware of how these behaviors may influence his or her responses when they are presented by patients. Part of this self-introspection process involves assigning ownership to the sexual "problem" identified in patient care: Is it the *nurse's* problem due to the way the behavior is labeled or perceived? Or is it a combination of both? By determining who owns an identified problem, the nurse can become clear about how the problem can be resolved; i.e., if it is a matter of prejudicial attitude applied to a normal expression of sexuality, then intervention will be directed toward the nurse.

Education

In addition to seeking self-understanding about sexuality, the nurse needs to receive education on the many components of human sexual behavior. Factual information on the anatomical and physiological aspects of sexuality can be presented as the basis for comprehension of more complex content. With this foundation of knowledge, the nurse can study such topics as the

1 Parameters of normal sexual behavior
2 Most common or frequently occurring sexual dysfunctions
3 Impact of illness on sexuality
4 Methods used to assess and treat sexual dysfunctions

Ideally, study of these and other aspects of human sexuality in health and illness contexts should be included in the nursing curriculum.

While nurse educators seem to agree that sexuality is an integral part of the patient's identity, minimal attention has been devoted to teaching about sexuality in schools of nursing. Few nursing schools have courses on sexuality. Those that include an emphasis on the topic tend to do so as part of other standard courses on the reproductive aspects of sexuality. A recent study of the knowledge and attitudes toward sexuality of nursing students, registered nurses (graduate nurses), medical students, graduate students, and college students found that

1 Nursing students were more knowledgeable about sexuality than graduate nurses.
2 Nursing students and graduate nurses were less knowledgeable and more conservative than graduate students.
3 Medical students were more knowledgeable than both nursing groups but less knowledgeable than graduate students.[1]

These results seem to support the notion that there is inadequate basic preparation on sexuality as well as insufficient continuing education on the subject among both levels of nursing.

A number of approaches may be used to remedy the educational lapse with regard to content on human sexuality. Courses designed to encompass the physiological, social, emotional, and psychological aspects of human sexual expression over the health-illness continuum can be included in nursing curriculums. At the same time, continuing education efforts can direct attention at raising the levels of consciousness of graduate nurses with respect to the issues of sexuality.

The methods used to teach about sexuality can range from didactic presentations to use of media. Role playing of patient-nurse interview situations can help to reduce anxiety aroused when sexuality is to be discussed. Videotaped exercises with patients or role playing can also assist nurses in developing interviewing skills and becoming desensitized to the anxiety surrounding the topic. Practice with the interview situation will prove to be most useful in future counseling sessions in which sexuality is discussed.

The role-playing experience also provides the nurse with an opportunity to analyze *how* he or she is perceived by the patient who wishes to discuss a sexual concern. One means of determining the impact of the nurse's attitude toward sexuality in the patient care context consists of asking such questions as "Do the patients or clients I care for have few or no concerns about sexuality?" or "Am I conveying nonverbal messages that interfere or discourage patients from sharing their concerns with me?" In answering these questions, the nurse can focus on the *manner* in which an open or closed attitude is expressed and how it impacts on the patient.

Both education on and self-awareness of one's sexuality fosters the nurse's ability to recognize and acknowledge sexual problems of patients cared for. With this degree of understanding, the nurse can then plan for meaningful interventions designed to resolve or reduce the identified problem. It must be remembered, however, that an open, accepting, and nonjudgmental attitude toward socially accepted human sexual behavior is a prerequisite to effective problem identification and subsequent intervention strategies.

SEXUALITY AND ILLNESS

Illness in general may affect a person's normal sexual patterns and sexual expression. When ill, the individual can feel tired, anorexic or feverish or experience a feeling of malaise. The symptoms of various diseases and illnesses may specifically alter sexual functioning by interfering with normal sexual responsiveness capacities. For example, diseases that reduce effective androgen levels tend to depress libido in both males and females and specifically impair the erectile response of males. Diabetes mellitus is another illness characterized by impairment of the male erective response. Persons with cardiovascular disease, such as hypertension, also may experience interference of usual sexual responsiveness. These and many other physical problems influence how one will be able to express certain aspects of sexuality. When illness is considered a stressor, therefore, the relationship between various sexual dysfunctions and the ill state becomes clear.

Sexuality also is influenced or disrupted by the patient's contact with the health care system. As a person enters an institutional setting to receive treatment for an illness, vestiges of sexual identity are stripped away. The person is questioned, poked, and prodded while being admitted and settled into the hospital room. Personal belongings are removed and stored. The person becomes a "patient" dressed in a relatively immodest gown that is usually unlike any garments the person normally wears. Because sexuality is composed in part of one's social identity, status, style of dressing, and physical appearance, the patient experience itself can greatly alter one's sexual self-concept and lead to sexual dysfunction in varying degrees of severity.

CANCER AND SEXUALITY

For most people, a diagnosis of cancer tends to be associated with fear of death, disfigurement, and chronicity. Sexuality, by contrast, tends to represent vitality, virility, energy, pleasure, and enjoyment. These two conditions of *living*—the disease of cancer and the various aspects composing human sexuality—would seem to be on opposite ends of the experiential continuum. The person with cancer frequently experiences disruption of sexual functioning and impairment of sexuality in general. As opposed to other illnesses or traumatic events, cancer is characterized by a number of factors that contribute to its intense impact on the individual and family unit:

1 Cancer may be viewed as the body's betrayal of the person. It arises from within the person unseen and unnoticed.
2 The progress of the disease may be short and curable or long and ultimately fatal, lending an air of uncertainty and insecurity to the experience.
3 The treatment for cancer can involve surgical intervention, chemotherapy, radiotherapy, and immunotherapy with no guarantee that a cure can be obtained.
4 The impact of cancer on one's sense of self-control and omnipotence is profound.
5 Sexually defined gender roles can become disrupted or destroyed over a long course of treatment for cancer.
6 Length of treatment may reduce economic resources and induce changes in family and social relationships.

For these reasons and others, the cancer patient's sense of sexuality may be altered as the treatment process begins and continues.

The meaning of cancer to the patient and mate also influences their sexual relationship. Interpersonal relationships with family or peers may be weakened if the cancer patient feels tired, is in pain, or fears contact with others when resistance to infection is lowered. The spouse or sexual partner of the patient, in turn, may reduce frequency of sexual contact because of anxiety about "touching" cancer or fear of harming the patient. In either case, the result is diminished sexual satisfaction and expression for both parties. In some cases, the sexual partner rejects further sexual intimacy following alteration of the patient's physical state, e.g., colostomy, mastectomy. (The specific problems associated with these conditions are discussed below.)

Other factors that interfere with the sexual expression of cancer patients include the following:

1 Potentially long periods of imposed sexual abstinence due to restrictions of institutional setting

2 Absence of one's sexual partner

3 Uncertainty about diagnosis by either the patient or sex partner, which blocks free expressions of sexuality

4 Grief or depression that interferes with libido or sex drive

5 Anxiety that blocks or impedes sexual responsiveness

6 Presence of pain due to disease process or treatment

7 Weakness associated with progression of disease or treatment

In addition to these factors, the common belief that the illness of cancer equals termination of sexual expression establishes an expectation for many people that interest in sexual contact vanishes when one has cancer, or any other illness for that matter. Sexuality does not extinguish when illness strikes; it simply takes other forms when the customary avenues of expression are blocked. In these situations, touch, hugging, kissing, intimate conversation, or teasing may represent sexual expressiveness and enjoyment between partners. Patients also may find that self-stimulation such as masturbation becomes more important and meaningful when they are deprived of interpersonal sexual union. These expressions represent normal modes of expressing sexuality.

The terminally ill cancer patient experiences a multitude of problems when seeking to retain a sexual identity. Because of anxiety about death and dying, the sexual partner may reject contact with one who is dying. A basic conflict may exist with regard to sexuality and terminality—perhaps the two most highly charged areas of human interaction. The patient may seek to retain a sense of sexual control and proficiency while living until death. The partner, however, may be grieving about the anticipated loss and be unable to maintain a satisfactory degree of sexual sharing. For other couples, the patient may deny sexual need while the partner continues to seek maintenance of the contact.

Another way of conceptualizing the terminally ill cancer patients's dilemma is in terms of the vitality epitomized by sexual expression in comparison with the debilitation anticipated with the dying process. While the patient may in fact be experiencing deterioration of certain physical and/or psychological capabilities, a fundamental need remains for sexual expression. For the dying person and sexual partner, the *methods* of expressing affection, closeness, and love can be altered to foster continued sexual need fulfillment. To accomplish this, the couple may need guidance and counseling, a component of the nurse's role to be discussed later in this chapter.

SEXUAL DYSFUNCTIONS AND THE CANCER PATIENT

Sexual dysfunction may be precipitated by biologic, psychologic, or social factors that (1) preexisted prior to onset of cancer, (2) developed in conjunction with cancer and its treatment, or (3) evolved following completion of treatment. "Dysfunction" consists of any disruption of the human sexual response cycle;

the response may be inadequate or nonenjoyable. The problems to be discussed in relation to the cancer patient do not include the sexual deviations that may be pleasurable but that deviate from social norms; e.g., inflicting of pain on others, exposing of oneself, fetish behavior.

According to Kaplan, "sexual dysfunctions are psychosomatic disorders which make it impossible for the individual to have and/or enjoy coitus."[2] The major sexual dysfunctions for male and female are listed below.

Male

Impotence: An inability to obtain or maintain a satisfactory erection for the purpose of intercourse. Primary impotence exists when the male has never been able to achieve an erection sufficient for intercourse. Secondary impotence occurs when the male is unable to obtain or maintain erection in 25 percent of coitus opportunities. Impotence may be situational, functional, or temporal in occurrence. Causes of impotence can be (1) medicinally or chemically induced, (2) brought about as a result of organic disease (e.g., trauma, hormonal deficiency, anatomic abnormality), or (3) related to psychologic factors.

Retarded ejaculation: Also referred to as "ejaculatory incompetence" by Masters and Johnson,[3] this condition consists of the intravaginal inhibition of the ejaculatory reflex. Ability to obtain and maintain an erection remains intact, while the person is unable to achieve orgasm. Etiology of retarded ejaculation may consist of depressed androgen levels, undiagnosed diabetes mellitus, or the rare adverse side effects of certain drugs (e.g., Mellaril).

Premature ejaculation: The male is unable to exercise voluntary control over the ejaculatory reflex, with the result that orgasm is quickly reached. Although men differ in the time it takes to experience premature ejaculation, the crucial variable is the lack of control over the behavior, which is distressful for the individual. Causes of this condition infrequently are organic. Rather, psychological factors play the major role in the etiology of premature ejaculation.

Female

General sexual dysfunction: Also referred to as "frigidity" or "orgasmic dysfunction," this category of sexual problems consists of an inhibition of sexual arousal, absence of erotic feelings, impairment of the lubrication response, or inhibition of the orgastic reflex. In terms of orgasm, the dysfunction may be primary, in which the female has never experienced orgasm, or situational, in which the woman has experienced orgasm by one means but at present not via intercourse. Causes of general sexual dysfunction may be functional (e.g., pituitary dysfunction affecting testosterone levels, or clitoral adhesions) or psychological (lack of stimulation or learned inhibition.)

Dyspareunia: Painful intercourse can occur when there is inadequate vaginal lubrication, vaginitis, endometriosis, or steroid starvation in the menopausal woman. Adhesions of the clitoral region or deep penile penetration during intercourse may also be responsible for the pain.

Vaginismus: This condition occurs when musculature of the perineum and outer third of the vagina contract spastically as opposed to rhythmically. When penile entry is attempted, the vaginal opening contracts tightly, preventing entry. Rarely, vaginismic women may be able to successfully insert tampons but be unable to accept sexual intercourse. Other aspects of sexual responding, e.g., orgasm by manual stimulation, often remain intact.

Both males and females may experience sexual dysfunction at various times during life. However, the cancer patient is subjected to a higher probability of experiencing such problems because of the impact of illness and treatment on one's sexuality and sexual functioning. The specific cancer-related sexual problems to be discussed have psychological, social, and physical components. Each aspect is identified in relation to specific cancer-related conditions.

Surgically Induced Sexual Dysfunction

One of the major forms of treatment for cancer is surgical intervention that seeks to remove the malignancy with a curative or palliative intent. Although surgery is applied to the eradication of many types of cancer, the emphasis here will be on several of the most frequently occurring types of surgical procedures. A discussion of the physical, psychological, and social aspects of the sexual dysfunctions is included.

Mastectomy   A woman who must have a mastectomy undergoes a major revision in her self-image. Because the body's appearance is altered permanently by loss of one or both breasts, the woman needs to integrate the new physiognomy into an acceptable body image. The mastectomy patient may be concerned or fearful that her

1   Feminity has been destroyed
2   Ability to be sexually responsive has been terminated
3   Enjoyment of sexual intimacy will be clouded by pain or discomfort at the operative site
4   Sexual stimulation during foreplay will be inadequate because of loss of the breast as an erogenous zone
5   Appeal to men will be obliterated and result in rejection

For some women, the mastectomy experience results in a complete cessation of all intimate sexual contact. Others, for whom sexual intimacy played a minor or unimportant role in life prior to surgery, find that the surgery provides an ideal reason not be resume sexual intercourse.

The loss of a breast may result in many of these possible outcomes. However, these negative consequences need *not* be predetermined as certainties. A woman's feminity and sexuality are *not* defined by the size, shape, or number of breasts that she has. Sexuality is an internal sense of self-worth and acceptance of oneself *as is*. Unfortunately, society has placed a great value on the female breast, as evidenced by media presentations of women prominantly displaying breast tissue. Yet while *sex* is promoted by these methods, a true sense of *sexuality* is not. Thus, the woman who must sacrifice a breast to be cured of cancer retains her sexuality and full gender identification. She is not less female!

Crucial to the rehabilitation of the woman who undergoes mastectomy is an understanding and empathetic sex partner, i.e., husband or lover. The woman who is experiencing insecurity about her femininity, a sense of low self-esteem, or fear of rejection can quickly regain confidence in her sexuality by the honest understanding and support offered by the sex partner. A sincere attitude of "I care for and love *you*, not breast tissue." by the spouse conveys an essential message to the woman who is struggling to feel whole. Witkin beautifully summarizes this attitude for both the male and the female:

> It is therapeutic in the best sense for the couple to learn that the woman is a whole person regardless of the quantity or quality of breasts she possesses, and the man is enough of a human being himself to respond to that women as a whole person and not as a display rack for secondary sex characteristics.[4]

The emotional suffering as well as the physical alteration associated with mastectomy surgery can directly influence how the woman responds sexually. A previously sexually functioning woman may experience general sexual dysfunction related to her fears of rejection, inadequacy, or grief over the loss experienced. These problems can be short-lived and resolved with education, counseling, and support from the sex partner and care givers.

First efforts toward resumption of sexual intimacy are critical periods for the couple. The sex partner may hesitate to initiate contact because of a fear of causing pain at the operative site. Any hesitation can be interpreted as rejection of the female. To prevent such occurrences, the partners each need to share feelings experienced or anticipated; e.g., the husband can convey to his wife that he wants to protect her from pain. The couple can then discuss different coital positions that would not necessitate pressure over the healing tissue.

In some cases, the sex partner is repulsed by the appearance of the mastectomy incisional area. These feelings can be so intense that the person is unable to overcome them. The woman may also experience such feelings. In addition, both partners may hesitate to resume sexual relations because of fear of awkwardness or embarrassment. Both partners may need assistance in learning how to adjust to the physical change of mastectomy. The couple should receive counseling prior to surgery which explores feelings and attitudes toward the woman's sexuality and loss of a breast. It is vital that neither partner put up a "brave front" or appear to be unaffected by the operation. Following surgery, counseling should be continued as the couple adapts to the resumption of regular sexual interaction.

Hysterectomy   Surgical excision of the uterus due to the presence of carcinoma may result in a number of psychological/emotional reactions that disrupt sexual responsiveness. When oophorectomy is part of the surgical procedure, the woman may experience reduced lubrication and a thinning of the vaginal wall if supplemental estrogen compounds are not used. Sexual intercourse when lubrication is insufficient can result in dyspareunia and eventually vaginismus. Women who receive radiotherapy for carcinoma of the cervix may develop pelvic fibrosis, vaginal narrowing, and eventually dyspareunia as the vagina shrinks.

Because the uterus may have an extremely high value to the woman, loss of this organ can precipitate grieving. The uterus is variously viewed as (1) being the woman's center of strength and energy, (2) epitomizing the reproductive function, or (3) representing an essential component of sexuality. Loss of this body part, although internal, may foster development of feelings of inadequacy and reduced feminity. Women who are no longer interested in the childbearing experience may perceive hysterectomy as a resolution to birth control responsibilities, while others who are postmenopausal may experience grief over loss of the "maternal" organ in spite of an inability to conceive.

Sexual dysfunction related to hysterectomy tends to be related to psychological or emotional stress factors in most cases. The sense of reduced or lost sexuality interferes with normal sexual responsiveness or leads to a depression of libdo. From a physiological viewpoint, the sensitivity of the erogenous zones (e.g., breasts and vaginal and clitoral areas) remains intact following hysterectomy. Full resumption of sexual behavior and enjoyment may be anticipated following adjustment to the loss. A recent study reported that 87 percent of hysterectomy patients reported no changes in coital position following surgery. In addition, 70 percent of the women reported as much or more desire for intercourse after treatment as before onset of illness.[5]

With support of the sex partner, the woman who has a hysterectomy can continue to function sexually. The male needs to convey empathy and understanding of the woman's sense of loss. Intense reactions to this loss are less likely to occur, because of the nonvisible nature of the organ, however. Couples who have placed a high value on the uterus as a symbol of fertility or sexuality, of course, will have more difficulty in adjusting to its removal. Again, the couples need to discuss feelings and attitudes as a means of expressing conflicting emotions that could lead to rejection and serious sexual dysfunction.

Ostomy Both males and females can experience sexual dysfunction following colostomy, ileostomy, or other ostomy procedures. For the male colostomate, impotence may occur if autonomic neural pathways serving the pelvic region are interrupted during the abdominoperineal resection portion of surgery. Estimates for complete loss of potency range from 15 to 90 percent for the male colostomate.[6] In one study it was found that 78 percent of the adult ostomates (male and female) had no disruption of usual sexual behavior and practices. While 22 percent reported an increase in sexual interest, 21 percent stated that a decrease in interest had occurred. Overall, 87 percent of this sample were able to achieve orgasm following ostomy surgery.[7]

The ostomate may experience numerous fears related to the altered method of elimination represented by the abdominal stoma. Primary fears are of spillage, gas, and odor. The anticipation of one or all of these events may prevent the ostomate from resuming or initiating sexual intimacy. Inability to accept the location of the stoma can result in termination of sexual contact by the ostomate or sex partner who is unable to adjust his or her self-image to the permanent surgical change. Ostomy surgery *is* radical in the alteration of body functioning that it creates. However, it need *not* be responsible for cessation or extreme curtailment of sexual activity. The male or female ostomate can resume normal sexual functioning without interference of the stoma.

Men who experience impotence following ostomy surgery may regain full potency if neural pathways were not severed. Female ostomates in the childbearing years seem to have no undue difficulty in conceiving, carrying, and delivering healthy infants. The orgasmic response in both sexes remains intact and functional with undamaged neural servicing. Sexual dysfunction, when it does occur, is related to emotional stress, fear of accidents (leakage, gas, odor), or difficulty in achieving a sense of sexual competence after surgery.

Ostomates are encouraged to resume sexual activity when weakness and operative pain subside. Prior to intimate contact, the person should bathe and care for the ostomy. Some people prefer to wear a modified girdle, or cumberbund-like covering over the stoma. When impotence is permanent, the couple should receive counseling on alternate ways of giving and receiving sexual pleasure and satisfaction. Booklets such as *Sex and the Male Ostomate; Sex, Pregnancy and the Female Ostomate;* and *Sex, Courtship and the Single Ostomate* (see Biblography) contain valuable information on ways to sexually adjust to ostomy surgery and life with a stoma. Patients who have a form of ostomy surgery can greatly benefit from the information contained in the pages of these booklets.

Surgically induced sexual dysfunctions can occur with males undergoing retroperitoneal lymphadenectomy for treatment of nonseminomatous testicular tumors. While absence of significant reduction in semen volume is anticipated in many cases, Bracken and Johnson[8] found that 7 out of 12 patients were able to father children after having the surgery. Men with inoperable prostatic adenocarcinoma can experience decreased libido and levels of circulating testicular androgens following bilateral orchiectomy or exogenous estrogen therapy. In these cases, the sexual dysfunction is related to an organic etiology. Total prostatectomy with seminal vesiculectomy interrupts the periprostatic plexes of nerves and usually results in impotence. Again, the patient's sexual dysfunction is organically caused but does not preclude development of alternate means of expressing sexuality.

Permanent alteration of the body image results in each of the cancer surgeries discussed. In order to reestablish a satisfactory and functional sense of sexuality, the person must resolve feelings of loss, fear, and anxiety about his or her self-worth and value to self and others. The nurse can play an essential role in fostering the development of this sense of wholeness as a sexual being.

Age-Related Sexual Dysfunction

Cancer often strikes those in the middle to elderly phases of life. For this reason, many cancer patients are in the sixth, seventh, eighth, or older decade of life when they are diagnosed and treated for cancer. These men and women can experience all the threats to body image, self-concept, and emotional stability that younger cancer patients undergo. The crucial difference, however, is that these people also are aged, and consequently the sexual dysfunctions that may be experienced can be attributed to factors that tend to be less prevalent for younger cancer patients.

Aging Process   The postmenopausal woman may experience some sexual dysfunction as a result of physiological changes related to cessation or reduction in sex steroid production. The vaginal walls begin to involute, and the length, width, and expansive ability of the vagina decrease. Lubrication is reduced, and this situation may result in urethral irritation following intercourse. Breast nipple tissue remains responsive to sexual arousal, but breast tissue may not retain similar qualities. In spite of these changes, the aging female need not experience any alteration at orgasmic response levels. The key element is a continued interest in sexual stimulation and intimacy.

Aging in the male sexual system tends to be less obvious than in the female. Degenerative processes inhibit sperm production, with the result that the seminal fluid is scanter and thin in consistency. Ejaculatory force and pressure are reduced, which may decrease sensual experience. With enlargement of the prostate gland, contractions of the organ are weaker during orgasm. Ability to obtain and maintain an erection often is intact well into the ninth decade of life.

Partner Availability   Many aging persons with cancer find that maintenance of sexual intimacy is blocked due to nonavailability of a partner. The widow or widower who has lost a mate may find it difficult to establish a new relationship after having shared life with the deceased for 30, 40, or 50 years. Aged individuals may experience conflicting emotions about *wanting* new intimate relationships, feeling that the deceased would not approve.

Social Values   Closely associated with partner availability is the problem of social values and attitudes toward the aged and sexually expressive behavior. Western culture tends to associate eroticism and sexual pleasure with youth and physical beauty. Aged persons can experience this societal value as a deterrent to a sense of continued desire and attractiveness. For the person who has been treated for cancer, the social bias is doubled. The person is not supposed to express sexuality not only because he or she is aged, but also because he or she has or had cancer. The previously stated equation of "cancer equals termination of sexual expression" can be enlarged to "age plus cancer equals termination of sexual expression" as a basic reflection of societal pressure applied to the aged who seek to maintain sexual behavior patterns.

Widowed cancer patients may experience familial pressure to "honor the memory" of the deceased instead of initiating a new intimate relationship. The patient usually feels guilt and embarrassment for wanting to continue a pleasurable part of life. Physically and emotionally, there should be no impediment to a renewal of sexual behavior after the patient has undergone a personally acceptable period of mourning.

Physical Impairments   Aged cancer patients with sexual partners may experience dysfunction in relation to other physical impairments found to be prevalent among the older age groups. Arthritis, diabetes mellitus, cardiovascular difficulties, or orthopedic problems can interfere with the physical activity associated with the person's customary sexual practices. Pain from any of these conditions can completely block desire for sexual contact.

The aged cancer patient faces many obstacles to maintenance of sexual expression. In spite of these problems, if the man or woman has led a sexually active life before cancer and the aging process begins, he or she is very likely to seek to retain this behavior pattern.

Drug-Related Sexual Dysfunction

Cancer patients may receive chemotherapy as a major form of treatment. In addition, they may take any number of nonchemotherapy compounds that have an impact on sexual desire and performance. Table 13-1 presents a summary of these chemicals and their known effects on sexuality. For a more in-depth discussion of the pharmacology of each drug, please refer to a text devoted to this content. Body size, age, dosage, and length of use will influence individual impact on sexuality.

Generally, sexual behavior and sexual dysfunctions are attributed to a number of factors, e.g., the chemical action of the drug, the psychoemotional expectation associated with the drug, one's basic values and attitudes toward sexuality, and the degree of stress experienced. While certain drugs may have pharmacological properties that inhibit or enhance sexually expressive behavior, the effect can often be modified by these other factors.

The cancer patient's sexuality is subject to numerous threats that can lead to sexual dysfunctions of varying degrees of intensity. How the patient responds to the impact of cancer on the sexual self-image may be influenced by the nursing care received from the time of diagnosis through the rehabilitation period.

THE ROLE OF THE NURSE

The cancer patient frequently has concerns about sexual integrity when in the desexualizing atmosphere of an institutional setting. Acknowledging the concerns and devising solutions that have the potential of reducing these feelings become the goals of nursing intervention. The nurse's role is composed of assessment, intervention, and evaluation.

Table 13-1   Effect of Drugs on Human Sexual Behavior

Drug category	Effect
Depressants	
Alcohol	
1 Low doses	Temporary increase in libido
2 Chronic usage (alcoholism)	Temporary or permanent impotence due to neurological damage
Barbiturates	
1 Low doses	Temporary increase in libido
2 Large doses	Depression of sexual behavior
Narcotics and mood-altering agents	
Hallucinogens } Marijuana	Subjective enhancement of coitus
Cocaine	Subjective increase in sexual enjoyment
Morphine, heroin, codeine, methadone	
1 Low doses	Subjective enhancement of coitus
2 Chronic usage	Depression of sexual behavior
Amphetamines	Subjective increase in libido and ability to perform sexually
Sex hormones	
Androgen (testosterone)	Increase in sexual drive/libido for males and females
Estrogen	Male decrease in libido and sex drive
Oral contraceptives (combinations of progesterone and estrogen)	Reduced anxiety of pregnancy; may enhance sexual enjoyment
Antihypertensives and antidepressants	Sometimes impotence or ejaculatory problems
Sedatives and tranquilizers	Enhancement of sexual enjoyment possibly due to reduction of stress levels
Phenothiazines	Sometimes "dry" ejaculation in which semen empties (refluxes) into bladder
Chlordiazepoxides	Sometimes increase in sexual interest as anxiety decreases
Aphrodisiacs	
Cantharides (Spanish fly)	Irritation of male GU tract; no sexual stimulant effect although erection occurs
Amyl nitrate	Enhancement of sexual pleasure at time of orgasm
Yohimbine	Erection may be stimulated, but is not a sexual stimulant
L-Dopa (levodihydroxyphenylalanine)	Temporary increase in libido and erectile ability; not a true aphrodisiac
PCPA (parachlorphenylalanine)	Questionable increase in libido not confirmed in humans

Assessment

Because sexuality tends to be a sensitive topic of discussion for many people, the nurse's assessment of this system can be assisted by the use of a sexual history format. Prior to gathering information on the patient's sexual patterns the nurse needs to

1 Establish rapport with the patient or couple, clearly establishing the purpose for such discussion

2 Clarify the nurse's role with respect to sexual behavior; i.e., the nurse is a professional who is concerned about care for the patient but who is not interested in sexual intimacy with the patient

3 Have a thorough understanding of the nature of the patient's disease stage and method of treatment to be used

The interview setting is a crucial component in determining how the patient will respond to assessment of sexuality. The atmosphere of the exchange should be quiet and private. During history taking, the nurse must attend to verbal and nonverbal cues emitted by the patient which reflect emotional reaction to the topics raised. By following the interview format presented below, the nurse can elicit specific concerns and problems.

The sexual history format presented is comprehensive in the content covered and may be modified to meet specific needs. With the information obtained in the history, the nurse will be in a position to establish goals for care during and following treatment. At the same time, identified problems can begin to receive attention early in the cancer treatment process, ideally precluding exacerbation of the difficulties anticipated by the patient. Remember, assessment is a *dynamic* process: the nurse needs to continually update or modify information obtained during the history-taking sessions to coincide with the patient's ever-changing needs.

Intervention

Nursing intervention for sexual dysfunction or problems of sexuality consists of three components. In order to carry out these interventions, however, the nurse must first have achieved a sense of self-awareness about his or her personal sexuality. With a sense of comfort and confidence in personal sexual identity, the probability of the nurse's interventions meeting with success is greatly increased.

Information The cancer patient who anticipates radical surgery, a long course of radiotherapy, or chemotherapy needs information in the form of anticipatory guidance. For example, the patient who is to receive chemotherapeutic agents may experience complete or partial loss of hair—alopecia—as well as unpleasant side effects. Alopecia can be a severe blow to one's sense of sexuality. As the nurse explains what might happen, the patient can be assisted to prepare for this possibility; e.g., by shopping for a wig or hairpiece before the loss is complete. Alteration of features due to steroid intake also needs to be discussed and resolved. Women who acquire a "moon-faced" appearance and increase in body hair, for example, can feel desexualized when the impact of these side effects is not considered.

Information on specific potential changes in sexual desire or functioning can be provided for those patients who have had or will have radical surgeries for cancer treatment. It is imperative that the nurse thoroughly evaluate the patient's attitude toward prior sexual behavior *before* providing information. For some people, the discussion of a *possibility* may establish a self-fulfilling prophecy: the possibility becomes an expectation that results in behavior change actualizing the prediction. Most patients, however, are greatly relieved to learn that sexual patterns may be maintained following physical recovery. The ostomate who anticipates rejection from female intimacy, for instance, can be greatly relieved to learn that most ostomates retain potency and masculinity following surgery. In all cases, the information must be factual and, where necessary, sanctioned by the physician.

During sexual history taking, the patient may reveal anxiety about a current sexual problem. In addition, the nurse may personally observe behaviors that the patient considers abnormal, e.g., masturbation. The information provided can focus on the naturalness or normality of the behavior for large segments of the population, thereby removing the fear of abnormality or deviance. Of course, not all sexual behaviors are socially sanctioned, and unsanctioned behaviors should not receive automatic legitimization because the patient is hospitalized. The patient who chooses to expose the genital area at inappropriate times and places needs to receive information that (1) the behavior is not acceptable in the present context, (2) the nurse is aware that the patient is experiencing unpleasant feelings, and (3) the nurse will assist the patient to identify concerns and seek assistance for them where necessary. A nonjudgmental attitude will assist the patient in discussing sexual problems.

Sexual History Format*

Instructions: In taking a sexual history, the nurse should first establish rapport with the patient or couple in a relaxed and private setting. History taking should be accomplished in a conversational manner starting with less threatening topics and progressing to more intimate informational areas. If hesitancy is encountered in answering a question or discussing a particular topic, skip it and return to it at a later time in the interview. More than one interview may be required to complete the format.

I. Physiologic information (largely obtained from patient chart)
    1 Medical evaluation for present illness:
        a Laboratory data
        b Treatment modalities being used:
           Chemotherapy—specify drugs used
           Radiotherapy—specify amount of treatment completed
           Other drugs prescribed—specify
    2 Menstruation: *(Obtain this and remaining information from patient)*
        a Length of cycle
        b Duration of flow
        c Discomfort
        d Emotional changes
        e Arousal fluctuations during cycle

*Adapted with permission from Jack S. Annon, *The Behavioral Treatment of Sexual Problems,* vol. 2, *Intensive Therapy,* Enabling Systems, Inc., Honolulu, 1975.

II.   Sex education and information
    1   Sources of knowledge and age at time information was received:
       a   Pregnancy
       b   Sexual intercourse
       c   Menstruation
       d   Contraception
       e   Male erection (females)
       f   Formal sex education
       g   Books read
    2   Parents' attitudes and information above
III   Current typical sexual behavior with partner
    1   Who initiates (what percentage of the time)
       a   How initiation takes place
       b   Consequences of refusal
    2   Feelings about nudity
    3   Preference for situation, place, lighting, devices, oils, and lotions, etc.
    4   Noncoital contact (frequency; attitude toward)
    5   Coital contact (frequency; attitude toward)
       a   Positions (percentage of each; preference)
    6   Orgasm, male
       a   Techniques
       b   Frequency
    7   Orgasm, female
       a   Techniques
       b   Frequency
    8   Behavior and feelings after orgasm or intercourse
IV   Ideal sexual relationship (situation; time; place; sequence of behavior; ending)
V   Problems anticipated or informed of related to present illness, its treatment, and outcome
VI   Current sexual concerns or problems (personal or of the couple)

Part of the information-giving process involves an acknowledgment of the patient's right to feel and express emotions about sexuality. Too often patients feel that such emotions should not be exposed to verbalization, much less discussion. The anxiety people experience about sexual problems can be compounded by the emotions aroused with a diagnosis of cancer. The nurse therefore needs to purposefully and compassionately encourage the patient to verbalize any concerns he or she may have about sexuality and cancer. In those cases in which the patient rejects such opportunities, the nurse can clearly state a readiness to resume discussion when the patient feels ready to do so.

Counseling   In addition to providing information on sexuality and how it relates to cancer and its treatment, the nurse may become involved in the counseling role. Prior to assuming this level of intervention responsibility, the nurse needs to:

    1   Understand the patient's disease process and how it may influence sexual behavior

    2   Develop a nonjudgmental, open, and honest attitude toward the topic of sexuality and persons who may have sexual problems

    3   Acquire knowledge of a wide range of methods to express physical love, affection, and intimacy

    4   Become comfortable with himself or herself as a sexually expressive individual

    5   Possess the educational or experiential training necessary to provide counseling services

Counseling may take place with just the patient, with the patient and sex partner, or in a group setting. Should psychological impairment or dysfunction appear which exceeds expected levels of anxiety, depression, or emotional turmoil associated with cancer and its treatment, the nurse should not hesitate to arrange for referral to a skilled psychotherapist.

Counseling services provided by the nurse may include ventilation of feelings, assistance with problem solving in a decision-making context, and support with reference to coping strategies. When a sexual problem has been identified, the nurse should make every effort to include the patient's sex partner in counseling session, i.e., conjoint counseling. In this way, the partner and patient can both seek solutions to problems in a less stressful and more supportive environment than may be found when hospitalization is over. During counseling sessions, the nurse can explore feelings and attitudes toward a wide range of sexually normal behaviors. In the more relaxed and open counseling setting, the couple can discuss which behaviors will be acceptable and pleasurable. Homework assignments can then be made in which the couple experiments with different sexual behaviors.

The nurse can consult the following very brief list of texts for specific techniques and information applicable to sexual counseling: *Human Sexual Inadequacy* by William H. Masters and Virginia E. Johnson, *The Behavioral Treatment of Sexual Problems: Volume 1–Brief Therapy* by Jack S. Annon, *The New Sex Therapy* by Helen Singer Kaplan, and *Perspectives on Sexuality* by James L. Malfetti and Elizabeth M. Eiditz. These references and many others will assist the nurse in enhancing counseling skills and capabilities. Reading assignments for couples and for the cancer patient also can be made by the nurse from the burgeoning collection of current literature on human sexuality.

Counseling conducted in a group setting with a number of cancer patients provides opportunities to explore sexual issues and problems within a context of safety and reduced feelings of self-consciousness. Patients often feel less anxious and distressed when they find that one or more of the group members also fear or have experienced the same sexual problem. The group atmosphere can assist patients to regain a sense of acceptance of their sexuality from the continued feedback the group can provide. On issues such as how to find a sex partner, group suggestions and problem-solving efforts create a supportive network for the cancer patient who is reestablishing sexual identity. Ostomate group members often help one another with helpful hints on enhancing sexual attractiveness and rekindling sexual interests. After mastectomy surgery, women can meet in a group to lend emotional support to one another. Recovered mastectomees can participate in the meeting and serve as role models for group members.

The variation in *how* the nurse develops the counseling role is endless. The need is present and continuous.

Support   As mentioned previously, providing support is an essential component of the nurse's role in cancer care. In the area of sexual dysfunction, cancer patients may need large "doses" of emotional and social support as they cope with threats to sexuality. By conveying an accepting attitude toward patients and a respect for their sexual identity, the nurse can facilitate their retention of a meaningful self-image.

Effort must be directed at maintaining standards of personal modesty and privacy for the cancer patient. Patients who are accustomed to controlling their destiny need to retain decision-making powers as much as possible within the parameters of treatment. Opportunities for undisturbed quiet time can be provided the couple who would normally have such privacy. Patients who wish to do so can be encouraged to individualize hospital rooms with personal effects and clothing as a means of maintaining gender identification. Patients of either sex should be supported in self-care efforts that reflect feelings of self-worth and attractiveness.

Evaluation

Throughout the nursing process, the nurse evaluates the accuracy of the assessment made and the effectiveness of the interventions undertaken. This evaluation process assists the nurse in preventing increase in problem intensity as well as in identifying areas of improvement. As evaluation progresses, the patient and/or couple need to receive feedback on *their* progress as it relates to the nurse's interventions. The ongoing nature of evaluation permits the nurse to retain perspective on the patient's overall condition and how it relates to sexuality.

SUMMARY COMMENT

This chapter has sought to provide an overview of the many issues related to human sexuality and the cancer patient. The topic is immense in scope and potential impact on both patient and nurse. It must not, however, be overlooked in the rush to care for and cure the disease of cancer. The *whole* patient—all systems of functioning—must be attended to.

REFERENCES

1   Harold I. Lief and Tyana Payne, "Sexuality—Knowledge and Attitudes," *American Journal of Nursing*, **75**(11):2026–2029, 1975.

2 Helen S. Kaplan, *The New Sex Therapy* (New York: Brunner/Mazel, 1974), p. 250.
3 William H. Masters and Virginia E. Johnson, *Human Sexual Inadequacy* (Boston: Little, Brown, 1970), p. 116.
4 Mildred H. Witkin, "Sex Therapy and Mastectomy," *Journal of Sexual and Marital Therapy*, 1(4), Summer 1975, p. 295.
5 Clark E. Vincent et al., "Some Marital-Sexual Concomitants of Carcinoma of the Cervix," *Southern Medical Journal*, 68(5), 1975, p. 556.
6 Barney Dlin and Abraham Perlman, "Sex after Ileostomy or Colostomy," *Medical Aspects of Human Sexuality*, 6(7):32–43, July 1972.
7 B. M. Dlin, A. Perlman, and E. Ringold, "Psychosexual Response to Ileostomy and Colostomy," *AORN Journal*, 34:77–84, November 1969.
8 R. B. Bracken and D. E. Johnson, "Sexual Function and Fecundity after Treatment for Testicular Tumors," *Urology*, 7(1):35–38, 1976.

BIBLIOGRAPHY

Allen, Andra J: "All American Sexual Myths," *American Journal of Nursing*, 75(10):1770–1771, 1975.
Annon, Jack S.: *The Behavioral Treatment of Sexual Problems: Volume 1–Brief Therapy*, Kapiolani Health Services, Honolulu, 1974.
———: *The Behavioral Treatment of Sexual Problems: Volume 2–Intensive Therapy*, Enabling Systems, Inc., Honolulu, 1975.
Barton, David: "Sexually Deprived Individuals," *Medical Aspects of Human Sexuality*, 6(2):88–97, 1972.
Binder, Donald P.: *Sex, Courtship and the Single Ostomate*, United Ostomy Association, Los Angeles, 1973.
Bracken, R. B., and Johnson, D. E.: "Sexual Function and Fecundity after Treatment for Testicular Tumors," *Urology*, 7(1):35–38, 1976.
Burnham, W. R., Lennard-Jones, J. E., and B. N. Brooke: "The Incidence and Nature of Sexual Problems among Married Ileostomists," *Gut*, 17(5):391–393, 1976.
Carey, Phyllis: "Temporary Sexual Dysfunction in Reversible Health Limitations," *Nursing Clinics of North America*, 10(3):575–586, 1975.
Elder, Mary-Scovill: "The Unmet Challenge. . . Nurse Counseling in Sexuality," *Nursing Outlook*, 18(11):38–40, 1970.
Ervin, Clinton V., Jr.: "Psychologic Adjustment to Mastectomy," *Medical Aspects of Human Sexuality*, 7(2):42–65, 1973.
Fort, Joel: "Sex and Drugs," *Postgraduate Medicine*, 58(1):133–136, July 1975.
Gambrell, Ed: *Sex and the Male Ostomate*, United Ostomy Association, Los Angeles, 1973.
Golub, Sharon: "When Your Patient's Problem Involves Sex," *RN*, 27–31, March 1975.
Grinker, Roy R. Jr.: "Sex and Cancer," *Medical Aspects of Human Sexuality*, 10(2):130–139, 1976.
Jacobson, Linbania: "Illness and Human Sexuality," *Nursing Outlook*, 22(1):50–53, 1974.
Kaplan, Helen S.: *The New Sex Therapy*, Brunner/Mazel, New York, 1974.
Kent, Saul: "Continued Sexual Activity Depends on Health and the Availability of a Partner," *Geriatrics*, 30(11):142–144, 1975.
Krizinofski, Marian T.: "Human Sexuality and Nursing Practice," *Nursing Clinics of North America*, 8(4):673–680, December 1973.

Lief, Harold I., and Tyana Payne: "Sexuality—Knowledge and Attitudes," *American Journal of Nursing,* **75**(11):2026–2029, 1975.

Malin, Joseph M., Jr.: "Sex after Urologic Surgery," *Medical Aspects of Human Sexuality,* **7**(10):245–264, 1973.

Masters, William H., and Virginia E. Johnson: *Human Sexual Inadequacy,* Little, Brown, Boston, 1970.

Norris, Carol, and Ed Gambrell: *Sex, Pregnancy and the Female Ostomate,* United Ostomy Association, Los Angeles, 1972.

Romano, Mary D.: "Sexual Counseling in Groups," *Journal of Sex Research,* **9**(1):69–78, 1973.

Sadoughi, W., Leshner, M., and H. L. Fine: "Sexual Adjustment in a Chronically Ill and Physically Disabled Population: A Pilot Study," *Archives of Physical Medicine and Rehabilitation,* **52**(7):311–317, July 1971.

Schon, Martha: "The Meaning of Death and Sex to Cancer Patients," *Journal of Sex Research,* **4**(4):288–302, 1968.

Smith, Jim, and Bonnie Bullough: "Sexuality and the Severely Disabled Person," *American Journal of Nursing,* **75**(12):2194–2197, 1975.

Vincent, Clark E., et al.: "Some Marital-Sexual Concomitants of Carcinoma of the Cervix," *Southern Medical Journal,* **68**(5):552–558, 1975.

Weinberg, Jack: "Sexuality in Later Life," *Medical Aspects of Human Sexuality,* **5**(4):216–227, 1971.

Witkin, Mildred H.: "Sex Therapy and Mastectomy," *Journal of Sexual and Marital Therapy,* **1**(4):290–304, Summer 1975.

Woods, Nancy F., and James S. Woods: *Human Sexuality in Health and Illness,* C. V. Mosby, St. Louis, 1975.

Yahle, Margaret-Ellen: "An Ostomy Information Clinic," *Nursing Clinics of North America,* **11**(3):457–467, 1975.

Yeaworth, Rosalee C., and Joyce S. Friedeman: "Sexuality in Later Life," *Nursing Clinics of North America,* **10**(3):565–574, 1975.

Chapter 14

Living until Death: Caring for the Dying Cancer Patient

Pamela K. Burkhalter

I've had a long, hard-working life. I just want to die now. No more of this chemotherapy or radium implants. I just can't take it anymore. . . . Every effort is painful—to talk, to swallow, to move. Just to be comfortable and at peace. . . . I'm not afraid of death; I want the release it offers.

Death, dying, and cancer often are thought of as a dreaded, tragic triumverate. Yet the patient quoted above has a somewhat different viewpoint. This 70-year-old lady with metastatic carcinoma of the bowel had made several crucial decisions that coincided with her avowed desire to die peacefully while controlling the manner of her death. She had clearly stated her refusal of further palliative therapy. Should bowel obstruction again occur, she would consent to surgical intervention designed to make her more comfortable during her dying process. She very competently made these decisions, and she experienced a great deal of grief as she did so.

Not all cancer patients with terminal disease are able or willing to make such life-controlling decisions. Many patients choose to overtly or covertly relegate such responsibility to the physician, nurse, or other care giver. And this choice to determine how one wishes to die or to seek assistance in deciding from others needs to be acknowledged and honored by those committed to adding quality and meaning to the life of the dying person. The purpose of this chapter, then, is to explore some of the crucial facets of caring for the dying cancer patient.

ATTITUDES AND THE DYING CANCER PATIENT

Nurse Attitudes toward Death

When the nurse is confronted with the challenge of caring for the cancer patient, many considerations about the hows, wheres, and whys of the disease and its victim arise. It seems to be a truism that "cancer not only implies death to most people, it symbolizes a manner and style of expected life toward death, and a death while in life."[1] The nurse is not immune to experiencing fear, frustration, and/or fatalism when confronted with the awesome task of accompanying a cancer patient on the path toward death. In many ways, the nursing care designed and administered to the terminally ill cancer patient can smooth the path, leave it untouched, or roughen it. It truly can be an overwhelming undertaking when viewed in this light.

Although demanding of the nurse's resources, working with dying cancer patients *does* provide numerous opportunities for personal growth and development of self-awareness and sensitivity. Each instance of caring not only provides an opportunity to facilitate the nurse's personal growth, but by virtue of the emotional investment required, also allows the patient to experience closeness and psychological intimacy during a time that is potentially lonesome and fearful.

Patient Attitudes toward Death

The manner in which a terminally ill cancer patient evaluates the situation and responds to it will be directly influenced by his or her attitudes toward death. In turn, attitudes are modified by the course of the illness, personal experiences, and environmental influences. While some patients may never be formally told that the disease process has become uncontrollable or incurable, most cancer patients do receive either direct or indirect information on their prognosis. As the patient integrates the information, many *fears* may come to the fore which are reflective of attitudes toward the process of dying and the event of death. Patients may or may not experience all of these fears, and those who do experience them in varying degrees of intensity.

Fears *Fear of Aloneness* Cancer patients very often will express a fear of being alone or deserted at the time of death. For some, the refusal of sedation or analgesia stems from this fear of not knowing when death may arrive and, concomitantly, not wanting to be alone should the end of life occur. Fear of loneliness is related to the fear of the unknown. . . . What lies beyond this existence, or what doesn't lie beyond the border between life and death? Many people evidence great apprehension about this unknown aspect of life.

The fear of aloneness is also associated with fears of abandonment, of being left alone by significant others. Abandonment may be experienced when interpersonal contact ceases as well as when the patient no longer is able to have a pet or valued objects near by. Because most people live their lives in close proximity to others, the prospect of death faced alone can indeed be fearful and, consequently, anxiety-provoking.

Cancer patients may express the fear of aloneness verbally or in covert, nonverbal ways. Some patients reverse lifelong sleep patterns such that sleep takes place during the daytime. At night they may seek attention and companionship by talking with the nursing staff. Unfortunately, such patients may acquire the label "bothers" or merely "attention seekers"—both terms connoting a negative evaluation of behavior. Yet for this dying person, interpersonal contact (even that considered to be negative) with the staff at night decreases the aloneness and the risk of dying at night . . . alone.

Other patients may refuse sleeping medication for similar reasons. Although continuous sleep through to the morning is sacrificed, the patients' awakenings or stirrings allows them to reaffirm their aliveness during the night. And in a sense, for the patient's peace of mind, this behavior ensures more frequent checks by nursing personnel in response to interrupted sleep.

Not all terminally ill cancer patients acknowledge or become consciously aware of the fear of aloneness at death. Many adhere to religious or philosophical tenents that describe the event of death as a pathway to other, more peaceful and desirious states of being. As a consequence, whether one is alone or in the company of others has no relevance to the crossing from life to death.

Still other patients express a desire *to be alone* when death comes. They may fear the aloneness, but express greater fear of others viewing their death. Patients have expressed sentiments such as "I want my husband to remember me as I am now, not what I'll look like when I'm dead." For cultural reasons, in addition, some patients will have specific preferences for company or seclusion when death takes place.

Fear of Powerlessness   People tend to possess ambivalent attitudes toward self-power, or the ability to control one's destiny. With reference to death, one study reported that more than two-thirds of the male and one-third of the female respondents wanted to die suddenly or unexpectedly when the time came.[2] All were healthy at the time of survey. These results are interesting in view of the continuing efforts made to *increase* control over natural events. A paradox exists, and several questions arise as a result.

Much of what leads to death is currently under the control of medical science. Yet for at least some people, the preference is for a sudden, unprolonged death when that portion of life's continuuum is reached. As control over death in general increases, control over one's own death seems to have decreased. The result: a feeling of powerlessness. For the dying cancer patient, the conflict is exacerbated. This person is near the end of the continuum and may express several viewpoints, e.g., (1) a desire to live as long as possible, making full use of medical technology, (2) a wish for a sudden, nonpainful demise, or (3) a desire to determine the time of death or to decide when intervention is no longer wanted.

The questions that arise can indeed be challenging to care givers. How much power *does* the patient have to determine his or her destiny? When should the patient assume or continue to participate in decision making about death? What, if any, limits should be imposed on the patient's power of self-determination? For most care givers, answers to these questions·can be formulated only on an individual basis taking into account each patient's needs and emotional status. And most likely, that is the most philosophically sound way to approach this problem.

At the bottom line, the dying cancer patient may be fearful of losing power over death, while at the same time knowing at a rational level that power over death was not an option that could be exercised for an indefinite period of time. This fear of powerlessness, then, may result in a self-reinforcing cycle of anxiety and fear; i.e., as fear of one's powerlessness is recognized, anxiety arises. Anxiety leads to discomfort and acknowledgment of one's mortality, which in turn may foster fear of death. And the cycle repeats.

These fears of powerlessness may be manifested by resistance to change. Patients may refuse to enter the hospital to die and thereby exercise control over where the event will take place. At the same time they control who will be nearby when death takes place by insisting on remaining at home. Refusal to adhere to treatment protocols is another means of exercising one's power and thereby reducing fear. The gamble the patient takes is generally considered in making such a decision; i.e., while retaining power, one also may hasten the event one tries to control.

Fear of Dependence   Attitudes toward death also are influenced by fear of dependence. As a highly valued social more, independence is exercised by people in innumerable ways ranging from far-reaching economic decision making to determining where one will bathe. As a person enters a terminal, or ending, phase of life, however, fear of losing this independence may loom. For example, a patient who has determined how his or her bowels will be moved finds that suddenly he or she no longer can control this. The colostomy changes the method and means. Because the person is weakened following surgery and is "connected" to IVs, oxygen equipment, or nasal gastric tubes, the patient must depend on others to ensure proper bowel evacuation.

Fear of dependence on others for physical need fulfillment is common among dying cancer patients. As independence is relinquished or divested from the patient, helplessness may fill the gap. Patients of all ages may rebel and express anger, resentment, and frustration. The mind continues to realize that independent functioning is the desired mode, but the body often cannot comply. Frequently cancer patients become depressed in response to loss of independence and the fear of dependence that is implied.

When a cancer patient knows she or he is to die within a short period of time, concern about death can become masked by the fear of dependence on others. It may take the form of fear of depending on care givers to determine when, how, and where death comes. It must be realized clearly that this fear often is justified—patients *do* depend on nurses, physicians, and others to determine need fulfillment. The question becomes, To what *extent* need a cancer patient depend on others? and To what extent can the cancer patient monitor the level of dependence he or she experiences?

Hopes   Attitudes toward death are shaped by the patient's hopes as well as fears. Hope represents the person's life for the future. A patient who has no future has no hope. How "future" is defined, therefore, becomes crucial. For those who confine the future to "life continued in the same fashion," a terminal prognosis may indeed demolish hope. Those, however who define future in a more limited or religious-philosophical framework may continue to be hopeful up to and including the time of death. Hope, then forms the basis for a positive or accepting attitude toward death. Loss of hope, conversely, would seem to imply an abandonment of life.

Belief in an afterlife fosters hope for a future, albeit an unknown future. Cancer patients with religious belief support systems often express reduced fear or absence of fear of death. The hope for a pain-free, peaceful existence assists them in facing death without fear. Of importance, however, is the fact that persons with no avowed religious beliefs can also experience a hopeful attitude toward death as a path to new experiences.

Patients who use denial as a means of coping with the fear of death are, in a sense, engineering the maintenance of hope. Logically, if one denies death, a future remains, and consequently there is hope for that future. Thus, denial need not be maladaptive under certain circumstances. (Denial as a coping strategy is discussed below.)

Dying cancer patients' attitudes toward death are not completely characterized by fears on one hand and hopes on the other. As with any person, societal values and belief systems about death influence cancer patients' attitudes on death. As society has become more open to discussing the issues surrounding death, so have fatally ill patients begun to express attitudes on their approaching death.

In addition to the two major attitudes discussed, there is the one of *wonderment* and *awe*. Death is viewed as one phase of a life cycle that is never-ending and self-rejuvenating. As one human ends one part of the cycle, a new human begins another. The energy that is human spirit thereby continuously cycles throughout time. This philosophical stance fosters a positive attitude toward death by emphasizing the endlessness of life, not the finality of death.

Social mores also are emphasizing a more open attitude toward discussion of death in general. Over the past decade, a plethora of books, movies, articles, and conferences have been presented devoted exclusively to increasing society's awareness of death and the issues associated with it. Cancer patients, as members of the society, therefore may also reflect these more open attitudes.

In caring for the dying cancer patient, nurses *must* become aware of the attitudes toward death possessed by their patients. It is these attitudes, and the belief systems and thought processes related to them, that shape the patient's responses to the illness. How the patient copes with the dying process will, in large part, be determined by general attitudes toward death as well as each person's unique attitudes toward it.

THE DYING PROCESS

Each person begins to die from the moment of birth. Yet the dying state or process is more clearly and acceptably attributed to the patient with an identified illness, such as cancer. This person's dying trajectory, or path to death, is defined as being shorter than the care giver's. For many cancer patients, the process of dying gives rise to more anxiety and fear than does the last phase of the process, death. It is *getting* to death that creates an entirely new set of experiences for which very few people are prepared. Each patient must rely on previously devised coping strategies that often are inadequate under the new conditions of dying.

Telling

As a cancer patient's disease reaches an incurable state, because of widespread metastasis or inoperable location, for example, the label "dying" or "terminally ill" is placed on the patient. Before this point is reached, there have been many opportunities to inform the patient of the diagnosis and prognosis. How the patient responds to treatment and the dying state will in large part be determined by the information possessed about the illness.

Telling the patient the diagnosis and prognosis legally falls into the physician's realm of responsibility. Often nurses, family, and friends of the patient become involved in the telling or not telling situation. For various reasons, those who have influence over the patient's life may decide that the patient should not be informed of the diagnosis or prognosis. As a result, a closed awareness context is created in which the patient is unaware of her or his condition while those caring for her or him are fully informed. Many health professionals question whether a closed awareness context can truly exist. Patients, it is argued, can see deterioration of physical capacities and can detect care givers' changes in attitude toward them. Nonverbal, covertly delivered messages about the truth can be conveyed while words are never spoken. Yet the patient seems to *know* she or he is dying. In those situations in which the body does not deteriorate visibly and in which severe pain is not present, it is possible that the dying cancer patient may not know that a terminal phase of life has begun.

Under these circumstances, an ethical issue arises: Should every cancer patient be told the diagnosis and prognosis of the disease? While many nurses and other care givers believe the patient *must* be informed, others hold opposing opinions. The American Hospital Association has clearly stated the patient's *right* to know diagnosis, treatment, and prognosis "in terms the patient can be reasonably expected to understand."[3] (See Appendix, "A Patient's Bill of Rights.") Herein lies the most reasonable course in telling. Each cancer patient indeed has a right to obtain information about the course of her or his life. How, when, and by whom the information is delivered, however, is subject to careful manipulation by those responsible for care. The patient can receive information in a number of ways:

1 At the time of diagnosis, the physician may choose to fully inform the patient and/or family of the nature of the illness as well as the proposed treatment plan.

2 At the time of treatment initiation, the patient may be informed as part of

the informed consent procedure. Here the "teller" has some latitude in determining the *extent* and *depth* of information provided.

3   The physician or other designated teller may give the patient *doses* of information over the full course of diagnosis and treatment. Thus, at each phase of intervention, the patient learns more about the progress of the disease.

4   The patient may "put the pieces together" herself or himself and arrive at a diagnosis and prognosis. Here the patient may not seek information from the physician, but chooses to find out on her or his own. The patient may then seek verification of the information from care givers.

5   As the patient initiates information-seeking behavior, the physician, nurse, or other person answers truthfully.

6   The patient makes comparisons between herself or himself and other patients or people who have had the disease. In addition, the patient may draw inferences about the body changes taking place or simply observe the behavior of self and others. Each method provides information on the dying process.

In either case, the informing or telling that takes place must be accomplished in such a way that *hope is retained*. While no guarantee can be given that cure is possible, the truth *can* be anchored in realistic, probable outcomes. For example, pain control and management becomes a realistic goal when the patient is dying. Telling the patient that the prognosis is grave *and* that all effort will be directed toward ensuring quality of living is a means of retaining hope.

At any point, the dying cancer patient can exercise the option of rejecting the information presented. For many, this self-monitoring process coincides with the person's individual tolerance for knowing that death is approaching. Fears about death and the manner of dying feed into the decision to accept or reject information.

In determining whether the patient should be told the diagnosis and/or prognosis, care givers, whether nurses, physicians, or family members, formulate a number of assumptions. From these assumptions, it is possible to hypothesize patient responses and interventions that may be necessary. As depicted in Figure 14-1, the patient and family need support whether or not the patient is informed. The patient may overtly or covertly convey a desire to know or not know the information. Patients who at one time reject the information may at another time need it. It is necessary, therefore, for the nurse to support the patient's need not to know while at the same time continuing to convey a readiness to talk when the patient is ready to hear the message. Of interest is the impact that the assumptions may have on determining the patient's access to an *opportunity* to cope with the "terminal" information. The decision makers, health professionals and family members, assume that the patient *wants* to live longer. Yet this assumption seldom is validated with the patient. It takes the form of a projection on the patient of what the healthy ones would want if they were dying. In viewing the flow diagram in Figure 14-1, it becomes imperative that the patient's decision makers consider the following: "So often people are just not protected from the truth that you think you are protecting them from; they are left alone with it instead."[4]

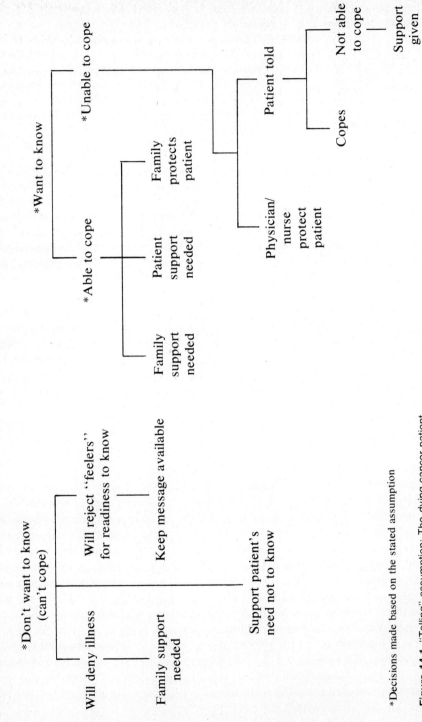

DIAGNOSIS AND/OR PROGNOSIS

*Don't want to know (can't cope)

Will reject "feelers" for readiness to know

Keep message available

Will deny illness

Family support needed

Support patient's need not to know

*Want to know

*Able to cope

Family support needed

Patient support needed

Family protects patient

*Unable to cope

Physician/nurse protect patient

Patient told

Copes

Not able to cope

Support given

*Decisions made based on the stated assumption

Figure 14-1 "Telling" assumption: The dying cancer patient.

282

In formulating assumptions about whether to tell or not tell a dying cancer patient the diagnosis or prognosis, the care giver must carefully evaluate the basis for the assumptions. The assumptions need to be validated or denied by communication with the patient. After all, the dying person *is* the one who is the center of the dying process. In some way, this person must become part of the decision-making process that concerns her or his very existence.

Coping Strategies

The dying cancer patient seeks to generate a coping strategy at the time of diagnosis and may modify it during the course of the illness. The strategy, or plan for coping with a new life experience or crisis, is subject to the influences of care givers, family treatments, and the response to intervention efforts. At certain times, the patient needs supportive assistance in continuing to cope. In itself, help seeking *is* a strategy and should be recognized as such. In other words, whatever the patient does in response to the dying state can be considered a coping strategy. Some strategies, however, are maladaptive: they aggravate rather than ameliorate the dying person's suffering. When this occurs, nursing interventions are designed to promote and facilitate the development of adaptive coping responses.

Coping strategies parallel the dying process; they represent the cancer patient's method of living until death. The strategies to be discussed are not mutually exclusive. Each is intertwined and interdependent upon the other. Some strategies are reflective of specific models, such as that presented by Elisabeth Kübler-Ross[5] and that of Weisman and Hackett.[6] While some patients may follow a sequence of five stages (denial and isolation, anger, bargaining, depression, acceptance) or three stages (reduced alternative, middle knowledge, countercontrol and cessation), respectively, others follow no identifiable progression. Skill in correctly identifying the stage the dying person has entered is extremely difficult when clear boundaries do not exist. As a result, the strategies discussed here are representative of landmarks that the nurse can identify while caring for a dying person. With identification of the patient's current experience, the nurse can intervene without labeling the patient or placing the person on a continuum she or he may not fit.

Seeking Self-Awareness   The dying cancer patient may cope with dying and death by seeking self-awareness or by being open to efforts to foster self-awareness. By developing an intense understanding of the feelings generated by dying, the person is able to decrease the amount of energy devoted to suppressing such insight. As the patient becomes sensitive to the dying experience and *acknowledges* the feelings, the person may begin to experience an enhanced sense of the worthiness, meaningfulness, or purposefulness of life. For some dying cancer patients, development of self-awareness and a heightened sensitivity to inner feelings may come about as opportunities for open, nonjudgmental discussion are provided by the nurse, chaplain, or physician. In these sessions, the nurse actively listens to the patient and acts as a counselor in problem-solving situations.

Development of self-awareness, however, does not preclude the appearance of depression, anger, or other feelings. It does help the patient get in touch with what is taking place; it fosters growth in dying. Patients who seek self-awareness generally are open to others; they are able to talk about life as well as death; they are more easily able to *be* a part of life while dying. It is essential that the nurse caring for the cancer patient who seeks self-awareness also seek such personal growth.

The nurse who seeks self-awareness in relation to feelings toward death and dying encounters new experiences of emotional intensity. The nurse participating actively in seminars, conferences, or classes devoted to self-awareness or personal growth at the same time becomes better able to relate to the dying person. Although the patient may not be at the same point of growth as is the nurse, the nurse is able to facilitate patient awareness when feeling comfortable and secure in her or his own level of development and sensitivity. Of course, many patients may never reach a stage of self-awareness in dying. And many nurses may choose not to enter this demanding and intense area of personal relationships. However, for those that do choose to struggle through personal fears concerning their own mortality, the rewards are immeasurably valuable to the dying patients cared for. These dying cancer patients will have an opportunity to share their dying experience while savoring the joys, pains, and gifts of each day of life.

Seeking Self-Protection As nurses learn during early educational experiences in nursing, self-protecting responses represent methods of defending oneself from stresses, whether internally or externally generated. Regardless of the psychodynamic model espoused, comprehension of the purpose of self-protecting mechanisms allows the nurse to pinpoint patient behaviors that may be maladaptive. It must be remembered that use of these mechanisms is common to all people in varying degrees and is not exclusively related to psychopathology. These responses constitute a primary coping strategy for the dying cancer patient.

Denial Cancer patients frequently go through a stage of denying the diagnosis either when first perceiving a physical malfunction or abnormality or when learning of the disease's presence from a physician. After the person enters a dying trajectory, maintenance of denial becomes more difficult as deterioration becomes inescapably obvious. Inspite of the facts, the patient may *need* to deny the inevitable—death. Acknowledgment of one's fast-approaching death when unresolved fears are looming may not be possible for some patients. In these cases, the nurse seeks to support the patient's denial in a neutral fashion, neither encouraging nor discouraging its continuation. When the patient indicates a desire to move away from denial by such actions as questioning the effectiveness of treatment, the nurse will be in a position to offer support for other emotional states.

Maintenance of denial throughout the course of illness may be maladaptive in that the patient also denies a need to deal with problems related to the disease. By denying dying, the patient sees no need to make out a will, settle business or employment affairs, or make plans for care of children or a spouse. Family members can react with anger toward the patient who denies the need to attend to such affairs, but seldom will force the patient to do so. As a result, family and care givers actively support the denial at a time when a more constructive approach is warranted. Dying patients who are denying in a maladaptive fashion can benefit from counseling focused on urging recognition of their condition. Again, as denial is reduced the patient continues to need hope. There must be a realistic expectation that hope exists for pain relief, comfort, dignity, and a sense of worthiness in simply living each day.

The positive aspect of denial of dying is in the strength to *resist* death that it can engender. By denying death, the cancer patient is able to actively cooperate in treatment protocols, to be optimistic in considering prognosis, and to exude a sense of strength—though often tenuous—to those around. Within this denial, however, lies a burden and dilemma for the patient: should the denial cease, the position of strength may diminish, leaving the person vulnerable to her or his fears. Here again, the nurse can assist the dying cancer patient to acknowledge the role denial has played while at the same time fostering awareness of feelings. In such an open context, the dying person can achieve personal growth through the dying experience.

Denial, then, may represent a positive or negative source of self-protection for the dying cancer patient. Throughout the illness the patient may adhere to denial as the primary coping strategy, or it may be used on a temporary basis. In either case, the nurse attempts to support the patient in coping with the ultimate threat to life.

Regression Cancer patients often regress as they enter the terminal phase of life. The person's life space is reduced and contracted in terms of interests and concerns. Daily activities assume greater relevance than extended future planning. Life in the future focuses on tomorrow or this week. For some patients, hours assume major significance in terms of planning or anticipating daily events. Regression to simpler times, interests, and concerns allows the patient to savor the less complex aspects of daily life: room arrangements, visits, meals, routines of self-care. For these patients, disruption or failure to adhere to what seem to be basic, uninteresting daily activities can represent a serious loss to the person.

With narrowing of the patient's perceptions and areas of interest, planned activities involving reexpansion of the patient's world to previously encompassed activities may be rejected by the patient. Nurses and family members, therefore, who project onto the patient needs for "usual" sources of stimulation may find that these overtures are ignored, passively accepted, or overtly refused by the dying person. As a consequence, care givers should carefully determine what the *patient's* desires are before attempting to impose experiences on the patient.

Patients who use regression as a self-protecting response to threat need not become childlike in behavior or consistently constrict their life space and interests. Many dying cancer patients regress on a periodic basis in conjunction with the ups and downs of treatments, the sense of physical well-being or painfulness, or the responses of significant others to the dying process. Regression serves as an adaptive strategy for patients who can and wish to enjoy and savor the intensity of a more circumscribed daily life. It becomes maladaptive when used exclusively and prematurely, thereby preventing a fuller enjoyment and participation in valued experiences.

Withdrawal   After learning that the prognosis is grave, the dying cancer patient may withdraw from interpersonal relationships, social contacts, career interactions, or life in general. Withdrawal can be adaptive by providing time for the person to focus on introspection, sorting things out unhindered by external demands. As a short-term means of maintaining one's sense of inner privacy, withdrawal can be a positive coping strategy. However, as a primary means of responding to stress, it is generally associated with depression, an intense feeling of sadness and loss. Withdrawal from interpersonal contact may isolate the patient at a time when maintenance of intimacy is crucial. Family or care givers who experience this form of rejection by the patient may not understand the meaning of the behavior.

The person who withdraws is unwilling or perhaps unable at that moment, to cope with the meaning and implications of dying. By pulling out, she or he does not face the problems for a time. Dying cancer patients tend to seek reestablishment of valued intimacies as they are able to reconcile the realities of their situation. Nurses, physicians, and family members who are aware of the patient's need to receive nonacknowledged support will maintain feelings of affection, love, and intimacy that the patient is temporarily unable to reciprocate. When the patient no longer needs to withdraw or has been helped by care givers to relinquish the behavior, the person will again need to experience interpersonal closeness or contact.

Anger   Dying cancer patients may at times cope by expressing and experiencing anger: anger at fate, at the betrayal of their body, at others who are healthy, at themselves for past behaviors currently reevaluated as detrimental. Anger is considered to be an intense emotional experience with negative overtones and is described as an unpleasant state of emotional arousal. During the dying process, most cancer patients experience a phase of anger that can range from intense rage externally directed to mild expression of dissatisfaction. Behaviorally, the person may verbalize the emotions to others. The person may strike out at other persons or at the environment with argument, rejection of assistance, or withdrawal from interpersonal relationships. For some patients, the very miracles of modern medicine that enable them to delay death through technological expertise become the actions at which anger is directed. Each innovation in treatment stimulates hope for cure or delay of death; each failure of treatment to achieve the goal stimulates despair and, sometimes, anger and frustration. The frustration experienced by the dying patient can be translated into anger: "Why isn't there a cure for *me*?" "If man can conquer space, why can't he conquer cancer?" The "why" questions asked by the dying patient are expressions of anger and despair.

As a coping strategy, anger often is viewed as maladaptive in that its expression frequently is misunderstood by family members and care givers; it can alienate those the patient may need for emotional support at a later time. Anger can be masked by other behaviors that may or may not be viewed in a positive or negative light by the patient or others. For example, the newly diagnosed patient with lung cancer defiantly refuses to stop smoking cigarettes. By continuing to smoke, the patient expresses anger and denial of any responsibility for the present condition. Other angry patients give vent to the emotion in a more passive way. The pleasant, seemingly cooperative patient with liver metastasis carefully attends to fluid-restriction instructions provided by the nurse. In response to questions designed to determine comprehension of the treatment, the patient correctly and accurately repeats the information given. A short time later, however, the patient is found at a distant drinking fountain consuming fluid in an unrestrained manner. When queried as to the reason for the detrimental behavior, the patient innocently states, "I didn't think *water* would hurt my liver." Here the patient clearly may be expressing pent-up anger and rage at a restriction felt by the patient to be unjust and symbolizing loss of control and of basic decision-making power. However, the nurse should ascertain, again, what the patient's understanding is of the treatment.

Anger can function like denial: it can stimulate defensive behaviors against a threat—death. While anger in this context is adaptive, it can truly sap the patient's strength and energy resources and serve to isolate the person from loved ones. Dying people who are angry, however, have a just reason to feel as they do. When viewed from the patient's perspective, it is reasonable and appropriate that the person experience anger, and even rage, at what is taking place.

Searching

At the time of diagnosis or before, the cancer patient begins the search for the "proper way" to respond to the illness. During treatment, the patient takes on the sick role and can usually quickly learn the rules and expectations of hospital care. When the person enters a dying trajectory, however, she or he often does not know the proper way of dying. The search for this "way" can take many forms and tends to be conducted in an unobtrusive manner by the patient.

How *does* the patient learn how to die? Past experience(s) with the dying and death of a relative or friend can provide some guidelines for socially acceptable behavior. The manner in which the person copes with dying, whether at home or in an institutional setting, can be examined and evaluated by the dying patient in an attempt to find a way that best suits the patient's own personality and values. The patient also can learn from the past experience what was *not* acceptable or which behaviors failed to bring peace and comfort to the dying person or family members.

A second way to search for the right way to die is composed of the idealized versions of dying presented in the media—books, movies, television. These sources of information reflect the pain, agony, and ugliness that characterize death in many contexts as well as an idealized, romanticized version of dying. From these often fictionalized accounts, the patient also gleans information about behaviors that may be used during the dying process.

Cultures tend to prescribe the acceptable behaviors for major life crises and events. Thus, the culture provides a third way for a patient to know how to die. Within a culture, religious belief systems may further specify behavior patterns to be followed at various times on the life/death continuum. These cultural expectations serve an extremely useful function by providing the dying person with a set of values and beliefs that can assist in determining behavior during the dying process. For this reason, the nurse should carefully evaluate the cultural heritage of the dying cancer patient as one means of determining how the patient will cope with dying.

A fourth method of searching for the way to die involves the day-to-day exchanges between the patient and the immediate environment. Each instance of verbal and nonverbal communication between patient and family, patient and nurse, or patient and other patients creates a situation in which the dying person learns what behaviors are and will continue to be acceptable "dying" behaviors. The patient learns which requests will be labeled legitimate or exaggerated by the type of response received from care givers. For example, the presence of pain and the way the patient seeks pain relief measures will often become a central focus of interchange between patient and nurse. Each time the patient makes a request for pain relief, she or he can evaluate the manner in which it is fulfilled. If it takes a seemingly long time to fulfill, the patient may surmise that the request, its frequency, or its delivery was unacceptable. Thereafter, the patient may "test out" other request strategies to determine the most effective and mutually acceptable one. This process, when it occurs, generally takes place at an unconscious level; i.e., the patient does not preplan specific approaches. When pain relief requests are quickly fulfilled, the patient may assume that the behavior is appropriate and meets one of the care giver's expectations. Such a trial-and-error process most likely takes place throughout the dying patient's illness career. Through these exchanges, the patient receives hints as to how dying people are expected to behave. During this process, however, the patient can experience frustration and uncertainty.

For the dying cancer patient, the search for the way to die represents a struggle to cope with the reality or unreality of the minute-by-minute situation. Having never experienced the dying process, the patient is thrust into uncharted territory of emotional upheaval. Never before or ever again will the person be so taxed to learn how to *be*. Ideally the patient *can* learn, by making use of inner resources and/or by accepting help from others to integrate a manner of dying into the "style, meaning, and sequence of that which has gone before."[7] To accomplish this must become a goal of the nurse who cares for the dying cancer patient.

Grieving

The cancer patient who knows she or he is dying experiences grief in relation to the anticipated and actual losses that will and have occured. "Grieving" consists of the process of coming to terms with loss, of letting go of the lost person or thing, and of resolving the feelings aroused by the loss experience. It is a basic life process: each person grieves at various times in life. For some people, the loss of a patient constitutes the initial experience with grieving. For others, loss of status due to job change, unemployment, or retirement fosters the beginning of grief work. The mother who has delivered a healthy baby experiences the loss of the fetus from the womb. There probably is no facet of living that is exempt from the loss experience—and the dying process is no exception.

Over time, the dying person may spend large portions of each day considering the losses that are occurring. Not only does the patient lose health, independence, and control over one's destiny, but the person also experiences loss of self as she or he knows it to be. In addition, whereas the family will lose the patient—someone loved and valued—the *patient* will lose everything: family, friends, pets, views of nature, waking up in the morning, feeling the warmth of sunshine, etc. The patient's anticipated losses are immense in number when compared with those of surviving family and friends. It is vitally important that nurses keep this perspective in mind when interacting with grieving family members. The focus should be on the patient and how the patient's grief work is progressing.

Separation Gaining insight into the physiological aspects of the terminal condition, the cancer patient at the same time is or will become aware of separation in many contexts. For some patients a psychological separation begins in which the patient emotionally dissociates herself or himself from the body when not in pain. In these cases, the patient becomes unconcerned with physical care and focuses on the inner world of memory and critical evaluation of past life experiences. Because part of the grieving process involves a breaking of ties with past, present, and future experiences, this evaluation of one's life forms one step in the sequence. No longer does the patient *need* to concentrate on righting past wrongs or be obsessed about what happened long ago. At this point, one can consider one's life and its accomplishments, determine whether one is satisfied or not with the life led, and begin to say goodbye to these memories. This detaching process allows the patient to bring closure to different parts of her or his being and identity. As this emotional work progresses, the patient can reduce the energy expended in maintaining these ties.

Separation from people in the patient's life also takes place. Frequently, as the patient's physical condition deteriorates and the patient nears an acceptance of death, the person ceases to want many visitors or contacts with family. In her or his own way, the patient has said goodbye to each person and no longer *needs* to see them. For family and friends, this termination by the patient can be extremely painful and upsetting. Yet from the patient's point of view, she or he has acknowledged, dealt with, and accepted the loss of these relationships. The patient's world is contracting into an ever-narrowing sphere of interest in preparation for the final separation from life.

Depression   Each person at various times in life can become depressed for reasons ranging from sadness for a specific loss, to hormonal cycles, to serious emotional dysfunctions. The depressed person's interests narrow, the ability to attend to others or activities is reduced, the person tires easily or experiences lethargy, and/or there is a tendency to withdraw from usual interpersonal relationships.

Depression is a lonely, isolating experience that often is misinterpreted by care givers. At times, there is a tendency on the part of the nurse, for example, to hesitate to interrupt or disturb the depressed person; e.g., "She seems so peaceful and relaxed." This *assumption* may reflect the nurse's feeling of insecurity or inadequacy in being able to relate comfortably to the depressed person's experience, i.e., to what might be said or acted out. From the dying person's point of view, however, it is sometimes essential that the nurse go beyond personal hesitancy to be *with* the patient, to acknowledge the sadness experienced by the patient and that which is aroused in the nurse.

The dying cancer patient will seldom state, "I'm depressed." More generally, the patient will express depression in overt behaviors such as decrease in talking, sleep disturbances, decrease or increase in appetite, decreased self-care, and lack of interest in surroundings. Basically, the usual expected behavioral patterns become depressed or reduced in frequency. Covert expressions of depression can consist of somaticizing emotional concerns into physical symptomatology such as headaches, backaches, upset stomach. In addition, the patient may behave in ways uncharacteristic of usual behavior, e.g., sleeping 12 hours a day, becoming compulsive about routines, or being unable to enjoy or follow the events in a favorite television program.

The person who is dying may experience depression in varying degrees of intensity, frequency, and duration. At the time of diagnosis or confirmation of a terminal prognosis, the person may become withdrawn and sorrowful while attempting to cope with the information. This episode may last a few hours, days, or weeks, or it can constitute a continuing pattern that will be maintained throughout the dying process. When depression is continuous, it acts as a barrier against the emotional growth that leads to a sense of wholeness and satisfaction with one's self-worth. By retaining a depressed emotional state, the dying person holds at bay this opportunity to savor each moment of life.

Patient depressive episodes that are short-lived should be anticipated by the nurse caring for the dying person. Feelings of sadness, quietness, and sorrow are associated with the self-grieving process, termination of relationships with loved ones, and the ups and downs of the treatment sequence for cancer. At times, the drugs administered for cancer treatment can facilitate the development of depression caused by negative side effects due to the action of these drugs on the body. Sometimes the patient can slip in and out of mild depression each day.

Because depression is generally considered to be an aversive emotional response, the depressed dying person may deny the experience when queried as to its presence or absence. It thus is important to remember that part of depressive behavior can include a superficial rejection of help at the very instance when the person deeply *needs* to be cared for. The depressed cancer patient may unknowingly create a self-perpetuating cycle in which assistance is refused overtly and refusal is complied with by care givers. As a result, the patient is further isolated with the depression. Interrupting this potentially harmful cycle represents a major area of intervention to be discussed below.

Certain patients present a "normal" behavioral appearance when interacting with others but retreat into overt depression when this mask is not required. Here the patient seeks to prevent others from being touched by the profound sorrow and sadness that is experienced. At the same time, the family, friends, and care givers may wear their own normal face masks to prevent the patient from becoming aware of their grief. Thus, a mutual game of "hide the real emotion from the other" gets played. The potential for harm to both parties is great. The energy expended in maintaining these facades could more effectively be channeled into open sharing and mutual support in a time of crisis.

Although the ethical, legal, and moral issues surrounding the termination of one's own life, or suicide, have not been settled with reference to the dying cancer patient, the possibility that such an attempt may be made by the depressed patient must be carefully evaluated by care givers. A profoundly depressed person who is aware of the terminal nature of the disease may choose to actively end life. Whether this action or option should be sanctioned or not will most likely be determined in the court system. Until that time, care givers will continue to experience a "tightrope" kind of position on the patient's right or lack of right to passively or actively end life.

During the dying process, depression may be a transient or continuous experience for the patient. To the extent that this emotional response reduces the dying patient's quality of life, it may become the focus of concentrated intervention efforts to alleviate its impact. As a short-term response, depression during the dying process can be anticipated and planned for so that when and if it does appear, the nurse can be prepared to recognize the behavior and offer meaningful support.

Sensitivities and Fears   In grieving for oneself, the cancer patient often takes into consideration what and who will be left behind, i.e., what the patient's legacy will consist of. In addition, the patient generally will take steps to ensure that the valued persons, objects, and/or pets will be adequately cared for after the patient's death. This sensitivity by the patient to consider and plan for the needs of others may reflect a need to safeguard the person's achievements. As such, these protective actions ensure a continued survival of portions of the patient's life and values; i.e., the patient can continue to live on in a philosophical sense through the continued life of others or the continued use of valued objects.

Many dying cancer patients develop an acute appreciation for the seemingly least significant aspects of daily living, those events and things that tend to be taken for granted when one is healthy. This savoring of life's simple treasures may extend to the finest nuances of vision, taste, color, smell, and touch. In a sense, the daily activities of living acquire a higher, more intense valence for the person who has realized that life as it is known is coming to an end. Concurrently, the dying person may appear to evolve a decreased sensitivity to the less enjoyable aspects of life and interpersonal relationships, e.g., arguments, manipulation of others. In these cases, the patient seems to *choose* where energy will be invested and enjoyed. It is at these times that the nurse sees the dying patient in a more calm, peaceful, and relaxed attitude toward life.

Grieving for one's own impending loss of life can also be accompanied by fears—fears of what will happen after death, to other persons loved by the patient, or to one's job or business or what will take place in treatment and care up to the time of death. The unknown aspect of each of these future events can foster anxiety as well as fear. For some people, a belief in an afterlife assists in reducing fear. However, religious or philosophical belief does not preclude feelings such as those expressed by Mrs. C.:

> I know I said before that I wasn't afraid to die . . . but . . . I . . . *am* afraid . . . now. I don't want to go to sleep at night. . . . I might not wake up. I'm so afraid to die, to be alone dying.

As this dying cancer patient related these feelings, she visibly shook and hyperventilated. She had been quite philosophical several weeks earlier as the treatment course and prognosis were discussed. With the onset of complications that precluded the administration of chemotherapy, however, the patient's deteriorating physical condition precipitated a change in the overt expression of feelings. Chemotherapy is often seen as the "last hope" by many cancer patients, and even though its usage is feared, when its covert promise for that last hope is withdrawn the patient feels the finality of his or her diagnosis. The patient whose chemotherapy regime must be withdrawn because of negative side effects is frequently precipitated into a major psychological crisis: the denial afforded by the use of such drugs is stripped harshly away. Anger is often felt by the patient and sometimes by the members of the health care team. The patient feels there is now nothing to stand between him or her and death: death as a potentiality has become death in reality, and this reality must be faced.

Patients who are not able to discuss their fears or concerns about life and dying may also be unable to bring satisfactory closure to some parts of their life, e.g., financial arrangements for survivors. Here it becomes most important for the nurse to facilitate the patient's ability to talk about the realistic situation and needs that require the patient's attention. By no means does this imply that the nurse should *force* the patient to "face the facts" regardless of the resistance or denial present. It is important to recognize that the patient's goal *can* be accomplished without undue emphasis on confronting a harsh reality.

Part of the dying process experienced by the cancer patient is grieving for the self. Grief work may begin at the time of diagnosis or at any time during the course of treatment. Patients vary greatly in reaching completion of grief work, which can culminate in a feeling of satisfaction, peacefulness, and calmness. Most cancer patients benefit from differing forms of nursing intervention during the dying process. Aspects of nursing interventions in the care for the dying cancer patient therefore constitute the final section of this chapter.

REACHING WHOLENESS

In caring for the dying cancer patient, the nurse seeks to design interventions that will promote a quality of *living* until the time of death. "Quality" can be defined in terms of fulfilling physical, social, intellectual, psychological and emotional needs that each patient may express in varying degrees of intensity. As care is designed and implemented, the nurse also seeks to continuously reevaluate the adequacy of actions taken. The most crucial ingredient in the care of the dying person is *caring*. Without a sense of commitment to promote quality living within the bounds of reality, the nurse may find that personal feelings of frustration, anger, and hopelessness dominate overall effectiveness. It is clearly recognized, however, that such feelings can and do arise in the most dedicated nurse as the dying person is cared for. Achieving a balance between an all-consuming involvement with each patient and a distant objectivity, then, is a major goal for the nurse.

Assessing Patient Needs

In-depth discussion of the assessment of physical needs of the cancer patient is discussed in Part Two of this book. For this reason, the focus of this section is on the social, emotional, and psychological assessment of the dying cancer patient.

Social Needs   *The Problem of Labeling*   A dying person may experience a kind of labeling by significant others. As the patient enters a dying trajectory, family, friends, or care givers may unknowingly begin to interact with the patient as if the person were already dead. Behaviors indicating this phenomenon include decreased visits by family or hospital personnel, exclusion of the patient from discussion of the person in her or his presence, or assignment of care of the patient to less trained nursing personnel. The patient may be related to as if she or he were a member of the "living dead." A major part of the nurse's assessment procedure, as a consequence, *must* focus on:

   1   Identifying one's attitudes and feelings toward the dying cancer patient
   2   Observing the style of interaction of other nurses caring for the patient
   3   Focusing on introspection about one's own behavior as the patient is cared for

Attention to these nurse-related assessments will allow one to become aware of how one is interacting with the patient and what one's personal emotional responses are. Because the nurse can represent a significant source of social need satisfaction for the patient confined to a hospital setting, it is imperative that the nurse recognize the extent to which this need fulfillment may be enhanced or thwarted by personal feelings and overt actions.

The Non-Talkative Patient   The dying patient frequently desires visits by family members during which the patient may say little. For the family, the lack of verbal communication and the strain of attempting to create it can result in feelings of helplessness and confusion. It is often of great assistance to family members to tell them that the patient may wish only to see them, hear them, and experience their nearness—not carry on social discourse. The nurse can discuss the feelings of family members with them as a means of reducing tension and promoting understanding of the patient's need to continue the visits. Many dying people, regardless of the level of physical deterioration or consciousness, receive much comfort in knowing that a loved one is near, silently conveying caring and affection. Words become superfluous in these situations.

Recognition of Special Social Needs   Although institutional rules and regulations frequently preclude patient contact with small children or pets, the dying cancer patient, in this writer's opinion, should be given free rein when it comes to bending these rules. Cancer strikes people of all ages, but it is the elderly person who may have developed social needs and dependencies that require rule bending. For example, the widower who lives alone with a cat, dog, or caged bird may want desperately to see the loved companion before death. If isolation does not prohibit such a visit, the nurse may seek to arrange this kind of reunion for the patient. In this way, a realistic, basic social need can be met following careful assessment of patient priorities.

For other cancer patients, social need assessment may reveal a desire to make one last visit home for Sunday dinner, to go to church, to attend a graduation or special event, or to be present at a child's wedding. As the nurse interacts with the patient, it is often very helpful to ask such questions as "What would you want to do or see or go to if you had the opportunity?" or "What would you like to have if you could have anything?" These open-ended questions are designed to elicit the patient's often unspoken desires and hopes. They should never be asked with an implied guarantee that the request will be granted regardless of its nature. One patient, for example, had been disoriented and confused for several days. Family members were concerned that she was "losing her mind." As this writer spoke slowly with the patient, alone, and waited for replies that sometimes came several minutes after the question, the patient was able to answer the "What would you like?" query. She wanted very simply to see a priest and a favorite sister she knew. This social need would not have been fulfilled if the assessment process had not included the time and interest to find out *overtly* what the patient might want. In general, the wishes and wants of the dying cancer patient are simple and easily attained once clearly identified.

Variation in Social Needs   The needs for social contact may become greatly constricted over the course of the dying process. The patient may state a preference for the number of visitors to be limited or for treatments and nursing care to be administered in more compact sessions instead of over longer periods of time. By reducing the number and frequency of all social interactions, the patient can control the quality and intensity of selected interactions. Other patients may want large numbers of visitors and become upset when this does not occur.

A relatively common concern of dying patients is aroused when they are told, "so-and-so came to visit but you were asleep." *Many* cancer patients have expressed a strong desire to be awakened when friends or family arrive. There is a feeling of urgency in ensuring that these contacts are retained. Of course, the nurse needs to *ask* the patient what the preference is—to be allowed to sleep and miss a visit, or be awakened to have the visit. Depending on the patient's physical condition, this question may need to be asked each day. At certain times, the patient's request may have to be modified to be in keeping with the patient's physical and emotional levels of tolerance for stimulation.

Influence of Ethnocultural Background   Cultural variation in the manner in which dying behavior is manifested also must be considered in the assessment process. For members of some cultural groups, it is required that the entire nuclear and extended family congregate around the patient or be near the patient at times of serious illness. Although this behavior may be stressful to nursing and medical personnel, depending on the nature of the behaviors exhibited by the visitors, the patient may receive considerable comfort from the support provided. The nurse, then, needs to carefully assess the patient's belief system and ethnocultural background to determine anticipated behaviors of visitors.

At the same time, while recognizing and respecting the patient's need for meaningful social contact, the nurse continues to act as the patient's advocate when stimulation from visitors appears to be harmful. Thus, the dying patient who fatigues easily or who becomes confused and disoriented with large amounts of auditory stimulation should probably have limits placed on the number, frequency, and duration of visits. Clear and mutually established agreements between visitors and nursing staff take into account the patient's needs for both social contact and rest and quiet.

Emotional and Psychological Needs   An experience with cancer arouses intense emotional responses in the majority of people. A dying cancer patient not only experiences these feelings but must also contend with the knowledge or suspicion that the future is limited. The focus of emotional and psychological need assessment is on determining:

1   The presence or absence of emotional responses such as fear, anger, anxiety, depression, elation, or hopefulness
2   The nature of the patient's past and present coping strategies as a means of anticipating patient needs for assistance
3   The patient's comfort in coping with these responses
4   The extent to which intervention that provides support or fosters development of more meaningful emotional adaptation may be required

Assessment takes place through (1) observation of patient and family behavior, (2) discussion with the patient which includes validation of suspected or probable modes of responding, and (3) direct interaction with the patient as nursing care is administered. Initial assessments are reevaluated as new information is obtained on the patient's emotional state.

Psychological assessment focuses on orienting the patient to time and place as well as identifying dysfunctional behaviors related to reality orientation. Patients must never be labeled "crazy" or "having a nervous breakdown" when aberrant behavior is presented. Instead, a formal psychological evaluation should be requested which seeks to determine whether organic and/or emotional factors are correlated with the unusual behavior. For example, patients who "see things that aren't there" may be hallucinating because of organic causes unrelated to the emotional stress experienced. Nursing assessment should include collection of information on the nature, onset, duration, and character of such patient behaviors.

Assessment Areas   Emotional and psychological assessment areas may include an emphasis on the following:

1   "On a scale of 1 to 10, how do you feel in terms of anxiety (depression, anger, hope, etc.) about your present situation?"

2   "What do you fear most about your illness?" The nurse can include an emphasis on the past, present, or future.

3   "Which emotion best describes your feelings right now?" or "How do you feel emotionally?" A question such as this also can focus on past or anticipated feelings.

4   "How do you think another person would feel if he or she were in your place?" Here the nurse may be able to get a response about someone else when the patient is not yet able to personalize the feeling level of the experience.

5   "If you have had a previous experience with serious illness, tell me how you responded then." "What did you *do*, how did you behave, what did you feel?"

These and *many* other questions or statements can be used as tools to gain an understanding of the patient's emotional and psychological state of being. At all times, the nurse must be clear on one thing: *Why are these questions being asked?* Is this information *necessary* or merely *interesting?* The purpose of assessment should always be to gain a fuller understanding of patient needs such that nursing care designed to meet the needs will have a high probability of meeting with success.

At various times during patient care activities, opportunities will arise to discuss with the patient her or his emotional status or needs. These opportunities are invaluable, for they frequently reflect the patient's *need* to communicate a feeling or emotion. The receptive and sensitive nurse will be able to respond to questions and statements with further queries for clarification and support when she or he is "tuned in" to this aspect of continuing assessment.

Assessment represents the foundation of purposeful and effective nursing intervention efforts. It is an ongoing, ever-varying process that provides the nurse with keys to the puzzle of patient need. With careful assessments, intervention becomes a meaningful nursing activity.

Intervening

Nursing interventions can be both passive and active in the manner of implementation. The goal(s) of nursing intervention may be

- To support identified patient coping behaviors
- To facilitate the development of effective coping strategies
- To foster patient growth and awareness during the dying process
- To modify maladaptive patient behaviors
- To promote a quality of living until the time of death

Goals for physical comfort also are included in nursing care planning. However, the emphasis here is on the social, emotional, and psychological aspects of nursing intervention.

Support of Coping Behaviors   Dying patients who are utilizing effective and meaningful coping strategies benefit from receiving nursing support for these behaviors. It is not necessary for the nurse to agree with the style of coping the patient uses, but it *is* important that the nurse be willing to recognize personal reactions and be able to offer emotional support to the patient. Providing support does not necessarily imply the active promotion of a patient belief. For example, the patient who seems to overtly deny the realistic situation of dying can receive neutral support from the nurse. In this case, the nurse can provide factual information to the patient regarding the situation and can acknowledge the patient's need to be hopeful. At the same time, the nurse can consistently attempt to avoid giving false reassurance. In this type of interaction, the patient receives emotional support but not encouragement to retain a potentially maladaptive coping style.

Adaptive coping behaviors frequently include aspects of denial, hopefulness, depression, anger, fear, and relief. As the nurse identifies these patient responses, it then becomes possible to offer support to the patient during the experience. Statements such as "Often patients with cancer feel sad at different times during treatment," represent an acknowledgement of a patient expression and at the same time act as permission to feel in a particular way.

At other times, support is provided by helping patients gain perspective on their overall situation. The patient who has been ill for many months, who has undergone extensive treatment, and who currently is experiencing anger can gain understanding of the situation as the nurse acknowledges the patient's *right* to feel angry and recaps the reasons for the anger. The nurse makes statements as

"You know, anyone who has been ill for——number of months and has under-gone surgery, radiation therapy, and chemotherapy might feel some anger about not being cured of the disease/cancer. That's a great deal of stress to handle. What's your feeling about what has been happening to you?" Some patients need to hear that their feelings are normal *and* that other people have felt similar-ly. In addition, as time passes and the patient undergoes numerous treatment procedures, it is very possible for the patient to lose track of the sequence of events. When the patient then feels confused and frustrated, a clear summary of what has occurred can be helpful in sorting through the facts.

Providing emotional and social support also consists of assuring patients that emotional responses and their expression are sanctioned behaviors. Pa-tients often feel embarrassed or guilty about expressing emotions in the presence of strangers—including the nurse. A nonjudgmental reassurance on the part of the nurse to the patient can reduce or eliminate the patient's self-consciousness or reluctance to express feelings. At the same time, it is important that the nurse determine what the patient's attitude is toward such expressions. Those who are extremely uncomfortable when others view their distress should be protected from such exposure as much as possible. The nurse may also want to create privacy for those persons who indicate a need for quietness.

Family members, friends, or job-related companions can also be sources of support for the dying patient. The nurse may find that it is necessary to carefully assess the capability of the significant other to provide the depth of support the patient needs. With receipt of emotional support from care givers, family mem-bers frequently can become the major emotional support resource for the dying person. As the patient expresses feelings or indicates their presence through overt behavior, the nurse seeks to determine who can best meet the patient's need. For some patients, a friend, spouse, or religious leader can fulfill the need for emotional support more effectively than can the nurse.

Patients who exhibit severe emotional disturbance or an inability to cope with the stress of living until death often require the services of a psychologist, psychiatrist, or social worker who is skilled in psychotherapy. In these cases, support from the nurse consists of seeking the necessary referral or consult and supporting intervention suggestions formulated by the consultant. Continuing psychotherapy may be necessary on either an in-hospital or outpatient basis. Persons with cancer who are in a terminal phase of living may openly respond to the therapist as a means of expressing personally unacceptable feelings, thoughts, and behaviors. Family members also may find it helpful to use such supportive services over the course of the patient's illness. As major support sources for the patient, the family can receive needed assistance from the therapist in order to continue their role and to gain an understanding of their own emotional experience.

Facilitation of Self-Awareness   Development of a heightened sense of self-awareness and sensitivity can occur, in varying degrees, in all dying cancer patients. The role of the nurse in this growth process may take many forms.

Imagery   One of the more recent approaches to working with the cancer patient has been developed by Simonton and Simonton.[8] Within a framework of fostering development of the patient's ability to be responsible for her or his body's reaction to the disease, imagery techniques are used to assist the patient in combating the disease. Patients are taught to visualize the disease, its treatment, and the action of the body's immune system against the cancerous growth. These exercises are conducted along with a relaxation sequence a prescribed number of times each day. No blame is cast on the patient for "getting" cancer. Rather, the emphasis is on facilitating the development of inner sensitivity to the manner in which the body and mind can interact in a mutually supportive and beneficial manner to help heal the body.

Group Discussion   In a group setting, several cancer patients and care givers (nurses, physicians, social workers, chaplain, family members) have an opportunity to experience personal growth and an increase in self-awareness via the interaction that takes place. The group format in which several cancer patients with differing or similar diagnoses participate allows for:

1   *Providing mutual support:* Patients with similar diagnoses can discuss common feelings with assurance that each will have the basis for understanding one another's experience to a greater extent than will nonill group members. Group members who have been ill for a longer period of time can aid group members who have been newly diagnosed. In these cases, the "old-timers" can truly empathize with the new member's feelings of fear, anger, frustration, and hopefulness. In addition, the old-timers can help the patient bridge the gap between being a healthy person and a cancer patient.

Although not the primary focus of group meetings, care givers also can receive support in the group setting. Patients may offer support to the nurse just as the nurse offers support to the patient. Care givers may find it helpful to express their own reactions and feelings about the patient's condition in such a way that the patient gains insight into the concern and depth of involvement that is present. Nurse-to-nurse support and understanding enhances the patient's sense of a team effort seeking ways to best care for the patient.

2   *Determining level of understanding:* As patients talk about their disease and the feelings associated with it, questions will arise which reflect the patient's understanding of treatment and prognosis. When the patient's knowledge is distorted or inadequate, the physician or other group member can provide the necessary information. Occasionally, patients will repeatedly receive the same requested information without really *hearing* what has been said. This selective listening usually is associated with denial. The nurse should plan one-to-one sessions with the patient as a means of gradually building up the patient's tolerance to *hear* what is said. With a clear understanding of the disease and its treatment, the patient can participate in the group in such a way that remaining emotional needs can be met.

3   *Learning to savor life:* Dying cancer patients often seek to restructure their lives once a terminal prognosis is identified. The patient's focus centers on the present, the day-to-day sequence of events and experiences. Many patients express an urgency to *live until they die*. This attitude is exemplified by the following statement:

> The most important time in anyone's life is right now. Regardless of age or condition, the present is the only time that counts, the only time we actually live in. The past is gone, the future is not yet here. Living in the past, or anticipating the future deprives us of energy and involvement in the present and destroys the very substance of our lives.[9]

While many patients may not express such an intense desire, many others do. The nurse may find that patients very much want to be productive and useful: they want to *live* the life that they have. Participation in a discussion group is one way for the patients to feel effective: they *are* effective and productive as they share feelings and support with other people. To ensure that the feeling of involvement and commitment continues for group members, the nurse may at times find it necessary to hold meetings in patient rooms when certain patients are too weak to attend at the usual location.

Patients also learn to savor life through the activities of other patients. This vicarious enjoyment of living can become especially significant for the weakened patient who is not able to pursue desired personal activities. Again, the group setting establishes a dependable time and place for this sharing to take place.

4 *Keeping priorities in order:* During the course of group discussions, patients may express many concerns, some of which do not coincide with the priorities established by care givers. This is where the nurse must actively *listen* to the patient: the nurse must learn to hear what is most meaningful and important *to the patient*. While care givers tend to focus on the "classic" problems of cancer management, such as pain, debilitation, or nutritional deficiencies, patients can have a different set of priorities. For example, the dying patient who has nausea and vomiting following meals may be more concerned with a difficulty in falling asleep at night than with the gastrointestinal problem. For this person, sleeping is more significant than food retention. Of course, attention must be directed at *both* problems. The important point is that the nurse attend to the patient's message as a priority item for the patient.

Family Conferences   Just as the patient needs an avenue for self-expression and a means to develop self-awareness, so does the family of the dying patient. Family conferences attempt to provide an opportunity for ventilation of feelings, expression of concerns, and sharing of support resources. In these meetings, the nurse, physician, and other care givers can (1) provide information on the patient's condition, (2) recognize the family's needs, (3) acknowledge the family's role in care giving, (4) make them a partner in supporting the patient, and (5) give support and understanding of the stresses experienced by family members. A family conference, ideally, can be a regularly scheduled event (often in the evening) and/or can be arranged to meet specific crises or family requests. As the family retains strength to cope with their stress, they will be able to more effectively do the same for the patient.

Literature   Achieving a sense of heightened sensitivity to life and self-awareness can be facilitated through the reading of literature on various topics related to philosophy and religion. For those patients who feel comfortable with exploring feelings via the simulation aroused by reading, the nurse can suggest meaningful reading materials. There are literally hundreds of books, magazine articles, and other types of reading media devoted to the issues of life and death. The nurse needs to become somewhat familiar with this body of literature so that recommendations can be made to interested patients and family members. For example, books such as *Life after Life* [10] provide a warm sense of hopefulness and comfort for the dying person who fears a nonexistence after death. While the patient need not accept the content of a suggested reading, it may provide stimulation to further thinking and discussion in a one-to-one or group setting. The patient may find that consideration of others' viewpoints on the living-until-death experience will assist in clarifying the person's own values and attitudes.

Through use of newly devised therapy techniques and group and one-to-one patient and family discussions, the nurse can facilitate the development of the dying person's self-awareness and emotional growth. In turn, the nurse will experience the stimulation of personal sensitivity and commitment to this intimate aspect of nursing care.

Being with the Patient   Perhaps the primary role of the nurse, and probably the most difficult to fulfill, is an ability and commitment to *be with* the dying cancer patient as care is administered. "Being with" the patient means a willingness to give of oneself to the patient, to empathize with the patient's emotional turmoil or steadiness, to be sharing of one's own emotional investment in another person. There is great risk in doing this, for in extending caring and involvement to the patient's living each day, the nurse can experience grief and loss when the patient dies. It is this element of involvement and empathy that creates a quality method of interaction between patient and nurse. The nurse who is able to be with the patient can experience considerable personal satisfaction and fulfillment with each patient contact.

Many nurses learn how to emotionally be with the dying patient through patient care experiences or previous personal experience. Others can acquire skill in this area through (1) introspection with regard to values and attitudes toward death and dying, (2) study of the literature on living and dying, and (3) participation in conferences, classes, seminars, etc., devoted to self-awareness and personal growth. There are no easy "rules" to learn: each person must develop a personal and satisfying style of interacting with the dying patient. By being attentive to one's attitudes and responses as care is given to the patient, the nurse can subsequently evaluate personal feelings and reactions. Often it is helpful to share these feelings with concerned peers, friends, or family.

In being with the dying cancer patient, the nurse needs to develop an ability to *let go* also. The nurse cannot or should not become so deeply involved with each dying patient that perspective on the patient's prognosis is lost. This, truly, is an extremely difficult ability to develop. It has many ups and downs as the nurse attempts to protect the self from emotional hurt and loss while at the same time seeking to provide the understanding and caring the dying person values. Because there are never any guarantees that one will *not* experience emotional pain by investing in another person, the nurse needs to carefully consider the extent to which she or he can allow herself or himself to become deeply involved with a number of patients. That is, by understanding one's own strengths and limitations, it is possible to acknowledge to oneself and peers that a particular emotional limit has been reached. The following example illustrates this point:

> Ms. B., the nurse, had cared for Barbara during her final hospitalization for multiple myeloma. When Barbara, who was about the same age as Ms. B., died, Ms. B. experienced acute grief. She had "been there" for Barbara: shared the patient's fears, supported her emotionally, talked about dying and what it meant to the patient. The emotional investment was heavy. A few days later, Mr. K., a terminally ill patient with lung cancer, was admitted and assigned to Ms. B. As she assessed the patient and learned of the prognosis, she was able to acknowledge a hesitancy to become deeply involved with this patient so soon after having undergone an intense loss experience. With this understanding of a personal limitation, Ms. B. requested that the patient be reassigned or that another nurse focus on establishing a close, emotionally supportive relationship with the patient. This request was honored.

This example reflects *one* way in which the patient's need for emotional closeness can be met when the nurse feels unable to fulfill the role. At other times, a family member or friend may become the patient's source of emotional intimacy.

In this writer's opinion, the nurse who cares for the terminally ill cancer patient can gain much in terms of inner growth and a deep sense of personal fulfillment by extending herself or himself emotionally. As the patient grows, so does the nurse who is willing to risk.

Fostering Behavior Change At times, the dying patient may exhibit maladaptive behavior that reduces the person's quality of living. Patients may develop manipulative, self-pitying, or generally uncooperative behavior patterns that impede effective nursing care. In these cases, the nurse needs to carefully assess the problem behaviors, determine causative factors when possible, and design interventions that can change the behavior. Behavior-modification techniques may be quite effective in altering behavior: as the undesired behavior is no longer reinforced, a more appropriate behavior receives noncontingent attention. In this way the "old" behavior decreases in frequency while another behavior increases. This approach is most beneficial when the nurse has gathered information on the rate, duration, intensity, and frequency of the target behaviors. As the behavior is disrupted, the nurse will be able to clearly define the impact of the intervention. Some of the problem areas that respond positively to the behavior-modification approach include eating, patient activity levels, modes of verbal communication, and self-care activities.

It is important that the nurse identify a reward or reinforcement system that is meaningful to the patient. Praise, attention, or access to special events or privileges can be very effective reinforcers. In addition, the patient often can take an active role in a modification program, depending, of course, on the nature of the problem behavior.

A second important point that deserves emphasis involves *ownership* of the problem. The nurse needs to carefully determine if the ''problem'' belongs to the nurse or the patient. Does the behavior reduce quality living for the patient? Is it annoying to the nurse but not to the family or other patients? Are there behaviors that the patient is concerned about but which the nurse finds acceptable? Once it is clearly established *whose* problem the behavior is, it is then possible to design interventions that will meet the identified need.

Behavior may also be changed as the patient develops a sense of self-awareness and is able to attend to inner responses and feelings. Patient behaviors that are inappropriate or maladaptive may change to more adaptive modes of expression as a function of the patient's emotional state of growth. In these cases, the nurse may wish to focus on providing support to the patient so that the person can develop a more useful coping strategy. At other times, the nurse may find that it is essential to overtly interrupt the patient's behavior pattern through confrontation. Patients can be unaware of the impact of their behavior on others and appreciate the nurse's feedback. Of course, confrontation does not need to imply a negative interaction. It can consist of straightforward communication to the patient of how the behavior impacts on those in the environment. It can take place in a one-to-one or group setting. It should *always* be done in a supportive, nonjudgmental manner. The patient needs to know that the nurse will not reject her or him, but will ''stick it out.''

In turn, the nurse will find it helpful to be clear on personal reactions to problem patient behaviors. One means of becoming clear on this issue is to identify whether the behavior is temporary or represents a long-standing style of behaving in stressful situations. In some cases, the patient's behavior *will not* be changeable, and the nurse may then want to consider seeking support in continuing to cope with the patient's problem behavior; this is an example of the nurse's ownership of the problem.

Retaining Perspective

Inherent in caring for the dying patient is much emotional stress as well as reward. For this reason, nurses often need to find ways of retaining enthusiasm and commitment to this form of oncology nursing. Retaining one's perspective in the face of repeated experiences with the care of terminally ill cancer patients can be accomplished in a variety of ways.

Grouping   The sharing of frustrations, fears, angers, and sadnesses with one's peers in a group setting is one of the most helpful means of retaining perspective. In a group, nurses who are involved with the care of particular patients or who are familiar with the case can express feelings and receive support from other group members. Each nursing unit that cares for dying cancer patients should establish an ongoing or periodic opportunity for nurses to meet in a group setting. Staff nurses as well as supervisory and ancillary levels of nursing can set up such an opportunity.

It is not important to have a group leader in this type of meeting, although the members may wish to designate such a position. The purpose of the group is threefold:

1   To ventilate and express feelings related to caring for the dying person
2   To develop a trusting, open support system that acts as a cushion for the emotional stress that can be experienced in oncology nursing
3   To foster problem-solving techniques when particular patient problems arise

As the group is initiated and formed, the nurses will need to focus on becoming a group, i.e., *grouping*. This is accomplished in an atmosphere that is accepting, honest, and trustworthy. At times it may be necessary to concentrate on group dynamics as grouping takes place. Members will need to develop a sense of comfort and trust in the other nurses before they are willing to expose inner feelings and emotions.

The oncology discussion group (a suggested name) represents a highly successful and meaningful method of retaining one's perspective as dying cancer patients are cared for. While it has some flaws, limitations, or drawbacks, it has the potential to become one of the nurse's strongest sources of support and growth.

Developing Staff Abilities   Another approach to retaining one's perspective consists of developing the nurse's ability to provide purposeful, effective, and satisfying nursing care to the dying person. Whenever possible, the staff nurse should seek to enhance ability to be with the dying patient. This can be accomplished in a variety of ways:

1   Attending seminars, workshops, conferences, and classes devoted to fostering self-awareness and sensitivity to the dying cancer patient's needs
2   Studying literature written on the various issues and aspects of caring for the dying person.
3   Initiating experiences that use exercises or games designed to heighten introspection and an understanding of one's feelings, attitudes, or values
4   Using films, video-tapes, slide-tape programs, or other audio-visual materials as stimulators to group discussion of living and dying
5   Seeking consultation from other health professionals, e.g., nurse clinicians, social workers, physicians, and psychologists, on how they deal with the issues of death and dying and the interface between the care giver's feelings and delivery of patient care services
6   Involving other care givers from all levels of educational background in discussion groups and programs on living and dying
7   Accepting "homework" assignments, either self-created or determined by a facilitator, that stretch one's intellect and emotional responsivity

It should be emphasized that any of these methods need not involve tremendous outpourings of organizational energy. The range of complexity can be from a spontaneously called team discussion to a well-organized conference. The *how* is less important than the *who* and *what* that needs attention.

SUMMARY COMMENT

This chapter has sought to provide an overview of the many facets of caring for the dying cancer patient. By no means is it exhaustive of all the issues and topics that constitute the area of living until death. Each nurse who interacts with a dying person will have many questions, responses, and reactions that can be addressed only by a deep personal involvement in this area of oncology nursing. As the nurse becomes involved and committed to a quality of living until death, the nurse's own feelings of accomplishment, challenge, and joy in living will be enormously enriched.

REFERENCES

1 Melvin J. Krant, "What Does the Patient Know?" *Proceedings of the American Cancer Society's National Conference on Human Values & Cancer* (New York: American Cancer Society, 1973), p. 48.
2 Gunnar Biörck, "How Do You Want to Die?" *Archives of Internal Medicine,* **132**(10):605–606, 1973.
3 American Hospital Association, "A Patient's Bill of Rights," approved by the association's House of Delegates, February 6, 1973.
4 Cicely Saunders, "A Death in the Family: A Professional View," *British Medical Journal,* **1**:30–31, January 6, 1973.
5 Elisabeth Kübler-Ross, *On Death and Dying* (New York: Macmillan, 1969).
6 Avery D. Weisman and Thomas P. Hackett, "Predilection to Death," *Psychosomatic Medicine,* **23**:232–256, 1961.
7 E. Mansell Pattison, "The Experience of Dying," *American Journal of Psychotherapy,* **21**(1): 32–43, 1967, p. 42.
8 O. Carl Simonton and Stephanie Simonton, "Management of the Emotional Aspects of Malignancy," *New Dimensions in Habilitation for the Handicapped,* symposium held in Forth Worth, Texas, June 14 and 15, 1974.
9 "Notes, Quotes & Postscripts," *JPN and Mental Health Sciences,* July–August 1974, p. 14
10 Raymond A. Moody, Jr., *Life after Life* (Atlanta: Mockingbird Books, 1975).

BIBLIOGRAPHY

Becker, Ernest: *The Denial of Death,* Free Press, New York, 1973.
Beverley, E. Virginia: "Understanding and Helping Dying Patients and Their Families," *Geriatrics,* **31**(3):117, 121–122, 127, 1976.
Burkhalter, Pamela K.: "Fostering Staff Sensitivity to the Dying Patient," *Supervisor Nurse,* **6**(4):54–59, 1975.
Corder, Michael P., and Robert L. Anders: "Death and Dying—Oncology Discussion Group," *JPN and Mental Health Services,* July-August 1974, pp. 10–14.

Davis, Barbara A.: " . . . Until Death Ensues," *Nursing Clinics of North America*, 7(2):303–309, June 1972.

Driver, Caroline: "What a Dying Man Taught Doctors about Caring," *Medical Economics*, January 22, 1974, pp. 81–86.

Epstein, Charlotte: *Nursing the Dying Patient*, Reston Publishing Co., Reston, Va., 1975.

Feifel, Herman, and Allan R. Branscomb: "Who's Afraid of Death?" *Journal of Abnormal Psychology*, 81(3):282–288, 1973.

———, Freilich, Jeffrey, and Lawrence J. Hermann: "Death Fear in Dying Heart and Cancer Patients," *Journal of Psychosomatic Research*, 17:161–166, 1973.

Fond, Karen I.: "Dealing with Death and Dying through Family-Centered Care," *Nursing Clinics of North America*, 7(1):53–64, March 1972.

Glaser, B., and A. Strauss: *Awareness of Dying*, Aldine, Chicago, 1965.

Gottheil, Edward, McGurn, Wealtha C., and Otto Pollak: "Truth and/or Hope for the Dying Patient," *Nursing Digest*, 4(2):12–14, 1976.

Hodge, James R.: "How to Help Your Patients Approach the Inevitable," *Medical Times*, 102(11):123–133, 1974.

Hunter, Pat: "Sharing the Fear—and Comfort," *Sunday Star-Bulletin & Advertiser*, (Honolulu, Hawaii), October 3, 1976, A-32, A-34.

Kastenbaum, Robert, and Ruth Aisenberg: *The Psychology of Death*, Springer, New York, 1976.

Koestenbaum, Peter: *Is There an Answer to Death?* Prentice-Hall, Englewood Cliffs, N.J., 1976.

Krant, Melvin J.: "Grief and Bereavement: An Unmet Medical Need," *Delaware Medical Journal*, 45:282–290, 1973.

———: "What Does the Patient Know?" *Proceedings of the American Cancer Society's National Conference on Human Values & Cancer*, American Cancer Society, New York, 1973.

Kübler-Ross, Elisabeth: *Death, the Final Stage of Growth*, Prentice-Hall, Englewood Cliffs, N.J., 1975.

———: *Questions and Answers on Death and Dying*, Collier Books, New York, 1974.

Liebman, Albert, Silbergleit, Inger-Lise, and Stuart Farber: "Family Conference in the Care of the Cancer Patient," *Journal of Family Practice*, 2(5):343–345, 1975.

Moody, Raymond A., Jr.: *Life after Life*, Mockingbird Books, Atlanta, 1975.

———: *Reflections on Life after Life*, Bantam/Mockingbird, New York, 1977.

Raft, David: "How to Help the Patient Who is Dying," *American Family Physician*, 7(4):112–115, 1973.

Reynolds, David K., and Richard A. Kalish: "The Social Ecology of Dying: Observations of Wards for the Terminally Ill," *Hospital & Community Psychiatry*, 25(3):147–152, 1974.

Silberman, Henry K.: "Appointment with Death: Attitudes and Communications," *Missouri Medicine*, 70:37–42, January 1973.

Simonton, O. Carl, and Stephanie Simonton: "Management of the Emotional Aspects of Malignancy," *New Dimensions of Habilitation for the Handicapped*, symposium, June 14 and 15, 1974, Fort Worth, Texas.

Skoog, Richard: "Death and the Problems of Honesty," *Wisconsin Medical Journal*, 74(2):11–12, 1975.

Sudnow, David: *Passing On: The Social Organization of Dying*, Prentice-Hall, Englewood Cliffs, N.J., 1967.

Verwoerdt, Adriaan: "Some Aspects of Communication with the Fatally Ill," *Proceeding of the American Cancer Society's National Conference on Human Values & Cancer,* American Cancer Society, New York, 1973.

Whitman, Helen H., and Shelby J. Lukes: "Behavior Modification for Terminally Ill Patients," *American Journal of Nursing,* **75**(1):98–101, 1975.

Zuehlke, Terry E., and John T. Watkins: "The Use of Psychotherapy with Dying Patients: An Exploratory Study," *Journal of Clinical Psychology,* **31**(14):729–732, 1975.

APPENDIX: A Patient's Bill of Rights*

1   The patient has the right to considerate and respectful care.

2   The patient has the right to obtain from his physician complete current information concerning his diagnosis, treatment, and prognosis in terms the patient can be reasonably expected to understand. When it is not medically advisable to give such information to the patient, the information should be made available to an appropriate person in his behalf. He has the right to know by name the physician responsible for coordinating his care.

3   The patient has the right to receive from his physician information necessary to give informed consent prior to the start of any procedure and/or treatment. Except in emergencies, such information for informed consent should include but not necessarily be limited to the specific procedure and/or treatment, the medically significant risks involved, and the probable duration of incapacitation. Where medically significant alternatives for care or treatment exist, or when the patient requests information concerning medical alternatives, the patient has the right to such information. The patient also has the right to know the name of the person responsible for the procedures and/or treatment.

4   The patient has the right to refuse treatment to the extent permitted by law, and to be informed of the medical consequences of his action.

5   The patient has the right to every consideration of his privacy concerning his own medical care program. Case discussion, consultation, examination, and treatment are confidential and should be conducted discreetly. Those not directly involved in his care must have the permission of the patient to be present.

6   The patient has the right to expect that all communications and records pertaining to his care should be treated as confidential.

7   The patient has the right to expect that within its capacity a hospital must make reasonable response to the request of a patient for services. The hospital must provide evaluation, service, and/or referral as indicated by the urgency of the case. When medically permissible a patient may be transferred to another facility only after he has received complete information and explanation concerning the needs for and alternatives to such a transfer. The institution to which the patient is to be transferred must first have accepted the patient for transfer.

8   The patient has the right to obtain information as to any relationship of his hospital to other health care and educational institutions insofar as his care is concerned. The patient has the right to obtain information as to the existence of any professional relationships among individuals, by name, who are treating him.

*Reprinted with permission of the American Hospital Association.

9   The patient has the right to be advised if the hospital proposes to engage in or perform human experimentation affecting his care or treatment. The patient has the right to refuse to participate in such research projects.

10   The patient has the right to expect reasonable continuity of care. He has the right to know in advance what appointment times and physicians are available and where. The patient has the right to expect that the hospital will provide a mechanism whereby he is informed by his physician or a delegate of the physician of the patient's continuing health care requirements following discharge.

11   The patient has the right to examine and receive an explanation of his bill regardless of source of payment.

12   The patient has the right to know what hospital rules and regulations apply to his conduct as a patient.

Chapter 15

Spiritual Ministries with Cancer Patients

David Y. Hirano

THE RELATIONSHIP OF MEDICINE AND RELIGION

The relationship of medicine and religion is prehistoric. From the beginnings of time religion and medicine have been partners in healing. Discoveries of the remains of Paleolithic humans show that they wore amulets and charms, presumably to ward off illness. Diseases of all kinds have been with humanity from the beginning, and people have dealt with them in many ways.

In the early history of medicine the healer was the religious person, who cured people of diseases through nonphysical means directed toward the mind and/or the spirit rather than the body. As one reads the religious history of peoples, one discovers in Buddhism stories of miraculous healings by those who have been enlightened; in Shinto the *shaman,* a person who works with the supernatural as both priest and doctor, was and still is an important figure; in Judaism great prophets such as Elijah are healers; and in Christianity there are many stories of how Jesus the Christ and his followers cured people of diseases and even brought people back from the dead.

Although there is a tendency of modern, technological persons to view faith healing skeptically, in America today there are Pentecostal and charismatic Christians who practice faith healing. Among the Japanese in Hawaii, the *odaisan,* a *shaman,* is still a popular person to seek when modern medicine fails. Catholic Christians are drawn to Lourdes and other sacred places to seek healing. Westerners wear amulets and charms to ward off illness or to seek some kind of magical cure. In the "primitive" cultures of the twentieth-century world, voodoo, the witch doctor, and the medicine man are still active.

Medicine and religion come from the same roots. Religion arose from emotions and instinct; medicine sprang out of magic and superstition. Emotions, instinct, magic, and superstition are intangibles. They are very difficult to explain and define. They deal with the subconscious, superconscious, and conscious states of the mind, or with the nebulous thing called "spirit."

With the advent of technology there came a cleavage between the religious and medical fields. Each became a speciality. Religion dealt with the spiritual world, with theology, and with faith. Medicine, with the exception of psychiatry, dealt with the physical and became a science, giving the appearance of exactness. In present-day society, in which science is God, things such as faith and spirit, whose existence cannot be proven, are not credible. Twentieth-century technological persons are less religiously oriented and more skeptical about religion; hence the cleavage.

There are attempts being made to close the gap between religion and medicine. Psychiatrists and clergy need to learn about one anothers disciplines. Perhaps the greatest impetus toward closing the gap began in the 1930s with the birth of the clinical pastoral education (CPE) movement. The CPE program is being adopted by many seminaries, and seminarians and clergy are being urged to enter the program.

The minister or seminarian in the CPE program works for 12 weeks in a hospital with physicians, medical interns, residents, and nurses. The author of this chapter spent his clinical education program in Boston City Hospital. He began his training by being an orderly on a surgical ward for several weeks, before being assigned a medical ward on which he was chaplain. His training included viewing several operations, watching an autopsy, attending lectures given by physicians, and reading books on psychology and healing. Thus he experienced the hospital from bedpan to operating room and from bedside to morgue. As more seminarians and ministers take the CPE program, the gap of understanding and cooperation between medicine and religion will close.

DEFINITIONS OF "RELIGION" AND "SPIRITUAL"

Up to this point, the words "religion" and "spiritual" have been used interchangeably. For the rest of the chapter a distinction is made between them. "Religion" and "religious" refer to beliefs about the nature of the universe, life, and the ultimate. Practices or systems of beliefs, such as Buddhism, Christianity, Hindu, or Islam, would be called religions. One who practices or believes in these systems would be called religious.

The word "spiritual" refers to a part of a person. It refers to the "essence" of a person. It is the nonphysical and nonmental part of the person. Determining the spiritual part of a person may be done in the following manner: One may ask, "Who are you?" The answer is usually a name, such as "Mary Ann Smith." The questioner presses, "Who is Mary Ann Smith?" Mary Ann probably responds with identification in terms of role, sex, historical data, and other things. The questioner persists, "Who are you?" When the answers reach the limit, Mary Ann may reply, "I am I." The definition of "I" is intangible, inexplainable, and incomprehensible. Yet each person has a uniqueness that is the I. The I is the essence of the person. It is the person's essence. That is the part of the person that is spiritual. The author of this article feels that all persons are spiritual in nature and that the universe is spiritual at its core.

SPIRITUAL MINISTRIES WITH THE CANCER PATIENT

The patient with cancer is a spiritual being and therefore has spiritual needs that must be treated. The cancer therapist should be concerned with the whole person: body, mind, and spirit. For the body there are physicians, for the mind, psychologists and psychiatrists, and for the spirit, the religious person. Giving spiritual therapy is not the clergyperson's duty alone; any religious person may be able to do it. However, the minister, priest, and rabbi are trained in dealing with spiritual matters. It is important that clergy be represented on the health care team. Instead of working independently, the religious professional and the members of the health care team (nurses, doctors, physical therapists, etc.) can work together so that the whole person is treated.

The Clergy and Psychosocial Needs of the Cancer Patient

The psychosocial needs of the cancer patient have been discussed in other chapters of this book. However, it is sometimes difficult to distinguish between psychosocial and spiritual needs. Because they are similar in nature, some of the needs that are hard to distinguish are discussed here from a clergyperson's point of view. It is well to keep in mind that spiritual or religious questions are those that deal with the meaning of life and death, with the nature of the universe, with the ultimate, and with life after death.

One of the fears the cancer patient faces is that of death and dying. There is anger, guilt, and loneliness along with the fear. The patient may ask a question such as "Why did God do this to me?" He or she may say, "I've lived a good life, I've cared for my family, I don't do 'bad' things; still I have cancer." Behind the question and statement is the fear, anger, guilt, and loneliness that accompany death and dying.

Here the clergyperson is a valuable asset. The clergy are people who will listen to the patient and help him or her to deal with the feelings. It must be noted that some clergy will give the cancer patient judgmental statements or pat answers. Therefore, it is important that the proper clergyperson be called. This issue is dealt with in a later part of this chapter.

The clergyperson may work with the patient in helping him or her find some hope of immortality. There is within almost every human being the quest for immortality, eternal life, or a life after death. Most religions have within their belief system some provision for life after death. These ideas are of comfort to the dying patient.

The minister, priest, or rabbi can help the terminal patient prepare for death. The clergyperson can assist in planning the funeral and the memorial services. Often the dying patient will confide in the clergy and reveal thoughts about death that have not been talked about even with the closest members of the family. In these moments the sensitive clergyperson will become a link between the patient and family. The clergyperson can also help the patient to find ways to handle finances, care for the survivors, and ease the sting of death.

Another psychosocial problem that is faced by the clergy in working with cancer patients is grief. Grief is usually associated with death; with the cancer patient grief often occurs with the loss of some part of the body. It is clearly evident when a woman has a mastectomy, when a young man has a leg amputated, or when there is a radical neck operation. It may not be as evident with someone who has had a gastrectomy, but the loss is felt. Other cancer patients lose hair from radiotherapy or chemotherapy or lose their own image of a healthy body. In any event, with all cancer patients there is grief.

The clergyperson will work with the patient through the grieving process. In rehabilitating the patient, the clergyperson will work toward helping the person to discover his or her own worth or at least to reaffirm that worth. Most clergy believe that the person is of infinite worth to God or some Supreme Being, and through listening, counseling, and presence will communicate that to the patient.

In the hospital, the cancer patient quickly becomes dehumanized. He or she is reduced to "Patient in Bed 217A." All the civilian clothes are taken away and replaced by a jonny. The belongings are put in a safe place. Instead of a familiar room, the patient is placed in a strange, bare room with a stranger. The nurses have no names; the doctor visits once in a while. Everything about the hospital is foreign. The clergyperson visits the patient because of a sincere interest in the patient's well-being. Thus the psychosocial need brought on by this depersonalization is partly met by the clergyperson.

Sometimes it is easier for a clergyperson to deal with the patient's psychosocial needs than it is for a psychiatrist, the clinical psychiatric nurse specialist, or the psychologist. When the psychiatric specialist introduces himself or herself, the patient may build immediate defenses. He or she may say, "I'm not crazy. I don't need a psychiatrist." Whereas the clergyperson does not encounter that response.

However, in some cultures the presence of a minister, priest, or rabbi may cause panic in the patient because they are called only in times when the patient is severely ill or on the deathbed. A sensitive clergyperson will ease the anxiety by introducing himself or herself and giving the reason for the visit.

Some clergy are trained in psychotherapy and thus can deal with the psychosocial needs of the cancer patient as well as the clinical psychiatric worker can. These pastoral counselors are valuable to the cancer care team. In most cases the clergy are trained in referral; thus when they are handling patients who have severe emotional problems, they will quickly refer to the proper resource.

The Clergy and the Sacramental Needs of the Cancer Patient

In addition to psychosocial needs, the cancer patient has sacramental needs. These are associated with various sacred rituals or pietistic practices of religious sects and denominations. For instance, the Roman Catholics have many sacraments, such as baptism, confirmation, ordination, marriage, healing (sometimes called "last rites"), and the eucharist; Protestants differ from having no sacraments—the Quakers—to having the same number as the Catholics do.

While technically the word "sacrament" is defined as "an outward symbol of an inward and spiritual grace," for the purpose of this chapter the word "sacrament" is used rather liberally. It refers to matters that people consider sacred. Thus sacramental needs include the need to pray, to meditate, to read the Bible, to read some sacred scripture, or to have performed one of the sacraments listed above.

Although the clergy are the primary persons who work with the sacramental needs of the patient, those needs can be met by nurses, doctors, family, and others who are religiously inclined. This function is discussed more fully in the section of this chapter, "The Role of the Nurse in Spiritual Ministries."

The administration of the sacraments to a patient is becoming known as highly effective among medical professionals. Prayer, for instance, is sometimes as effective as medication in the relief from pain or anxiety. When the author has prayed with a patient, though in severe pain prior to the prayer, he or she has seemed relaxed and eased after the prayer. The effect of meditation on cancer therapy is now being tested by Dr. Carl Simonton at the Cancer Counseling and Research Center in Fort Worth, Texas.[1] His research indicates that meditation is effective in the therapy of cancer patients.

A 41-year-old man was dying from a recurrence of cancer in what was left of his intestines after a total gastrectomy with colectomy. The clergyman visited the patient on his daily rounds to hospitals. Hs listened to the needs of the patient and found that he wanted to become a Christian. The proper ritual was performed, after which he said, "I want the whole treatment." The clergyman, through listening, discovered that what the man wanted was baptism and communion. While the wife was in the room the minister took some water, touched the man's forehead, and baptized him. The man turned to his wife and said, "I feel at peace; it really makes a difference." When communion was served at bedside with his mother and in-laws present, with tears in his eyes he said, "Now I know that I have not missed any part of being part of God's family." Several weeks later he died after having made peace with his friends, family and God.

The Clergy and the Family

In addition to the patient, the patient's family also has psychosocial and sacramental needs that the clergyperson can assist in meeting. Like the patient, the family goes through the stages of death and dying outlined by Elisabeth Kübler-Ross.[2]

From diagnosis through rehabilitation and/or death, the family finds itself on a roller coaster. When the patient is without pain, the family is optimistic. When the patient is in a great deal of pain, the family is depressed. The family members go from despair to hope to despair. They experience the stages of dying, but rarely in the progression suggested by Dr. Kübler-Ross. Sometimes they miss a stage. Often the stages are scrambled.

With the terminal patient's family, the sensitive clergyperson will work so that the family members accept the inevitability of death. One of the tasks he or she tries to accomplish is to have the family members express their feelings to the dying patient, especially those feelings of love and caring.

At times the clergy person will serve as an interpreter and mediator between the family and the patient. A man and his sister came to a group meeting of people with cancer. The man had lung cancer. When he came to the group his face was ashen, his posture bent, and his breathing heavy. His sister brought him to the group because he was terribly depressed. He would lock himself up in a closet and stay there for hours. His depression was compounded by his mother, who was elderly, had a weak heart, and had not been told of his ailment. He felt he needed to hide his ailment from his mother, with whom he lived. In counseling, the sister heard the brother's predicament and the causes of his depression. She found a way to tactfully tell the mother of the son's condition, which she accepted. The mother found him some meaningful things to do while rehabilitating from his surgery and therapy. Remarkably, he snapped out of his depression. His face colored, his posture improved, and his walk livened. The clergyman who led the group was the catalyst in enabling the family and patient to communicate their feelings and come to a meaningful resolution.

In the traumas that surround the diagnosis of cancer and its treatment and subsequent rehabilitation or death, the clergyperson gives support. With the wife of the 41-year-old man who died from cancer, the minister, while visiting with the patient daily, made it a point to also speak to the wife. At least twice a week he met with her so that she could ventilate her feelings of anger, despair, hope—in short, the whole gamut of her experience surrounding her husband's dying. When he died, the minister met with the family, prayed with them, and wept with them; and he still maintains a relationship with the family. In this particular case the minister helped the family through anticipatory grief, the stage of preparing for the death of a loved one, and then through the grief that comes at the death. The clergyperson is a valuable resource to the family.

Even as the patient needs hope, so does the family. Sometimes that hope consists of holding on to the threads of a miracle cure. At other times it is facing the inevitable and hoping for eternal life, immortality, or the promise of a presence that shall always be remembered. In the last moments of life, it is hoping that in death the loved one will not be alone.

For those cancer patients who have had surgery, chemotherapy, and/or radiotherapy and are in the stage of rehabilitation, the clergyperson can help the family to face the issue of living with one who is deformed, weak, or changed in some way. He or she can work with the family members so that they will enable the patient to live the kind of life he or she wants to live given the limitations of the disease and its treatment.

In cases where there is the loss of a limb, breast, or part of the face, the clergyperson aids the family in seeing the patient as a person, as someone who may have been disfigured but is still in essence the same person they knew before the operation. The clergyperson can help the family to accept the patient with the disfigurement as a person and to treat him or her normally.

Often a husband is repulsed by his wife's mastectomy. The wife may feel that she is less of a woman. The clergyperson, through counseling the couple, can enable them to see each other as persons male and female and accept that the loss of a breast does not diminish the woman as woman. If the couple are familiar with talking about God, the clergyperson may also point out that to God all people, healthy or sick, whole or disfigured, are still precious in His sight.

When death comes, the clergy is there to work with the family and friends through the grieving process. Prior to the funeral, there is grief counseling in which the clergyperson listens to the family members as they remember the deceased. He or she may also validate the feelings of anger or guilt that come and especially the tears that flow freely. At the funeral the clergyperson will share his or her feelings about death and eternal life. In the poems and scripture read, life will be affirmed, the deceased remembered, and comfort given. Also, words of hope are offered through the reading of scriptures and the recitation of beliefs about eternal life, immortality, or life after death. This author in the text of the funeral again validates the feelings of the bereaved—anger, guilt, hope, sadness—as being okay.

In the days after the funeral, the clergyperson often follows up and cares for the family. In some churches, grief recovery groups have been established. In these groups persons who have suffered from some traumatic loss, such as the death of a loved one or a divorce, come together under the leadership of a counselor and by sharing their experiences support each other. The group becomes therapeutic. In other churches, laity become involved in the aftercare of the bereaved.

The clergy see the patient and family in all the stages of life. They are with the family in the joy of childbirth, in the celebration of marriage, in the anxiety of sickness, and in the pain of death. For many families the clergyperson is a part of their group. Therefore, for the religious family the clergyperson is very important. For families without religious backgrounds, the clergyperson can be an uninvolved but concerned person who ministers because he or she cares and who usually ministers without a price tag.

Clergy help prepare people for death and dying. Through sermons, study groups, and religious education, the clergy communicate their beliefs of the relationships of life and death and life after death. Some religions, such as Buddhism, stress the oneness of life and death. Christians sometimes focus on life after death more than on life itself, but nevertheless death is seen as an inevitable event. Thus the cancer patient who has had religious training does have a system of beliefs that can help him or her to face death and dying, and likewise the family has a crutch to lean on when death strikes.

The Role of the Nurse in Spiritual Ministries

The nurse is a key to helping patients find the resources for spiritual ministries. The physician is concerned with the physical well-being of the patient and rarely discusses spiritual matters. The nurse is also busy but spends at least 8 hours a day with the patient. He or she knows better than anyone else the moods, pains, and hour-by-hour condition of the patient and therefore has more opportunities to help meet the patient's spiritual needs.

Sometimes the patient and/or his or her relatives or friends call the clergyperson, but when there is a reticence on the part of the patient or when the patient does not know whom to call, the nurse becomes a primary resource for getting the patient and the spiritual counselor together.

Most people know that talking helps to relieve tension and to solve problems. But many people feel that they can handle their psychosocial and spiritual problems themselves. Sometimes patients need an extra nudge from the nurse to get help. The sharing of personal experiences or the experience of other patients might be helpful. The nurse may say: "I've found it helpful to talk about some of the things that make me anxious. If I had cancer I would be anxious. My minister is one that I talk to often, and he helps me with my feelings. Can I call your minister for you? If you don't have one, I'll be glad to call one for you." If the nurse has not had an experience like that, he or she may say: "People say that talking helps to relieve anxiety. Many people call on a minister, priest, or rabbi; can I call one for you?"

The nurse may wonder, "How will I determine what religion the patient belongs to?" Many hospitals indicate the religion of the patient on their admission chart. But in many cases this indication is not specific enough. People indicate their religion with "Christian," "Protestant," "Buddhist," "Roman Catholic," or whatever. If the chart indicates "Buddhist," "Roman Catholic," or "None," the nurse will not need to press. However, if the chart says "Christian" or "Protestant," the nurse will have to determine more specifically what denomination the patient belongs to, since there are some 200 Protestant denominations. After the determination of religious affiliation has been made, the nurse can link the patient to the proper spiritual resource by looking in the Yellow Pages, by calling the local council of churches, or by consulting a clergyperson.

If a hospital has chaplains assigned to it, linking the patient with a clergyperson can be done by calling the chaplain's office. The chaplain will determine with the patient the appropriate course of action. Some communities have a rotating chaplaincy service with the hospital, so that various clergy in the community call on the patients in the hospital at given times. In these cases, a call to the local ministerial association will get the nurse in touch with the proper clergyperson.

Some hospitals have protocols for meeting the spiritual needs of patients. The nurse might check with his or her supervisor or the administration to learn the protocol.

Cancer patients have spiritual concerns. Sometimes they are masked in statements such as "I wonder why life has been so rotten for me" or "Why is life treating me so badly?" or "What shall I do with the rest of my life?" Some questions and statements leave no doubt about the spiritual concern. Patients say: "Will you answer some questions I have about the Bible?" or "Why does God make me sick?" or "What do you believe about eternal life?" If the nurse can handle these questions, then no clergyperson need be called. However, if he or she is not willing or able to answer the questions, a clergyperson ought to be called.

It is helpful when the nurse prepares the way for a visit from the minister, priest, or rabbi. In some cultures people associate the presence of a clergy-person with death or imminent death. To avoid the resultant panic, the nurse might indicate in a tactful manner that the clergyperson is coming because he or she cares and because he or she is someone who might help in alleviating the patient's anxiety.

When the clergyperson has been contacted, the nurse can brief him or her about the patient's condition and, if the minister, priest, or rabbi is a stranger to the patient, introduce him or her. Helpful information about the patient includes the diagnosis, the prognosis, the immediate condition of the patient, and the treatment the patient is receiving. For instance, if the patient is undergoing radiotherapy and therefore is nauseated, the clergyperson needs to know that. If the patient is getting chemotherapy, the visiting clergyperson needs to know the effect of the treatment on the patient. If the patient has been given pain medica-tion and that is making the person drowsy, the clergyperson needs to know. A sensitive clergyperson will take the information given and tailor the visit to the needs and conditions of the patient. Because the clergyperson is not usually medically oriented, any help the nurse can give prior to the actual visit will be useful.

There are times when the patient experiences some trauma and no minis-ters, priests, or rabbis are available. At these points the nurse may mobilize his or her own resources to deal with the situation. When in depression, the patient may ask: "Why did God give me this cancer? Why didn't He just kill me? I wish I could die." Normally one would respond to the words and give a theologi-cal dissertation. However, this response may miss the need of the patient. An alternative response is to help the patient to find the statement behind the questions. The statement may be "God gave me this cancer." or "I know that God didn't give me this cancer, but I'm so mad I could die." or "I'm just going to sit around and vegetate until I die." The nurse can then help the patient work with the feelings behind the statement.

A better way of dealing with the spiritual questions that arise is to deal with the feelings behind the questions. With cancer there are feelings of anger, guilt, and confusion. The nurse can help the patient to identify these feelings and to affirm that they are all right. Then the nurse can help the patient deal with them in constructive ways.

There are other ways through which nurses can help to meet patients' spiritual needs. Nurses who are religiously inclined have prayed with their patients. This is a practice in some Roman Catholic hospitals, where the nurses are nuns. Some lay persons feel that praying is best left to the religious professional because he or she has a closer relationship with the Almighty. It is the author's belief that this is not so. Everyone, whether a professional or a lay person, has the same line to God. If the nurse wants to pray with a patient and feels comfortable doing this, it is permissible. Likewise, if the patient wants to have the Bible read, the nurse can do that also.

Within religious traditions such as Roman Catholicism, in which the sacrament of baptism is important, it can be administered by lay persons. If the patient is dying, a priest is not available, and the family wants the patient baptized, the nurse can do it. He or she takes water in the palm of the hand, places the palm and the water on the forehead of the patient, and says, ''I baptize you in the name of the Father, and of the Son, and of the Holy Spirit.'' The administration of the sacrament needs to be recorded on the patient's chart.

If the nurse is *not* a religiously inclined person, and the patient asks for some kind of spiritual ministry, the nurse needs to be honest. He or she can say: ''I am not a religious person, but I see that you have a need for spiritual help. I will find someone to help you.'' The patient needs to know that when a request for help is made, someone will meet it.

The nurse is essential in meeting the spiritual needs of the cancer patient. From admission to discharge, the nurse can assist the clergyperson in giving spiritual counsel and in meeting the needs of the patient.

THE RELATIONSHIP OF THE CLERGY AND THE PHYSICIANS

The predominant modality of giving health care is centered around the physician as the head of the health care team. Thus nurses, aides, orderlies, and others are supportive to physicians, who prescribe therapy and supervise it. However, there are many times when the physician and nurse do not communicate. Likewise, the physician and the patient and/or family may not communicate. When this happens, the clergyperson can help.

In professional status the clergyperson is a peer of the physician. A mystique surrounds the clergyperson so that the physician often does not know what a clergyperson does as a part of the healing team. Some physicians know the value of the clergy on the team, and these physicians value their services. This mystery and the peer status help to create problems that center around communication.

Sometimes nurses who are with the patient all day see problems that the physician misses. The nurses usually report them to the physician. However, in haste or because of other conditions, the physician may not hear the problems. If the problems are critical to the patient's emotional, spiritual, and physical well-being, and the phsyician fails to hear the problems, the clergyperson may be a resource to helping the physician to hear the nurses.

When the clergyperson is questioned by the patient about medical problems, it is not the clergyperson's task to answer those questions. However, the clergy can refer the question to the physician or encourage the patient to ask the physician. If the patient does not get the answers to the questions, then the clergyperson may step in and ask the questions for the patient or at least call to let the physician know that the patient has unanswered questions.

If the patient has not been told that the condition is critical and death is imminent, the clergy can intervene on behalf of the family and the patient. In conference with the doctor and family, a decision to tell or not to tell can be made. When the patient is told the news, the clergyperson can help the patient and family through the processes of dying and grief.

THE CLERGY AS A PART OF THE HEALTH CARE TEAM

Unlike other health care professionals, the clergy see patients and their families in good times as well as bad. They see the patients in healthy surroundings as well as in the hospital. Thus the clergypersons' perspectives are vitally needed on the health care team.

For the patient who is church-related, the clergyperson is like a part of the family. He or she is the one to whom the patient goes when there are problems, when there is a celebration, or when there is a need to worship and pray. The clergyperson is an integral part of the person's world. Therefore, for these persons it is important that the minister, priest, or rabbi be called in times of crisis.

Every person is a composite of body, mind, and spirit. When one part is not functioning well, the other parts are affected. Thus when there is a physical injury, the mental and spiritual functions are affected. When there is anxiety, it manifests in psychosomatic symptoms. When there is lack of a reason for living, the body and the mind suffer. If the whole person is to be treated, then the clergyperson as the religious professional, trained in spiritual therapy, needs to be consulted and to be a part of the health care team.

SELECTING THE CLERGYPERSON WITH THE CANCER PATIENT

In selecting the clergyperson for the cancer patient, one needs to collect certain information. Those familiar with the religious spectrum in America know that there are a wide variety of religions and clergypersons. Among Christians there are three major branches: Roman Catholic, Eastern Orthodox, and Protestant. The Roman Catholics are monolithic; the Eastern Orthodox have several branches: Greek Orthodox, Russian Orthodox, Armenian Orthodox. The Protestants are a complex group. There are at least 200 Protestant denominations.

Some of the major ones are American Baptists, Southern Baptists, National Baptists, Presbyterians, Lutherans, Methodists, Episcopalians, United Church of Christ, and the Disciples of Christ. Judaism has three major branches: Reformed, Conservative, and Orthodox. Within Buddhism there are various types: Theravada, Mahayana, Japanese Buddhism (part of Mahyana), and others. This listing does not encompass the kinds of religion existing in America. In addition, within each religion or denomination there are fundamentalists, conservatives, and liberals. Therefore, the process of collecting information is very necessary.

When the patient has no preference as to a clergyperson, then someone who has had clinical pastoral education or has done work in pastoral psychology may be consulted. The pastoral counselor is trained in the fields of theology and psychology. Course work involves marriage and family, group dynamics, and individual psychology. Practical training involves many hours of supervised counseling. The trained pastoral counselor is able to do psychotherapy.

As with any other referral, the nurse needs to be sensitive to the needs of the patient and then to match the clergyperson to the patient's need. Always the health of the whole patient will need to be the motivating factor.

REFERENCES

1 Jeanne Achterberg, O. Carl Simonton, and Stephanie Matthews-Simonton. *Stress, Psychological Factors, and Cancer*. Fort Worth, Texas: Cancer Counseling and Research Center, 1976.
2 Elisabeth Kübler-Ross. *On Death and Dying*. New York: Macmillan, 1969.

Part Four

Unique Roles in
Oncology Nursing

Chapter 16

Chemotherapy and the Nurse's Role

Diana L. Donley

Chemotherapy, the treatment of a disease by use of naturally occurring or synthetic products, was initiated as a treatment modality for cancer during World War II. It was found that men who had been exposed to mustard gas had a decreased white blood cell count. Researchers realized that this response might be used to good effect on the elevated white blood cell counts found in leukemia. Since mustard gas is very toxic, the derivative used was nitrogen mustard. Nitrogen mustard also has severe toxic effects of nausea and vomiting, so researchers looked for similarly effective, but less toxic, drugs. There are now more than 60 drugs currently in use, with effects that range from prolongation of the disease-free interval to palliation and side effects that are more controllable than those of the earlier drugs.

The role of the nurse in chemotherapy was originally to observe for side effects and to give the patient emotional support. Now the nurse's role has expanded far beyond this. Nurses administer chemotherapy orally and parenterally. They support the patient physically, psychologically, educationally, and socially. It is essential that accurate records be kept, and these, too, are within the nurse's role. Patients on chemotherapy must be helped to learn to live with an uncertain future and to hope realistically while keeping fears of the disease and its treatment at a manageable level.

The first half of this chapter will focus on the chemotherapy drugs themselves: what they are, how they work, why they are used in combinations, when they are effective, and who can benefit from them. Many patients on these drugs either fear them unrealistically or hope they will provide a magical cure. One tends to fear less what one understands, and with understanding comes realistic hope. Nurses who can cogently and coherently discuss the rationale for using these drugs at the patient's level of understanding will help the patient understand them and thus have realistic expectations of the outcomes.

The second half of this chapter will focus on the nurse's role and responsibilities in the care of the patient on antineoplastic agents. The physical, psychological, emotional, and educative aspects of chemotherapy nursing will be covered. A table that summarizes specific nursing interventions is presented.

CHEMOTHERAPY: THE RATIONALE

Chemotherapy is given for the prolongation of the disease-free interval in some diseases, such as Burkitt's lymphoma, choriocarcinoma, acute lymphocytic leukemia, Ewing's sarcoma, rhabdomyosarcoma, embryonal testicular carcinoma, Wilm's tumor, and retinoblastoma. It is given as an adjuvant with surgery or radiotherapy in colon or breast cancer and in leukemia.

Chemotherapy is given when there is systemic disease that is incurable by surgery or radiation therapy alone. When it is given postoperatively to those with breast or colon cancer, it may not be known that there is definite systemic disease. The adjuvant effect desired here is preventative in its goal. Palliation is the effect most often achieved for most patients, given the current state of knowledge. "Palliation" means that there is a temporary reduction in tumor mass or a relief of symptoms such as obstruction.

HOW NEW DRUGS ARE DEVELOPED

Researchers throughout the world are constantly looking for new drugs. If a new drug seems promising, studies are done on animals first. In the United States, all testing is supervised by the National Cancer Institute. Phase I of testing the drug on humans is restricted to a few institutions in which strict controls can be maintained and life-support systems are available if severe unexpected toxic reactions occur. It is oriented to finding the correct dosage level in humans with minimal side effects. Phase II of human testing is limited to selected investigators throughout the nation. Its focus is to discover which tumors the drug is effective against. Concurrently, in vitro testing continues to discover the biochemical reactions of the drug in tissue culture. Phase III trials are comparative, testing the efficacy of the new drug against more established ones. The final phase before general distribution is a search for the best way to use the new drug's potential. This may be in combination with other drugs; singly; or in combination with surgery, radiotherapy, or immunotherapy. The Food and

Drug Administration can then allow the drug to be generally distributed. Some drugs never pass the animal stage of testing, while others are found to be more effective in the treatment of diseases other than the one being tested for. The toxicities of some drugs preclude their use in humans, so ways to alter their biochemical structure are devised to retain the antitumor effect while decreasing or eliminating toxic effects.

In each of the experimental and clinical testing phases, reports in medical journals enable the physician to keep abreast of the progress of the researchers.

HOW CHEMOTHERAPY IS CHOSEN AS TREATMENT

Tumor conferences at local hospitals or regional tumor conferences are held at regular intervals to present additional data on these new drugs or on older drugs used in new ways. Another goal of tumor conferences it give the non-oncologist an opportunity to present the case history and physical findings of a patient whose treatment regime concerns him or her. In areas geographically distant from metropolitan areas, telephone conferences may be held. A surgeon, pathologist, oncologist, and radiotherapist confer with the consulting physician.

The diagnosis may be clear-cut, and the patient may present no unusual management problems. Then the selection of drugs is based on the cell type and location of the tumor. Certain drugs are cell-type–specific. For example, 5-fluorouracil (5-FU) is most effective against adenocarcinoma, a glandular tissue tumor, while bleomycin has been shown to be effective against tumors of squamous cell origin. The site is also a factor in determining what drug will be used. A tumor of the brain, regardless of whether it has metastasized from an adenocarcinoma of the breast or of the prostate, will not be touched by 5-FU, since this drug cannot cross the blood-brain barrier, as most drugs cannot. Thus, the location of the metastases also determines which drugs will be used.

The method of administration depends in part on the absorption of the drug and also on the desired effects. For some drugs, the oral route is preferred, and for others oral absorption is too unpredictable. Intra-arterial infusions are used to treat a cancer in an isolated organ, such as the liver, while perfusions are used to treat disease of an extremity, and malignant effusions are treated by instillation of the drug into the body cavity. In general, localized disease gets localized treatment, while systemic disease gets systemic treatment.

WHO IS ELIGIBLE FOR CHEMOTHERAPY

When the possibility of chemotherapy treatment is considered, one must also consider if the patient is eligible for chemotherapy. Not all patients who have systemic disease are capable of receiving these drugs without experiencing more harm than good. Keeping this in mind, a list of eligibility criteria has been developed. These criteria were originally developed for experimental trials of chemotherapy and may not be observed in day-to-day clinical practice.

Histologic Proof of Diagnosis

Histologic proof of a diagnosis of cancer is needed to prevent chemotherapy from being given for a nonmalignant disease or to determine if the patient has a second occurrence of cancer, called a "second primary." This may be of a different cell type or site of origin than the original tumor. Histologic proof is additionally needed to prove that a bowel obstruction or similar complication is due to a cancer recurrence and not to adhesions or some other nonmalignant process.

Bone Marrow Function

The patient should have adequate bone marrow function as evidenced by adequate hemoglobin levels and adequate white blood cell counts (WBC). In cases in which a decrease in these counts is due to overcrowding of the marrow by tumor, the drugs can still be given on the premise that removal of the tumor by the drug will allow the marrow to reexpand and replenish itself. One cannot determine if giving the drug will be beneficial in such a situation by examining the peripheral blood alone, and a bone marrow aspiration must be done.

In addition to the WBC, the lymphocyte count should be high enough to protect the patient against infection. The platelet count should be of adequate levels to prevent bleeding. It is essential to note these levels before treatment begins, especially when the drugs cause myelosuppression, as vincristine may do in a sensitive patient. Unfortunately, there is no way to determine before therapy who is sensitive and who is not.

Observation of Lesions

If the patient has measurable lesions, they may be measured directly, as with skin lesions, or indirectly, as with masses located in the lung or liver and visualized only by x-rays. Another indirect method of observing the efficacy of chemotherapy is to follow laboratory data, such as alkaline phosphatase, acid phosphatase, carcinoembryonic antigen (CEA), and others. It is not always possible to measure tumor growth or regression by either direct or indirect methods, and so the presence of measurable lesions is not a strict criterion except in clinical trials.

Nutritional Status

The patient who is to receive chemotherapy must have an adequate nutritional status, which is evaluated by (1) the patient's normal weight, as compared with the current level, (2) dietary habits, and (3) if there is a question of protein deficiency, the serum albumin-globulin ratio. The state of hydration should also be good, with a normal skin turgor, allowing for age differences. Since chemotherapeutic drugs are not taken up by fatty tissue, edema, or effusions, the amount of weight occupied by these substances is ignored when the drug dosage is calculated. If the patient is overweight or edematous, the dosage is based on the patient's ideal weight for height and age. If the patient is edematous but underweight, the dosage is based on estimated dry weight; for the underweight patient, it is based on actual weight.

Because of their action on the gastrointestinal mucosa, methotrexate and some other drugs may decrease absorption of nutrients, vitamins, and water.

Life Expectancy

The criterium of life expectancy is followed more often during experimental trials than in clinical use. Usually, it is preferred that the patient have a life expectancy of more than 4 weeks. While difficult to predict, this estimate is made for two reasons. First, chemotherapy given to a moribund patient will not prolong life, but may hasten death. Second, the side effects that accompany some drugs will only make the last few days of life miserable. When clinical studies or trials are in progress, a third reason for this criterion is to prevent the researchers from being uncertain as to whether the drug caused the death or the death would have occurred anyway. Occasionally, the reader may see chemotherapy being given in the terminal phase. It is usually being given to satisfy the psychological needs of the patient, the family, or on occasion the physician. It is difficult to know if the patient would benefit from an increased life span, or if life would only be prolonged without its quality being improved. If life is lengthened, the nurse can do much to improve its quality by her rehabilitative efforts.

Liver and Renal Function

The blood chemistries of the potential chemotherapy patient should reflect adequate liver and renal function. The majority of these drugs are detoxified or deactivated by the liver and excreted by the kidneys. If these organs function poorly, the drugs will be retained in a nearly active state; this situation may lead to overdosage.

Concomitant Illnesses

There should be no infection, bleeding, or other serious illness present which may be aggravated by the drugs. Most chemotherapy drugs lower immune resistance and affect the healing process. Bleeding tendencies could be enhanced by myelosuppression or by the effects of the drug on the liver. Ideally, there should be no serious emotional illness. This precaution is necessary to prevent possible overdosage of oral medications by the patient, to spare the patient the psychologic effects of treatment, and to prevent possible psychosis that can accompany some drugs (see Table 16-1).

Previous Therapy

There should be no chemotherapy in the 4 to 8 weeks preceding onset of a new chemical treatment regime, so that additive effects of the toxicities can be prevented. In cancer care centers that have life-sustaining facilities, such as cell separators to harvest and transfuse white cells into leukopenic patients, and isolation techniques, such as laminar airflow rooms, this criterion is frequently

Table 16-1 Chemotherapy Drugs

Drugs	Uses	Side effects	Lab	Special considerations
Antimetabolites				
5-FU (Fluorouracil)*	Cancers of GI tract, breast, lung, uterus, ovary, liver, skin, prostate, bladder, oropharynx.	Anorexia, nausea, vomiting, diarrhea, stomatitis, alopecia, bone marrow depression, skin sensitivities, dermatitis, nail changes, cerebellar dysfunction.	CBC, platelets.	Drug is most effective when given to mild toxicity. Stomatitis indicates impending bone marrow depression.
Cytosar (ara-C) (cytosine arabinoside)	Acute granulocytic leukemia, lymphomas lymphocytic leukemia, herpes zoster.	Bone marrow depression, nausea, vomiting, diarrhea, stomatitis, liver dysfunction fever, thrombophlebitis, esophagitis.	CBC, platelets, liver enzymes.	Is excreted rapidly through the kidneys. Crosses the blood-brain barrier.
6-MP (mercaptopurine)	Acute leukemia, chronic granulocytic leukemia.	Bone marrow depression, liver damage, occasional nausea and vomiting, stomatitis, mouth ulcers.	CBC, platelets, uric acid, liver enzymes.	If Zyloprim is given, the dose of 6-MP must be reduced to 1/3 or 1/4 the usual dose, since Zyloprim blocks the enzyme that destroys 6-MP. Is not given to alcoholics or if liver dysfunction exists.
Methotrexate (amethopterin, MTX)	Acute leukemia, choriocarcinoma, lymphosarcoma, CNS leukemia, most solid tumors, psoriasis, mycosis fungoides, osteogenic sarcoma.	Bone marrow depression, pruritis, urticaria, acne, stomatitis, chills, fever, nausea, vomiting, diarrhea, cystitis, diabetes, liver atrophy and necrosis, alopecia, photosensitivity.	CBC, platelets, liver enzymes, renal enzymes.	Methotrexate is excreted through the kidneys, so if renal function is impaired, the drug should not be given. Antidote for Methotrexate is Leukovorin (folinic acid). Is not given to those with liver dysfunction. Effect of MTX is decreased by salicylates, sulfonamides, aminobenzoic acid. Do not give with vitamins, vaccines, tetracyclines, chloramphenicol, Dilantin.

*The drug name in most common usage is listed first. Drugs are also known by the names in parentheses.

Drug	Indications	Side effects	Monitor	Notes
Thioguanine (6-TG)	Acute leukemia, chronic granulocytic leukemia.	Hepatic dysfunction, bone marrow depression, nausea, vomiting, skin rash, stomatitis, jaundice, photosensitivity.	CBC, platelets, liver enzymes.	Is metabolized by liver.
Alkylating agents				
Myleran (busulfan)	Chronic granulocytic leukemia, polycythemia vera, primary thrombocytosis.	Bone marrow depression, nausea, vomiting, testicular atropy, amenorrhea, gynecomastia, pulmonary fibrosis, skin hyperpigmentation.	CBC, platelets.	Is excreted by kidneys.
Leukeran (chlorambucil)	Chronic lymphocytic leukemia; Hodgkin's disease; lymphoma; CA of breast, ovary, testis.	Bone marrow depression, occasional gastric discomfort.	CBC, platelets.	None
Cytoxan (cyclophosphamide)	Acute lymphocytic leukemia, lymphoma, Hodgkin's myeloma, lymphosarcoma, most solid tumors, Wilm's tumor, rhabdomyosarcoma.	Bone marrow depression, mild nausea, occasional vomiting, stomatitis, alopecia, hemorrhagic cystitis, anaphylatic reaction, immunosuppression, liver dysfunction.	CBC, platelets, liver enzymes.	Cytoxan is excreted almost unchanged through the kidneys, so if the paient is dehydrated, the concentration of drug in the urine will cause irritation of the kidneys and bladder and so cause hemorrhagic cystitis.
Mustargen (nitrogen mustard)	Hodgkin's lymphoma, control of most effusions, CA of ovary and breast, bronchogenic cancer.	Severe nausea, vomiting, bone marrow depression, alopecia, jaundice, vertigo, tinnitus, decreased hearing, weakness, diarrhea.	CBC, platelets.	Vomiting may be so severe that if the patient has a tendency for a CVA, he may have a CVA while vomiting. Will cause severe damage to the skin if infiltrated or if spilled on skin; use sodium thiosulfate to reduce reactions.

Table 16-1 *(Continued)*

Drugs	Uses	Side effects	Lab	Special considerations
Mitomycin C	Gastric carcinoma, colon and pancreas, cervical, breast, bronchogenic, head and neck cancers; malignant melanoma.	Nausea, vomiting, bone marrow depression, severe skin reaction if given subcutaneously, severe malaise, fever, stomatitis, pruritis, alopecia, paresthesias, renal damage.	CBC, platelets, renal enzymes.	Vitamin B6 may reverse skin reaction if given immediately after extravasation intradermally.
Alkeran (melphelan, L-PAM, L-Phenylalanine mustard)	Myeloma; cancer of breast, ovary, or testicle.	Unpredictable bone marrow depression, nausea, vomiting, stomatitis.	CBC, platelets.	Tendency for nausea occurs if patient is fasting at the time of administration.
Thio-TEPA (triethylene thiophosphoramide)	CA of breast, ovary, lungs; lymphoma; control of effusions.	Potential allergic reaction, bone marrow depression, local pain, nausea, vomiting, dizziness, headache, anemia, GI perforation.	CBC, platelets, renal enzymes.	Is excreted by kidneys. If they are impaired, use with caution.
DTIC (imidazole carboxamide, imidazole mustard)	Sarcoma, malignant melanoma, Hodgkin's disease.	Severe nausea and vomiting, usually greatest on first day of therapy; fever; confusion; bone marrow depression; liver toxicity; flulike syndrome with headache, myalgia, malaise.	CBC, platelets, liver enzymes.	May give the patient a metallic taste. Burns on injection.
Plant extracts Oncovin (vincristine)	Acute lymphocytic leukemia, choriocarcinoma, lymphoma, most solid tumors, neuroblastoma, Wilm's tumor, rhabdomyosarcoma, CA of testes.	Rarely, leukopenia and thrombocytopenia; alopecia, peripheral neuropathy, paresthesias, loss of deep tendon reflexes, constipation, muscle wasting, upper-colon impaction, impotence, visual disturbance, seizures.	Neurological exam., CBC, platelets.	Patients on this drug should be placed on prophylactic laxative or stool softeners. Dosage is limited by neurotoxicity. Is very toxic to skin if infiltrated. Is used with caution in patients with preexisting neuropathies.

Drug	Uses	Side Effects	Monitoring	Comments
Velban (vinblastine)	Hodgkin's and other lymphomas, breast and reticuloendothelial malignancies.	Bone marrow depression, nausea, vomiting, constipation, vesiculation of mouth, diarrhea, abdominal pain, alopecia, stomatitis, paresthesias, headache, depression, loss of deep tendon reflexes, ileus, pain in tumor site, urinary retention.	CBC, platelets, neurological exam.	If splashed in the eye, this drug can cause corneal ulceration. Is very toxic to skin if infiltrated. Has cumulative toxicity.

Antibiotics

Drug	Uses	Side Effects	Monitoring	Comments
Cosmogen (dactinomycin, actinomycin D)	Wilm's tumor, sarcoma, choriocarcinoma, testicular CA, oat cell CA of lung, rhabdomyosarcoma.	Bone marrow depression, malaise, fatigue, lethargy, proctitis, nausea, vomiting, abdominal pain, alopecia, acne, diarrhea, dermatitis.	CBC, platelets, renal and liver function.	Is very toxic to skin if infiltrated. If given when the patient has chicken pox, patient may get CNS chicken pox with death resulting. If given after radiation therapy, may reactivate radiation site.
Daunorubricin (daunomycin)	Acute lymphocytic leukemia, neuroblastoma, acute granulocytic leukemia.	Bone marrow depression, mild nausea and vomiting, diarrhea, fever with skin rash, alopecia, mouth ulcer, possible cardiac toxicity leading to heart failure.	CBC, platelets, cardiac enzymes, EKG.	Dose is limited to 600 mg/m². Urine turns red, but not because of hematuria, as the drug is red.
Mithracin (mithramycin)	Testicular CA, malignant hypercalcemia, trophoblastic tumors.	Hypocalcemia, hypokalemia, severe bleeding that may begin with epistaxis or hematemesis, nausea, vomiting, diarrhea, stomatitis, change in liver and renal function with increased SGOT and BUN, thrombocytopenia, drowsiness, depression, headache.	CBC, platelets, liver profile, kidney function, prothrombin time, bleeding and clotting times, calcium and potassium levels.	Also is toxic to skin if infiltrated. Watch for signs of hypocalcemia: weakness, loss of muscle tone strength, signs of bleeding. Patient should not drive or operate heavy machinery after the dose

Table 16-1 *(Continued)*

Drugs	Uses	Side effects	Lab	Special considerations
Doxorubricin (adriamycin, ADRIA)	Sarcoma; Hodgkin's disease; acute leukemia; breast, genitourinary, thyroid, lung cancers; neuroblastoma.	Nausea, vomiting, congestive heart failure, alopecia, GI mucositis, myelosuppression.	Cardiac enzymes, EKG, CBC, platelets, liver enzymes.	Drug is very toxic if infiltrated. Observe for signs of cardiac decompensation (dyspnea, edema of legs, increased pulse, weakness, etc.) Dose is limited to 550 mg/m². Drug is red and causes red urine; not due to hematuria. Is metabolized by the liver.
Bleomycin (Bleaoxane)	Epidermoid cancer lymphoma, testicular carcinoma, urinary tract CA, soft-tissue sarcoma.	Pneumonitis followed by pulmonary fibrosis, fever, nausea, vomiting, increased pigmentation of skin, nail changes. May have pain and hemorrhage from tumor site due to rapid destruction of tumor tissue. Anaphylactic reaction. Rarely, stomatitis and myelosuppression.	Chest x-rays, blood gases, lung function studies, CBC, platelets, uric acid levels.	If fever occurs, it is on the day of administration and usually subsides with Tylenol. It may be necessary to give prednisone to subdue the fever. Watch carefully for signs of pulmonary fibrosis, i.e., cough, hemoptysis, exertional dyspnea. Dose limit is 400 mg. total. Test dose is given before first dose.
Hormones Prednisone (Sterane, Deltasone)	Acute and chronic leukemia; malignant hematologic disease; myeloma; any CA that is influenced by hormones, i.e., breast, ovary, prostate, etc; Hodgkin's and other lymphomas.	Muscle weakness, purpura, myopathy, euphoria, diabetes, psychosis, hirsutism, suppression of adrenal function, peptic ulcer, acne, electrolyte imbalance, spontaneous fractures of hip, hip necrosis, hypertension, pancreatitis, increased intraocular tension, alopecia, erythema of face, ulcerative esophagitis, headache, immunosuppression.	Periodic electrolyte checks.	Patients who have diabetes are harder to manage while on prednisone. It may induce diabetes if there is a tendency for it. Do not give with herpes simplex, keratitis, acute infections, or acute psychosis. Prednisone masks signs of infection. Give low-salt, low CHO, high-potassium diet. Monitor weight. Avoid salicylates. Drug is always given with antacid.

Drug	Use	Side effects	Laboratory monitoring	Nursing considerations
Androgens (Halotestin, testosterone)	Breast CA, if disseminated and post-menopausal or post-castration.	Hirsutism, fluid retention, nausea, dyspepsia, acne, increased libido, deepening of voice, salt retention, hot flashes, hypercalcemia if bone lesions present.	None.	Monitor weight. Give low-salt diet.
Estrogens (estradiol, stilbestrol)	Metastatic prostatic cancer, breast cancer if the woman is post-menopausal.	Fluid retention, nausea, vomiting, diarrhea, breast tenderness, vertigo, headache, rash, insomnia, changes in calcium and phosphorus metabolism, feminization, muscle weakness libido changes, polyuria, polydypsia.	Periodic checks of calcium and phosphorus.	Give low-salt diet. Monitor weight.
Progesterones (Delalutin, provera, megace)	Metastatic endometrial cancer, renal and breast cancer.	Nausea, vomiting, fluid retention, libido changes, occasional thromboembolitic disorders, depression, backache, breast tenderness, hypercalcemia.		Give low-salt diet. Monitor weight.
Miscellaneous agents Procarbazine (Matulane)	Hodgkin's disease, ovarian and oat cell cancer, myeloma, non-Hodgkin's lymphomas.	Nausea, vomiting, sedative effect, myelosuppression, myalgia, CNS irritability, inhibition of monoamine oxidase, rare psychosis, orthostatic hypotension.	CBC, platelets, liver and renal enzymes.	Is metabolized by liver, excreted by kidney. There is synergy with phenothiazines, barbiturates, and narcotics and alcohol intolerance with headache, facial edema, diaphoresis. Crosses blood-brain barrier. Seems to enhance effect of other drugs and radiotherapy. Since drug is MAO inhibitor, avoid cheese, alcohol, yogurt, antihistamines, narcotics, sedatives, sympathomimetics, tricyclic antidepressants, bananas.

Table 16-1 *(Continued)*

Drugs	Uses	Side effects	Lab	Special considerations
Hydroxyurea (hydrea)	Chronic granulocytic leukemia, malignant melanoma.	Nausea, vomiting, myelosuppression, rarely alopecia, skin rash, oral and GI ulcerations.	CBC, platelets, liver and renal enzymes.	Is synergistic with radiotherapy and may cause erythema. Crosses blood-brain barrier. Give with caution if liver or kidneys are impaired.
Mitotane (O, p′ DDD, lysodren)	Adrenocortical cancer after excision	Nausea, vomiting, GI toxicity, anorexia, diarrhea, CNS depression, dizziness, tremors, altered steroid metabolism.	17 OHCS, Liver and renal enzymes.	Instruct the patient to use care if coordination or concentration is needed. Steroid replacement may be needed.
Carmustine (BCNU), Lomustine (CCNU)	Primary and secondary brain tumors, Hodgkin's, lymphomas, gastric and renal cell cancer, melanoma.	Delayed myelosuppression, nausea and vomiting, diarrhea, mild hepatotoxicity.	CBC, platelets.	Crosses the blood-brain barrier.
Streptozotocin	Pancreatic insulinoma, carcinoid tumor, Hodgkin's disease.	Nausea; vomiting; renal tubular defects; stomatitis; abdominal cramps; diabetogenic; may cause hypoglycemia, nephrotoxicity.		May cause burning on administration. Test urine for glycosuria.
L-asparaginase	Acute lymphoblastic leukemia.	Minimal effect on bone marrow and GI tract but causes severe hepatic dysfunction; pancreatic, renal, and clotting dysfunctions; azotemia; possible anaphylaxis, blood dyscrasias; malaise; hypoalbuminemia, hyperglycemia; reversible encephalopathy.	CBC, platelets; liver, renal, and pancreatic enzymes; clotting studies; uric acid level; glucose level; serum albumin; MCV, MCHC, MCH.	Shaking vial harms enzyme.

not observed. In smaller institutions lacking such support systems for the patient who develops a total myelosuppression, it is necessary to consider the previous therapy criterion.

It is ideal that the patient have no major surgical procedure or radiotherapy in the 4 weeks preceding chemotherapy, except when chemotherapy is used in an adjuvant capacity. Patients who have undergone such therapy will have decreased nutritional status and may be in negative nitrogen balance. Chemotherapy can also cause decrease wound healing. These factors are considered when chemotherapy is used as an adjuvant with surgery or radiotherapy.

HOW CHEMOTHERAPY WORKS

Chemotherapy works on the cellular level. The action depends to a great extent on the type of drug used and on the timing of the administration according to the cell cycle. The cell cycle as presented here is in simplified form.

Review of the Cell Cycle

Normal cells grow and divide in an orderly fashion. The cell, in the normal metabolizing state called G_1, reaches a point at which division is needed either to ensure the cell's survival or to replace lost tissue. It then goes through the S phase, which refers to the synthesis of DNA (see Figure 16-1). A period of quiescence, called G_2, then follows. In G_2 the cell builds up energy reserves in preparation for the next phase, designated by M for mitosis. During mitosis, the parent cell in normal tissue divides into two daughter cells. The cancer cell

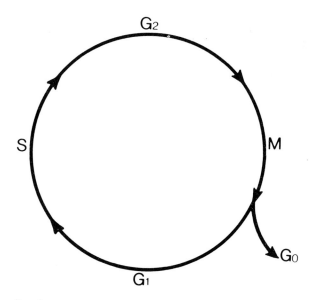

Figure 16-1   The cell cycle.

occasionally divides into three or four daughter cells. The new cells may go directly into the G_1, or active, state or may go into G_0, an inactive resting state. A cell in G_0 will go into the active state when signaled to do so by mechanisms not clearly understood. One such mechanism may be the presence of other cells around it. Normal cells have such a quality, called "contact inhibition," in which they sense the presence of other cells around them and stop their growth and division. Cancer cells lack this quality, and growth continues even though the cells are already crowded. The presence of cells in the pool called G_0 creates a problem when drugs that are given are active in the cell only when it is growing or dividing. This is one reason that many cycles of drugs are given and the main basis for combining drugs in a treatment regime.

DRUG TYPES AND THEIR ACTIONS

Each classification of drug has a different mode of action and works during a different phase of the cell cycle (see Figure 16-2). The diseases each is effective against are listed in Table 16-1, as are the toxic effects and special considerations for each drug.

Antimetabolites

Antimetabolites interfere with the metabolic pathways of dividing cells, usually with DNA synthesis. They can interfere with the biosynthetic enzymes, or they

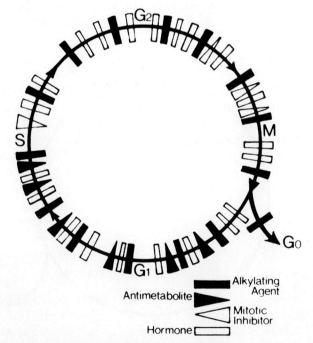

Figure 16-2 Action of chemotherapy drugs during the cell cycle.

can become incorporated into abnormal and nonfunctional products which are lethal to the cell. The cell takes these drugs into its interior, since they closely resemble normal metabolites that can be used to produce the proteins needed for division. As the cell tries to produce the proteins, it is unable to do so and dies. These drugs are effective during the S and G_2 phases.

Antifolics

Methotrexate is a folic acid antagonist. It blocks the conversion of folic acid to tetrahydrafolic acid, a substance needed for DNA synthesis and mitosis. Leukovorin is a derivative of tetrahydrafolic acid. When given after lethal doses of methotrexate have been given, it eliminates the need for the cells to convert folic acid into tetrahydrafolic acid. Normal cells recover rapidly, while cancer cells take much longer to recover. Methotrexate is also used in the treatment of severe psoriasis.

Antipurines

Mercaptopurine (6-MP) is a purine antagonist. Purines are proteins needed for DNA synthesis. If allopurinal (Zyloprim) is given with this drug, the dosage of 6-MP must be reduced one-third to one-fourth the normal dose, since allopurinol destroys the enzyme that inactivates 6-MP. If the dose is not reduced, there will be rapid accumulation of 6-MP to toxic levels. Mercaptopurine is not given to those with obvious liver dysfunction or to alcoholics because of its hepatotoxicity. A single dose given to these patients has been known to precipitate hepatic coma.

Antipyramidines

Pyramidines are another type of protein needed for DNA synthesis. In this category are fluorouracil (5-FU) and cytosine arabinoside (Cytosar or ara-C). Fluorouracil is a very versatile drug, since it can be used topically, orally, intravenously, or intraluminally for a wide variety of solid tumors.

Cytosine arabinoside (ara-C) is a drug with a wide variety of uses as well. In small doses it has proven effective in shortening the duration and severity of herpes zoster. The herpes zoster virus is a normal inhabitant of most people and usually causes disease only when the immune system is depressed. It is wise to give ara-C only to those who already have been diagnosed as having cancer. Nearly all the cancer chemotherapy drugs may *cause* cancer due to the immunosuppressive effects they have. Ara-C is especially immunosuppressive. Another drug, idoxuridine (IUdR), is just as effective in treating herpes zoster without having the immunosuppressive qualities of ara-C.

Alkylating Agents

The action of an alkylating agent is to directly attack the DNA and biosynthetic enzymes. It binds the chains of DNA together, preventing replication, or it can break the chain (see Figure 16-3). These drugs act independently of DNA synthesis and mitosis, earning them the name of non-cell cycle–dependent.

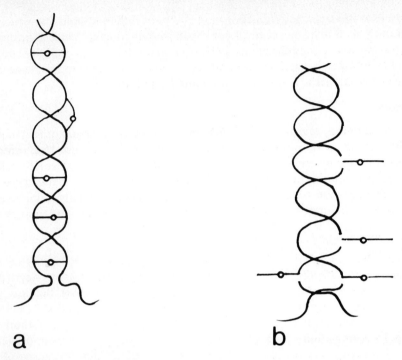

a   b

Figure 16-3   Effects of alkylating agents on DNA. (*a*) Bind chains together. (*b*) Break chains of DNA.

They are therefore effective against the nondividing population in the G_0 phase. The drugs included in this category are mechlorethamine (nitrogen mustard or HN_2), cyclophosphamide (Cytoxan), melphalan (Alkeran), chlorambucil (Leukeran), triethlyenemelamine (TEM), triethylene thiophosphoramide (Thio-TEPA), busulfan (Myleran), Imidazole carboxamide (DTIC), and the nitrosurea group, which includes carmustine (BCNU), lomustine (CCNU), and semustine (methyl-CCNU). The nitrosurea group is of special interest because of its unique ability to cross the blood-brain barrier, apparently due to its lipid solubility. The alkylating agents as a class share the common toxicity of bone marrow depression, nausea, and vomiting.

Natural Products

Antibiotics seem to have different types of effects on the cancer cell. Actinomycin D (Dactinomycin or Cosmogen) inhibits DNA synthesis. Daunorubricin (Daunomycin or DAU), doxorubicin (Adriamycin or ADRIA), bleomycin (Blenoxane), and mitomycin C act as alkylating agents. Mithramycin (Mithracin) acts by inhibition of RNA synthesis. All these drugs were first thought to be useful in treating bacterial infections, but were found to be too toxic for that purpose. However, they were found to be effective in the treatment of cancer.

The vinca alkaloids, extracted from the periwinkle plant, are vincristine (Oncovin) and vinblastine (Velban). These drugs act by inhibiting mitosis and are cell-cycle–specific, i.e., active only when the cell is in the mitotic phase of division. One toxicity consists of numbness and tingling of the extremities, loss of deep tendon reflexes, and ataxia.

The enzyme L-asparaginase inhibits protein synthesis and has as a direct toxicity hepatic failure, plus pancreatic and renal damage.

Hormones

The hormone group includes the adrenocorticosteroids, most notably prednisone, the progestins, estrogens, and androgens. It is not clear how these agents affect tumor growth rates. For some tumors that are hormone-dependent, such as prostatic or postmenopausal ones, or postcastration breast cancer, giving the opposite sex hormone changes the hormonal input into the cell and creates an unfavorable hormonal setting for tumor growth.

Miscellaneous Agents

Hydroxyurea (Hydrea) inhibits DNA synthesis, while procarbazine (Matulane) inhibits DNA, RNA, and protein synthesis. An investigational drug used to treat adrenocortical tumors, mitotane (O,p'DDD or Lysodren) is chemically similar to DDT. Its mechanism of action is as yet unknown.

COMBINATION CHEMOTHERAPY

The rationale for combination chemotherapy is based on the cell cycle and differing toxicities. A drug that is active at one point in the cell cycle is combined with another drug active at a different point in the cycle, with the additional criterion that all drugs in the combination be active against the cancer in question. Drugs with differing toxicities are usually combined, or the dosage is decreased when two drugs with the same toxicity must be given together. For example, COAP is an acronym for a combination of drugs used to treat acute leukemia. It is composed of (1) cyclophosphamide, an alkylating agent active during the entire cell cycle, with the major toxicities being myelosuppression and gastrointestinal disturbances; (2) vincristine, a mitotic inhibitor having neurotoxicity as its major toxic effect; (3) cytosine arabinoside, an antimetabolite active mainly during the synthesis phase, with the major toxicity of myelosuppression; (4) prednisone, a corticosteroid hormone that potentiates the other drugs and changes the hormonal milieu of the body, with the major toxicities of immunologic and adrenocorticosuppression. Doses are adjusted to give maximum effectiveness with minimal myelosuppression (see Figure 16-4).

Sequential administration takes full advantage of the cell cycle. On day 1, vincristine and cytosine arabinoside attack the cells in the mitotic and synthesis phases, respectively. Cyclophosphamide and prednisone are given daily to damage each cell that develops. It is estimated that by day 8, cells that were in the G_0 phase have entered the active phase, and the drugs active in the synthesis and mitotic phases are given again. After 14 days the patient rests, and in 2 weeks the course of drugs is begun again if the white counts show that the patient can tolerate it.

DAY	1	2	3	4	5	6	7	8	9	10	11	12	13	14
Cyclophosphamide (given po)	X	X	X	X	X	X	X	X	X	X	X	X	X	X
Vincristine (Oncovin) (given IV)	X							X						
Cytosine Arabinoside (ARAC) (given IV)	X							X						
Prednisone (given po)	X	X	X	X	X	X	X	X	X	X	X	X	X	X

Figure 16-4 An example of combination chemotherapy (COAP).

TOXICITY IN CHEMOTHERAPY

The toxicity for each of the chemotherapy drugs is presented in Table 16-1. Since a comprehensive discussion of each toxicity is beyond the scope of this chapter, each of the mechanisms will be discussed in general terms according to body system.

Gastrointestinal Toxicity

Gastrointestinal toxicity occurs as a result of the drug's effect on the rapidly dividing cell population of the mucosa. It is estimated that the cell population of the mucosa replaces itself every 3 days. Thus drugs given on day 1 will show an effect on the mucosa from day 3 on. Once stomatitis appears, the drugs should be withheld or ulceration may line the entire gastrointestinal tract. Nausea and vomiting are common GI toxicities. Caution in the choice of antiemetics is recommended. Compazine and Thorazine should not be used because of their effects on the liver, especially when drugs that are detoxified in the liver are given. Tigan and Vistaril seem to have less effect on the liver and are just as effective in controlling nausea.

Myelosuppression

The population of the bone marrow also rapidly divides. The estimated life span of the WBC is less than 24 hours, but there are usually adequate marrow reserves for another 8 to 10 days. The life span of the platelet is about 10 days, and the RBC lives for about 120 days. Hematologic effects of the drugs will appear in the peripheral blood in 7 to 10 days for the WBC, depending on the marrow reserves; in 10 days for the platelet; and in 3 months for the RBC. The depth of marrow suppression will not be known until this time. A patient who has few marrow reserves will begin to show leukopenia on 1 day. It is wise to check the WBC every 1 to 3 days for a patient on an oral myelosuppressive agent until the patient becomes stabilized, then once a week. For a patient on intravenous therapy, the WBC count should be done at least before each dose of medicine is given. These drugs are cellular poisons that cannot be counteracted. With the exception of methotrexate, once the drug is given, the myelosuppression will run its course.

Neurotoxicity

Neurotoxicity accompanies vincristine and vinblastine administration, and impulse conduction is slowed. The first symptoms of neurotoxicity are decreased deep tendon reflexes. Toxicity then progresses to loss of deep tendon reflexes, with foot and wrist drop. Parasthesias may be noticed early in the history of the toxicity, and eventually ataxias may develop. These losses may be reversible if the drug is stopped soon enough or if the dose is decreased at the first signs of numbness and tingling. Males may experience impotence. With other drugs, the nervous system effect may be one of psychosis, as with prednisone, or of cerebellar dysfunction, as with fluorouracil.

Hepatotoxicity

Hepatotoxicity, as caused by 6-MP, methotrexate, mithramycin, and ara-C, may be first manifested by changes in liver enzymes. The possibility for liver damage is increased if the patient has a history of alcoholism or increased alcohol consumption. For a patient who has been an alocholic, use of these drugs can precipitate an irreversible hepatic coma. The consumption of alcohol while on these drugs is contraindicated.

Cardiotoxicity

Cardiotoxicity occurs mainly with the use of doxorubricin (Adriamycin) and to a lesser extent with daunorubricin (Daunomycin). It is manifested by reversible right-sided heart failure. If the drugs are stopped when changes in cardiac enzymes, physical findings, or the electrocardiogram are noticed, the heart failure will not progress to left-sided failure.

Alopecia

Alopecia occurs because the hair cells grow rapidly and so are affected by chemotherapy drugs. The hair follicle itself may be undamaged, but the shaft of the hair has an indentation to indicate drug insult. When the hair is brushed or the patient moves his or her head on the bed, the hair breaks off (see Figure 16-5). Usually the hair will continue growth after cessation of therapy, but may continue to grow again while therapy continues, as the body adjusts to the drug's presence. Hair loss may be permanent.

Pulmonary Toxicity

Pulmonary toxicity when caused by Myleran takes the form of a cough and when caused by bleomycin takes the form of pneumonitis followed by pulmonary fibrosis. A cough may be the first sign that bleomycin toxicity is appearing. A cough can also indicate pressure on the recurrent laryngeal nerve from an

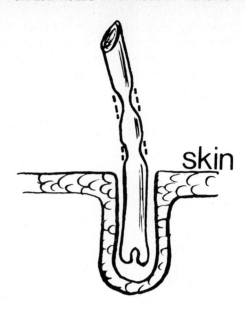

Figure 16-5 Effect of some chemotherapy drugs on the hair shaft.

enlarged right atrium or pressure on a bronchus from a tumor. If bleomycin is being used, an x-ray can usually readily differentiate between toxicity and progression of disease, although the cough of toxicity may appear before signs of pneumonitis are apparent on the x-ray. This toxicity may be reversible if the drugs are stopped before fibrosis appears.

DIFFERENTIATION BETWEEN DISEASE PROGRESSION AND TOXICITY

Some of the most critical observations the nurse can make in the care of the patient on antineoplastic therapy involve differentiation between toxicity and progression of the disease or appearance of another disease process. For example, a patient with pulmonary carcinoma received vincristine as part of the treatment regime. The first symptom of vincristine toxicity was numbness and tingling, and the dose was decreased. The patient soon developed severe constipation in spite of prophylactic stool softeners and began to lose deep tendon reflexes in spite of the fact that the vincristine had been stopped. Only after the patient had developed a right-sided weakness was the possibility of disease progression explored. A brain scan revealed left-sided cerebral metastasis, for which radiation therapy was then given.

This example is not a rare occurrence. A patient who has had abdominal surgery, is on a drug that causes nausea and vomiting, and develops vomiting without other signs of gastrointestinal toxicity, such as stomatitis, irritation of a stoma, or diarrhea, should be evaluated for another source of the vomiting, e.g., adhesions.

The clues for accurate symptom differentiation lie in the total assessment of the patient, a subject that is more full developed in Chapter 5, "Nursing Assessment of the Oncology Patient." It should be remembered that a diagnosis of cancer does not preclude the development of any other diseases, including another occurrence of cancer.

SEX AND CONCEPTION IN THE CHEMOTHERAPY PATIENT

All drugs are capable of causing sexual difficulties if one remembers that sexuality is 90 percent mental and 10 percent physical. The worries that most patients have while on these drugs can cause temporary frigidity or impotence. This topic is more fully discussed in Chapter 13, "Sexuality and the Oncology Patient." Some of the drugs can cause libido changes (see Table 16-1), and the patient should be notified that this can occur. It is possible for all drugs to cross the placental barrier and cause fetal abnormalities. All patients on chemotherapy should practice some form of birth control, with the exact method being decided upon by the oncologist or attending physician. Use of birth control pills, with their hormonal composition, may adversely affect the growth of the cancer or the treatment. Males should not attempt to father children unless the oncologist or attending physician gives permission, as nearly all the drugs can cause abnormal sperm production.

ANAPHYLAXIS

As with all drugs, there is a potential for anaphylaxis with chemotherapy drugs. This reaction has been observed with Thio-TEPA, bleomycin, and cyclophosphamide. Test doses are routinely given before Thio-TEPA and bleomycin therapy is begun. Anaphylaxis has been observed only infrequently with cyclophosphamide, but any of the drugs have such a potential. Anaphylaxis due to chemetherapy drugs should be treated as any anaphylactic reaction would be.

CHEMOTHERAPY: THE NURSE'S ROLE

The role of the nurse in cancer chemotherapy has greatly expanded. With the multidisciplinary approach being used more widely, the nurse's contribution to patient care has become increasingly more valuable. Of all the members of the multidisciplinary team, no one spends more time in direct contact with the patient than the nurse. As researchers expand nursing knowledge, more techniques are found that are beneficial in the prevention or alleviation of the patient's discomfort. The nurse administers chemotherapy, prevents the side effects where possible, and alleviates others. Through counseling, the patient can be spared much mental anguish and family unity can be preserved.

First and foremost, the nurse is concerned with the patient's safety during the administration of chemotherapy. Nursing interventions to prevent or alleviate toxic effects will be discussed and will be presented in table form for ready reference. The role of the nurse in education of the patient will be discussed. Some patients who do not know their diagnosis are given chemotherapy, and hints on how to handle this situation are given. Nursing interventions for patients on chemotherapy will be included in Table 16-2.

Table 16-2   Nursing Intervention

Symptom	Cause	Nursing intervention
Gastrointestinal toxicity		
Anorexia, nausea, emesis.	5-FU, Cytoxan, nitrogen, mustard, bleomycin, 6-MP, Imidazole carboxamide, Alkeran, Leukeran, Thio-TEPA, Cytosar, mithramycin, Actinomycin D, androgens, estrogens, progesterones, Thioguanine.	Provide good mouth care, encourage fluids, give appetizing meals. Foods should be bland, not highly spiced. Antiemetics such as Atarax, Vistaril, or Tigan may be given, though these drugs should be used with caution in patients who have liver disease or obstruction. IVs may be necessary.
Stomatitis (oral or stoma), GI ulcerations.	5-FU, Cytoxan, Imidazole carboxamide, nitrogen mustard, Cytosar, 6-MP, Thioguanine, Daunomycin, mithramycin, adriamycin, prednisone.	Provide good mouth care using swabs stead of toothbrushes. Give soft, bland foods. Drugs will be stopped. Mineral oil or Vaseline may be used to soothe the lips. Mouthwashes will only be irritating; may be 1/2 H_2O 1/2 H_2O_2, followed by water rinse. If severe pain exists, Xylocaine viscous may be used before meals, or Chlorseptic mouthwash.
Diarrhea.	5-FU, Cytoxan, nitrogen mustard, Actinomycin D, Imidazole carboxamide, methotrexate, estrogens. May also be caused by some antacids.	Usually drugs will be stopped if there are more than three diarrhea stools a day. Encourage fluids. Kaopectate, Lomotil, or antispasmodics may be given. (Patient should be checked for impaction if he or she has been constipated prior to ceiving chemotherapy.) IVs may be needed to replace fluid loss.
Dehydration, electrolyte imbalance.	Any of the above drugs, especially those leading to diarrhea.	Give serum electrolytes, IVs, electrolyte replacement therapy. Patients with dehydration are much more susceptible to hemorrhagic cystitis if on Cytoxan. They are also more likely to get obstructive uropathy if their uric acid level is high.
Gastric ulcers.	Prednisone.	Antacids must be given with steroids and continued for at least 1 week after discontinuance of the drug.
Constipation.	Vincristine, vinblastine.	Stop drugs. Laxatives and stool softeners are used as preventatives when patients are placed on these drugs.

Table 16-2 (*Continued*)

Symptom	Cause	Nursing intervention
Bone marrow depression		
Leukopenia.	Nitrogen mustard, 5-FU, methotrexate, Cytoxan, Imidazole carboxamide, Actinomycin D, vincristine, vinblastine, Alkeran, 6-MP, Cytosar, Thioguanine, Myleran, Leukeran, Daunomycin.	Reduce exposure to infection: give IV care, care for skin lesions, keep infected people away from the patient. If any signs of infection appear, stop chemotherapy drugs, begin antibiotics. May need reverse isolation.
Thrombocytopenia.	Same drugs that cause leukopenia.	Take bleeding precautions: patient should shave with an electric razor. Care must be taken with IV or IM injections, and pressure must be held over an injection site for 3–5 min. Requisitions for blood work should have "Bleeding Precautions" written on them. Aspirin in any form should never be given to any chemotherapy patient. If bleeding occurs and is not controlled by pressure dressings Collodian may be applied with a few fibers of cotton and then pressure dressing applied. Platelet transfusions may be given.
Anemia.	Same drugs that cause leukopenia. Hemorrhage due to hemorrhagic cystitis or due to mithramycin. Hemorrhage may also be due to GI ulceration from any of the drugs listed under GI ulcerations.	If there is active bleeding, cause must be found and eliminated. If drug-induced, stop drug and give transfusions while awaiting repopulation of the bone marrow. If due to GI bleeding, surgical intervention may be necessary.
Alopecia	Mithramycin, Cytoxan, nitrogen mustard, 5-FU, vincristine, vinblastine, Actinomycin D, Daunomycin, Adriamycin, prednisone.	Hair loss is usually temporary, and hair will grow again when the drug is discontinued. With some drugs, hair is lost initially but begins to grow again as therapy continues. There is no way to prevent hair loss, but keeping hair clean and neat will help the patient's morale. The patient may wear a hairnet to prevent it from falling all over the bed or floor. Wigs or caps may boost the patient's morale.
Skin sensitivities		
Increased pigmentation, acne, itching, urticaria, nail changes.	5-FU, methotrexate, Myleran, Actinomycin D, Daunomycin, prednisone, bleomycin, androgens.	If urticaria or itching is severe enough, drug may be stopped. Soothing lotions such as Alpha Keri or Caladryl may be used.

Table 16-2   (*Continued*)

Symptom	Cause	Nursing intervention
Genitourinary toxicity		
Hemorrhagic cystitis.	Cytoxan.	Stop drug immediately. This symptom is caused by high concentrations of drug in the urine due to dehydration. Encourage fluids, give IVs, insert Foley to watch the progress of the bleeding and to get an accurate output. Care must be taken to prevent fluid overload, especially in patients who have preexisting coronary disease. Transfusions may be needed if patient becomes anemic.
Pulmonary toxicity		
Pulmonary fibrosis, cough, hemoptysis.	Bleomycin (fibrosis and hemoptysis), Myleran (cough). Irritation of bronchus by tumor.	Drugs must be stopped. Fibrosis is irreversible, and steroids may be given to suppress symptoms. Cough may be controlled by codeine.
Cardiac toxicity		
Congestive heart failure (peripheral edema, lethargy, drowsiness, etc.).	Adriamycin, Daunomycin.	Stop drugs immediately, and it will be reversible if caught in time. To be treated as is failure caused by any other disease.
Neurotoxicity		
Tingling of fingers and toes. Loss of deep tendon reflexes.	Vincristine, vinblastine. May also be caused by tumor infiltration into area, e.g., in leukemia.	Stop drugs. If caught early enough, may be reversible. If not caught in time, may progress to irreversibility.
Hepatic toxicity		
Jaundice, lethargy, weakness, pruritis, coma.	Cytosar, 6-MP, methotrexate, mithramycin.	Drugs must be stopped. Give IVs, antibiotics as indicated, supportive care.
Blood chemistry changes		
Hypocalcemia.	Mithramycin.	Stop drug. Give calcium gluconate IV.
Hypercalcemia.	Increased bone destruction from any metastatic disease. Adrenal cancer.	Give Mithramycin in low doses. May also use x-ray therapy to the bone lesions to destroy the cancer and promote healing.
Hyperuricemia.	Increased cell death, whether due to tumor destruction or to normal tissue destruction.	Give Zyloprim (blocks the formation of uric acid). Force fluids or patient can go into renal shutdown from uric acid crystals.

Table 16-2 (*Continued*)

Symptom	Cause	Nursing intervention
Endocrine toxicity Diabetes.	Prednisone.	Drug must be stopped. Condition is then reversible. Control of preexisting diabetes is made much more difficult when prednisone is given.
Additional toxicity Constipation.	Vincristine, vinblastine.	Stop drugs. Laxatives and stool softeners are used as preventatives when patients are placed on these drugs.
Psychological changes Dizziness, headache, confusion, lethargy, euphoria, depression, psychosis.	Nitrogen mustard, Thio-TEPA, Imidazole carboxamide, vinblastine, Actinomycin D, prednisone, estrogens.	Dosage must be adjusted or drug may be stopped.
Fever	Cytosar, Imidazole carboxamide, bleomycin, Daunomycin. Infection. CNS leukemia.	If drug-induced, may give Tylenol or steroids to suppress the symptoms. If patient is on chemotherapy and develops any fever, he or she may be placed on appropriate antibiotics as a precautionary measure after cultures are done. If fever is caused by CNS leukemia, the disease may be controlled by methotrexate given intrathecally.

Patient Safety

Regardless of the setting the nurse may be in, he or she can do much to assure the safety of the patient before, during, and after the drugs are given. Before drugs are given, the patient should be checked on the following points.

Nutritional Status If the nutrition of the patient is abnormal, the cause could be drug toxicity; tumor involvement; emotional distress; recent surgery; post radiation effects; concomitant illness; side effects of other than antineoplastic drugs; inadequate food intake due to food dislikes, poverty, etc.; or malabsorption syndrome. Theoretically, if the patient, and therefore the cancer, is inadequately nourished, the cancer's growth rate will be impaired. There will also be, however, poor uptake of the drug by cancer cells, with poor cancer destruction. If the cancer does not take up the drug, more of the drug may be available to cause systemic toxicity. If the patient is poorly nourished, his or her normal cells will be unable to recover from the drug.

Hydration Status   Good hydration is important to help the body get rid of the detoxified drug, since many drugs are excreted through the kidneys. Increased uric acid levels combined with inadequate hydration can lead to obstructive uropathy. Cyclophosphamide and its metabolites are excreted through the kidney. If there is poor hydration, there is prolonged contact of the drug with the lining of the kidneys, ureters, and bladder, and hemorrhagic cystitis can result.

Oxygenation Status   The state of oxygenation may be impaired by the obstruction of a bronchus by cancer, by a coexisting condition such as emphysema, or by the toxicity of a fibrogenic drug such as bleomycin. Poor oxygenation retards cancer growth and results in less uptake of the drug by the cancer; thus more free drug can cause potential systemic toxicity. Respiratory function studies may be part of the workup done before bleomycin is given if there is doubt that the patient can ventilate his or her tissues adequately.

Fever   The absence of fever is desired. Any possibility of infection must be ruled out before chemotherapy is continued. Fever may result from tumor necrosis due to the action of chemotherapy. As tumors grow, they may occlude the blood vessels to normal tissue or to the tumor itself, and necrosis may result. Fever accompanies some types of cancer, such as lymphomas, leukemia, Hodgkin's disease, and hepatomas, or it could be caused by the drug itself (see Table 16-2).

The Presence of Toxicity   The presence or absence of toxicity from drugs previously given should be determined. This was discussed in the first half of the chapter.

Other Assessment Measures   Laboratory findings should be evaluated with particular attention to the WBC and platelet counts. Uric acid levels should be done once a week and other laboratory data as indicated by the patient's condition and drug regime (See Table 16-1 for lab data suggested for each type of drug.) Unusual findings should be discussed with the physician before chemotherapy is administered. Tumor measurements, unless done by indirect methods such as x-rays, should be done at least once a week. Tumor measurements should be done before every course of therapy is begun. Bleeding tendencies should be ruled out. The patient's emotional status should be stable. Nearly all patients need some education and reassurance each time the drugs are given. The nurse will want to schedule duties so that discussion time will be available to the patient.

Dosage of drugs should be recalculated periodically. Nearly all medications are calculated on the basis of milligrams per kilogram or per squared meter of body surface. The loss of as little as 1 kg of body weight can cause the dosage to be readjusted.

It is essential to be sure that the patient has not received an identical dose of the drug earlier in the day. Some patients are so conditioned to accept whatever treatment given them that they may not report it was given by another nurse or the doctor. If there is a possibility of this occurring, the pharmacist may send up only one dose at a time. Investigational drugs are kept in a locked cabinet and signed out as narcotics are.

Patient identification must be affirmed. It is possible to have more than one patient with the same—or nearly the same—name, with identical diseases, being cared for by the same doctor. When one of the house staff is to give the drug, he or she may be rushed and/or unfamiliar with the patient. These precautions are based on personal observation of the author, having seen both types of errors made.

An attitude of realistic hope can be maintained when giving or talking about these drugs. Patients sense the attitudes of those around them. If the nurse has no realistic hope and confidence in the treatment regime, the patient will sense this and doubt the outcome as well. Research is being done to determine the effects of patients' attitudes on the outcome of their illness. While no definite conclusions can be made as yet, it does seem that the maintenance of a positive attitude helps the patient in the battle against disease. Those who give up the fight may die sooner.

Since the majority of patients know what kind of drugs they are receiving, they are understandably apprehensive about their reactions to the drugs. The patient will appreciate having the nurse return after the treatment just to see how he or she is doing. It gives a concerned patient a sense of security to know that the nurse who cares about the person's welfare and feelings is nearby.

The dosage and administration of the drug must be recorded as well as communicated to other members of the team. Since one limits the total dose of some drugs before signs of irreversible toxicity appear, accurate recording is essential. For drugs such as bleomycin, daunorubricin, and daunomycin, a running dose total from onset of therapy must be maintained. These records must follow the patient from the acute care setting to the home, doctor's office, or clinic. With drugs such as fluorouracil, this precaution is not necessary as long as accurate records are kept throughout each course of therapy. These points must be considered regardless of who administers the medication and are similar to, although more thorough, than the precautions used before administration of digitalis, rauwolfia products, or some antipsychotics.

When the drugs are given intravenously, both the nurse and the patient can work together to minimize vein trauma. The following suggestions may help in keeping veins patent. A double-needle technique may be used. With this method the medication is drawn up with a needle of convenient size, such as an 18-gauge. It is then administered with a 23- or 25-gauge needle. This procedure serves the double purpose of minimizing the size of the hole made in the vein wall and reducing the nearly universal tendency of injecting the drug too rapidly.

The use of the tourniquet may be eliminated unless it is absolutely necessary. Doing this decreases the tendency for blood to leak from the wound once the needle is withdrawn.

Alleviation of the patient's fear will decrease sympathetic stimulation of the peripheral blood vessels of the skin. This stimulation causes vasoconstriction, so the patient who has less fear will have less constriction of the superficial blood vessels.

Use a heparin-locked needle or syringe for intermittent injections (see Figure 16-6). This prevents wear and tear on the patient's veins and emotions as well as the nurse's emotions. Because it can be very frustrating for the nurse and the patient to give or get intravenous injections every 6 hours, the lock can serve a dual purpose. Patients who may need injections twice or three times daily may be taught care of the heparin-lock unit so that they can self-administer medications at home. The ability to participate in one's own care provides a valuable psychologic benefit in addition to decreasing the costs of hospital, clinic, or office visits, of visits from a home care nurse, or of hospitalization.

An intra-arterial needle with an obturator may be used to prevent repeated venous trauma of laboratory tests.

When the hand or arm is warm, there is improved venous filling. Placing the extremity in warm towels or in warm water 15 to 30 minutes before attempting the venipuncture will help in vein filling. This will be of especial value to the older patient who is in an air-conditioned environment.

The leg or foot veins should never be used for chemotherapy injections, since the drugs are irritating and may increase a tendency for thrombosis formation.

The patient aids in this method of administration by ventilating concerns before the injection is attempted to decrease fears and also by remembering which vein was used last and asking to have the blood pressure checked or blood drawn from the opposite arm for a day or so. This allows for the healing process to occur in the vein wall without the venous distention putting more pressure on the wound. If a radical mastectomy has been done, usually only the unaffected arm is used for all blood pressure checks or for all venipunctures. The nurse who does not give the chemotherapy should be alert for potential venous scarring or incipient infections. If given adequate time, a scarred vein will heal itself to some degree. Infections will cause venous scarring, making the vein unusable for some time.

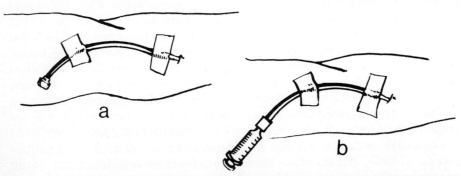

Figure 16-6 Two methods of giving intermittent venous injections (a) Winged needle with tubing and rubber stopper. (b) Winged needle attached to syringe filled with 1:1000 NS/heparin solution.

Nursing Interventions for the Patient on Chemotherapy

Many nurses who do not administer chemotherapy come in contact with the cancer patient. These nurses must be aware of which interventions are effective in prevention of toxicity and which toxic effects cannot be prevented but can be minimized. Many of the smaller institutions do not yet have a nurse who administers chemotherapy. While the drugs may be administered by a physician, it is the nurse at the bedside who must be aware of the effectiveness of the various measures to eliminate or decrease toxic effects. It is not possible to list every measure that will be effective for every patient. What works for one may not work for another. The use of an innovative approach is recommended while one remembers the potentiality for drug interactions or food-drug interactions. A summary of nursing interventions is presented in Table 16-2.

Measures for Nutritional Support   The physical measures of nutritional support are first, prevention or reduction of anorexia or nausea. Proteins in the form of eggs or milk products (for example, milk shakes) may be substituted for meat or fish if these are not well tolerated. Although it requires more energy expenditure by the body, the body can produce all but two of the proteins it needs for growth and repair of tissues from other substances. As a consequence, a very high protein diet is not needed. Food that is ethnically and esthetically pleasing should be offered to the patient. Food such as hamburgers from a favorite eating establishment may be more pleasing to the younger patient than routine hospital fare. The patient's ability to assist in the preparation of food may or may not be an aid to the appetite, depending on whether smelling food cooking is more nauseating than eating food already prepared. Ideally the food should be nonirritating, and few acidic foods should be given to reduce oropharyngeal irritation. Fluids can be offered in a variety of ways, from fruit juices to popsicles to nonalcoholic cocktails, to lessen chances of hemorrhagic cystitis for the patient on cyclophosphamide or of obstructive uropathy for the patient with elevated uric acid levels. A diet that is well balanced in protein and vitamins will help increase the patient's resistance to infections as well as aid the normal cells to recover from chemotherapy effects.

The patient who is nauseated may benefit from the use of antiemetics, but one must keep in mind the possible interaction of the antiemetic with the chemotherapy drug. One way to reduce nausea that occurs a few hours after injections is to give the drug after the evening meal. This is not true of all drugs or of all patients, but may help some of them, especially in the case of nitrogen mustard.

Once vomiting begins, it is the usual practice to withhold drugs until the vomiting can be controlled. When diarrhea begins, the drugs may be continued unless there are more than three diarrheal stools per day. Antidiarrheal drugs may be effective in controlling the symptoms once the drug is stopped. Many doctors hesitate to give antidiarrheal drugs until it is celar how many stools occur and until the extent of gastrointestinal toxicity can be evaluated.

Measures to Enhance Immune Resistance The measures to enhance immune resistance include all of the nutritive measures listed above, for good nutrition is essential to a well-functioning immune system. (See Chapter 17, ''Immunology and Immunotherapy: New Frontiers in Nursing,'' for further discussion of this topic.) Wound care should include daily inspection of traumatized sites to note and treat incipient infections early. A small bandage with an antibiotic ointment may be applied to fresh venipuncture sites. The patient should be kept apart from those who have infections, and the patient's room should be kept free of fomites.

The patient should be encouraged to obtain adequate rest and relaxation and to eliminate the use of nonprescribed substances, such as alcohol, marijuana, or heroin, as these have a tendency to decrease immune resistance.

Measures to Prevent Bleeding These measures are essential for one who has decreased platelets or deficiencies of the clotting mechanism, but may be of value for all patients. Beneficial measures include decreasing trauma of the skin and intestinal tract, using small-bore needles to minimize vein trauma, and administering medications by the oral route whenever possible. The laboratory department can cooperate in reduction of venous trauma by drawing blood with small-bore needles or by asking its more experienced personnel to draw the patient's blood. Writing ''Bleeding Precautions'' on the laboratory slips will help the technician recognize these patients. The presence of petechiae on the patient's body should alert one to the possibility of a bleeding disorder. If no obvious platelet or clotting disorder is present, one should remember the necessity for vitamin C in reduction of the fragility of the capillary walls and assess the patient's diet to ascertain if the intake is adequate.

Measures to Prevent Alopecia Few measures have been devised to prevent alopecia entirely, but some measures may help to reduce it. A scalp tourniquet applied to the head just below the hairline before therapy is given may be of benefit. This reduces the amount of blood carrying the active drug to the hair follicles and theoretically would work well for those drugs that are rapidly metabolized. If the drug remains in the blood in its active state for longer periods, a fair percentage of the drug will still be carried to the hair follicles. Braiding the hair or using a stocking cap will not reduce hair damage but will reduce hair loss. Many patients are able to adjust to their changed body image by using a wig to cover their hair loss. Keeping the bed and floor as free of the fallen hair as possible will help to spare the patient unnecessary mental and emotional trauma.

Measures for Emotional Support Provision of emotional support for chemotherapy patients is an ongoing process. Multidisciplinary team conferences are invaluable to assess fully the patient's emotional needs and level of functioning. Most patients in such a position go through a period of testing the nurses and the physician. The nurse will be asked the same questions the patient knows the doctor or another nurse has just answered. The patient may hear the reply of the first person asked, but either is unable to grasp the answer or must check with another person to be sure the answer is a truthful one. Cancer is one disease in which the public knows full well that all the truth is not always told to the patient. Each of us knows personally at least one individual, whether a friend, relative, or acquaintance, who has been in such a situation. The great majority of patients have had similar experiences, so during the testing phase the patient tries to find out who can and who cannot be trusted. This information will come not only from the words spoken but also from the manner in which they are spoken. The patient gradually learns who he or she can talk to about which subjects and who is unable or unwilling to discuss certain topics. The patient learns who among the nursing staff has the ability and/or time to discuss each topic he or she needs to discuss. The patient forms a support system within the institution, and the nurse can better tolerate this phase by knowing that it is temporary.

The appearance of ambivalence, confusion, depression, or euphoria may be due to physiologic processes such as drug toxicity, electrolyte imbalance, or brain mestastases as well as to psychologically oriented processes such as defense mechanisms, sensory deprivation, or sensory overload.

A patient whose chemotherapy must be withheld because of toxicity may become more fearful as a result of this situation, feeling that the last hope has been taken away. When the drugs fail, the person is sure that he or she is doomed. This is not necessarily so, for a period of rest may enable the doctor to restart therapy, or a combination of different drugs may be used. The patient will need diversional therapy as well as help to talk about fears at this point.

Measures for Educational Support   The educational support of the patient can be simply summarized: Tell the patient what the person wants to know when the person wants to know it. Some patients desire to know all they can assimilate about how the drugs work, how and why they are combined, and what can reasonably be expected from their use. These patients desire to handle this knowledge on an intellectual basis. A patient may begin therapy this way but have the need to ventilate fears later on. The opposite may also be true. When therapy begins, the patient may be able to respond only on a gut-level basis. As the needs to communicate on one level are met, different needs emerge. It is wise to allow the patient room and psychological space to move in either direction by supporting but not overreinforcing a particular behavior pattern or making it the only behavior that can lead to the patient's needs being met.

Some patients may fear knowing about the treatment, feeling it to be a mystical process. These patients may be looking for a miraculous cure, a state that seldom occurs with chemotherapy. Cancer does not develop in a day and, except for successful surgical intervention, cannot be cured in a day. A little knowledge of the disease and its treatment will aid in fostering a healthier and more realistic attitude in the patient.

Patients Who Do Not Know Their Diagnosis   Some doctors feel it wiser to withhold all news of a cancer from some patients or to use euphemisms to tell a patient of the diagnosis. The patient may not realize the "tumor" or "growth" in reality means "cancer." The doctor may say that the patient "knows" or "doesn't know" the diagnosis, but the nurse still must ask the patient what he or she knows. The nurse who knows what was actually told the patient can then compare it with the patient's verbalized concept of his or her illness. Denial may not be an unhealthy process, for it allows the patient to temporarily suppress certain facts until they can be integrated into the patient's self-concept. The key word here, of course, is temporary. Denial is healthy for a time, but eventually it becomes unhealthy. If the patient cannot express anger or move into other stages of grieving because of excessive use of denial, the patient may benefit from the interventions of a psychiatric nurse clinician, psychologist, or psychiatrist.

The denial of cancer presents a problem to the nurse expected to give antineoplastic therapy. Many patients will avoid asking questions simply because they already know on a subliminal level. Patients can sense the difference in the way others respond to them once the diagnosis of cancer has been established. The doctor may elect to inform the patient of the diagnosis when chemotherapy is initiated. This must be so if the drug or combination of drugs is experimental, since informed consent forms must be signed so that the criteria for use of the drug(s) can be met. If the patient is on previously established drugs and because of his or her own denial still does not know, the reality of the routine intravenous injections and the bodily changes experienced will soon crumble the defense of denial.

While the question of giving drugs to the patient who does not know what they are for poses a moral and ethical dilemma for the nurse, the nurse must realize that today it is legal to do so and that the responsibility for making the decision is the physician's alone. The patient's questions can and should be referred to the physician. If the nurse feels strongly enough about the issue, the nursing supervisor should be advised of the problem. The supervisor can then consider available alternatives. The nurse should consider that patients on antineoplastic therapy often know more about the drugs they receive than do patients on antibiotic therapy. Patients, regardless of the knowledge of their condition, can and should still be given emotional and physical support. One can still discuss one's fears even if the diagnosis is not known.

SUMMARY

Chemotherapy can be a beneficial treatment modality. Although survival can be measured in years for some patients, these patients are not often the ones seen in acute care settings, in clinics, or by the home care nurse. Instead, the patients seen are the ones whose survival can be measured in months. Until recently, chemotherapy was considered a "last-ditch" effort to stop disease progression. Now most physicians use it to increase the quality and the quantity of life.

Chemotherapy need not produce severe toxic reactions when management by both medical and nursing staff is appropriate, although in some patients they may occur. In the last few years there has been an increasing move to view chemotherapy in the light of a combined approach. Chemotherapy, surgery, radiation therapy, immunotherapy, and psychological counseling are being seen not as separate modalities in the treatment of cancer but as a combination of modalities that compliment each other for the ultimate benefit of the patient.

BIBLIOGRAPHY

Bouchard, Rosemary, and N. Owens. *Nursing Care of the Cancer Patient*. 2d. ed. St. Louis, C. V. Mosby. 1972.

Bruya, Margaret, and Nancy Maderia. "Stomatitis after Chemotherapy." *American Journal of Nursing*. **75**(8). August 1975. pp. 1349–1352.

Calabresi, Paul, and Robert Parks. "Chemotherapy of Neoplastic Diseases." In Goodman, Louis, and Alfred Gilman (eds.), *The Pharmacological Basis of Therapeutics*. 5th ed. New York, Macmillan. 1975. pp. 1248–1308.

Chabner, Bruce, et al. "The Clinical Pharmacology of Antineoplastic Agents. Part I." *New England Journal of Medicine*. **292**(21). May 22, 1975. pp. 1107–1112.

———. "The Clinical Pharmacology of Antineoplastic Agents. Part II." *New England Journal of Medicine*. **292**(22). May 29, 1975. pp. 1159–1168.

Cline, M. J. *Cancer Chemotherapy*. Philadelphia, W. B. Saunders. 1971.

Craytor, Josephine and Margot Fass. *The Nurse and the Cancer Patient*. Philadelphia, J. B. Lippincott. 1970.

DiPalma, Joseph. "Cancer Chemotherapy." *RN*. **39**(4). April 1976. pp. 85–88.

Dole, David, Anthony Fauci, and Sheldon Wolff. "Alternate Day Prednisone: Leukocyte Kinetics and Susceptibility to Infections." *New England Journal of Medicine*. **29**(22). November 28, 1974. pp. 1154–1158.

Herbst, Suzanne. "A New Approach to Parenteral Drug Administration." *American Journal of Nursing*. **75**(8). August 1975. p. 1345.

Holland, J., and E. Frei (eds.). *Cancer Medicine*. Philadelphia, Lea and Febinger. 1973.

Hubbard, Susan, and Vincent DeVita. "Chemotherapy Research Nurse." *American Journal of Nursing*. **76**(4). April 1976. pp. 560–565.

Marino, Elizabeth, and Dona LeBlanc. "Cancer Chemotherapy." *Nursing 75*. **5**(11). November 1975. pp. 22–33.

Mazzola, Rosanne, and George Jacobs. "Brain Tumors: Diagnosis and Treatment." *RN*. **38**(3). March 1975. pp. 42–45.

McMullen, Kathleen. "When the Patient Is on Bleomycin Therapy." *American Journal of Nursing*. **75**(6). June 1975. pp. 964–966.

Patterson, W. Bradford. "The Quality of Survival in Response to Treatment." *Journal of the American Medical Association*. **233**(3). July 21, 1975. pp. 280–281.

Payne, Johnnie, and Harold Kaplan. "Alternative Techniques for Venapuncture." *American Journal of Nursing*. **72**(4). April 1972. pp. 702–703.

Rodman, Morton. "Anticancer Chemotherapy: Part I—the drugs and what they do." *RN*. February 1972. pp. 45–56.

Rubin, Philip, and Richard Bakemeier. *Clinical Oncology for Medical Students and Physicians: A Multidisciplinary Approach*. 4th ed. Rochester, N.Y., American Cancer Society. 1974.

Seidler, Florence. "Innovative Approaches in Cancer Nursing Management." *Proceedings of the National Conference on Cancer Nursing.* New York, American Cancer Society. 1973. pp. 18–24.

Skipper, Howard. "Thoughts on Cancer Chemotherapy and Combination Modality Therapy (1974)." *Journal of the American Medical Association* **230**(7). November 18, 1974. pp. 1033–1035.

Somerville, Eileen. "The Nurse's Role in Cancer Chemotherapy." *Proceedings of the National Conference on Cancer Nursing.* New York, American Cancer Society. 1973. pp. 83–86.

Chapter 17

Immunology and Immunotherapy: New Frontiers in Nursing

Diana L. Donley

Immunotherapy was first used in ancient times in India and China to treat smallpox. Live, nonattenuated organisms from disease pustules were injected into those who had not yet had the disease in an effort to prevent it. Doing this caused as much disease as it prevented. In 1798, Edward Jenner used cowpox organisms to vaccinate people against smallpox. The first antibodies, against diphtheria, were discovered in 1890, and antigen-antibody interactions were explored in more depth in 1930. The field of immunology grew slowly until the 1950s. Now the expansion of knowledge is occurring at a more rapid rate.

Immunotherapy against disease is not new. For example, more than 100 years ago, heat-treated cancer cells were reinjected into the original host in an effort to control the disease. Since a high rate of infections accompanied an equivocal success rate, the project was shelved until more advances in the field had been made. In the preantibiotic era, the causative organism of an infectious disease was isolated, cultured, attenuated, and reinjected into the host. This procedure was abandoned in favor of the safer and more effective antibiotic therapy.

Knowledge of immunity and immunotherapy has advanced to the point that now patients with many diseases can benefit from alteration of the immune system. Those who have autoimmune diseases, such as lupus erythematosis, those receiving allograft transplantations, and cancer patients all benefit from the knowledge slowly and painstakingly garnered by the pioneers in immunology.

The first part of this chapter will give an overview of the development of the immune system. Since it is immunologic depression that contributes to the development and rapid growth of the cancer, the aspect explored in the second part is the depressed, rather than the overactive, immune system. The third part of the chapter will cover immunotherapy of cancer, while the fourth will explore nursing interventions for both the immunologically depressed patient and the patient on immunotherapy.

DEVELOPMENT OF THE IMMUNE SYSTEM

One of the first discoveries made by living organisms was that essential nutrients could be obtained by the ingestion of another organism. But ingestion resulted in the death of the ingested organism and forced the ingestor to find another source of nutrients. Another discovery was made when one organism learned to live on or within the tissues of a host and absorb the nutrients that would otherwise be used by the host.

> The invader evolved many structural and functional changes to allow it to survive at the expense of the host, who was also evolving to prevent its own destruction. Cell membranes and skin provided partial but not total protection. Many invaders could still gain access to the host's interior by natural or traumatic openings, or by creating their own openings. Most invading organisms live in a parasitic relationship with their hosts. Diseases such as herpes simplex, which cause the host little damage and are able to persist for long periods, show the adaptability of the parasite to the host. Other parasites caused greater damage to the host, so for further protection, the host developed the immune system.*

As organisms grew larger and more complex, the function of the immune system in protecting from invaders became of secondary importance, yielding to the more important function of protecting against somatic mutation.

The immune system consists primarily of the thymus gland, the tonsils, and the gut-associated lymphoid tissue, or Peyer's patches. The thymus is a lymphoepithelial structure arising from the ectoendodermal junction in the embryo. It develops from the third branchial pouch in most mammals and migrates into the mediastinum. It was previously thought that the thymus disappeared from the body after childhood. Now, however, it is recognized that while being most active during the first 4 years, the thymus is active throughout life.

"Stem cells," a term used to refer to the parent cells of any given population, are the precursors of all blood cells. To reach the final stage of a functioning blood cell, stem cells go through a process of differentiation, or maturation (see Figure 17-1). One of the first stages of differentiation is to the hemopoietic stem

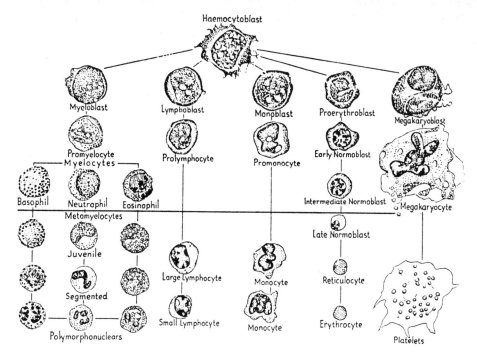

Figure 17-1 All cells below the horizontal line, with the exception of the late normoblast, may be found normally in the bloodstream. All cells above the horizontal line and the late normoblast may be found in normal bone marrow. *(Table I. The Origin of Blood Cells. Taken from L. E. H. Whitby and C. J. C. Britton, Disorders of the Blood, 10th ed.; Grune and Stratton, New York, 1966, p. 6.)*

cell, which requires further maturation before becoming a functioning immunocyte, leukocyte, or erythrocyte. The hemopoietic stem cell arises in the bone marrow and migrates to the thymus, where it undergoes transformation to an immunocyte. The term "immunocyte" refers to any cell, either plasma cell or lympocyte, that is capable of reacting in a specifically immunologic manner. For reasons that are currently unknown, many of these immunocytes do not survive. The thymus fulfills its role in the development of the immunocytes by being the only site at which these cells can be produced from the stem cell and by not releasing to the general circulation any immunocyte that can destroy the body itself. The immunocyte that has been modified by the thymus is known as a "thymus-dependent lymphocyte" (T-lymphocyte or T-cell).

The bursa-dependent lymphocyte (B-lymphocyte or B-cell) is also a product of the stem cell. It, however, undergoes the process of differentiation in the "bursa" tissue found in the tonsils and gut-associated lymphoid tissue (GALT). (This type of tissue is named "bursa" because it was first discovered in the chicken's bursa of Fabricius.) Both the B-cell and the helper T-cell are necessary for the production of antibodies, the T-cell cellular immune response, and the immunologic memory cell.

Antigen enters the body and is carried to the lymphoepithelial tissue of the lymph nodes, spleen, tonsils, or gut-associated lymphoid tissue. Once in these organs,

> the antigen is phagocytized by a macrophage [see Figure 17-2]. A T-cell and a B-cell then interact on the surface of the macrophage. A complex is formed which is either messenger RNA or an RNA/antigen complex. The complex then interacts with a small lymphocyte that has developed in the bone marrow but has not received immunologic stimulation up to this point. In the presence of this complex, the small lymphocyte becomes an immunoblast. A lengthy interaction time causes the immunoblast to become a plasma cell, capable of producing antibodies. A shorter interaction time causes the small lymphocyte either to become active in the cellular immune response (delayed hypersensitivity) or to become an immunologic memory cell. A second exposure to the messenger RNA or RNA/antigen complex will cause the memory cell to complete its maturation. It will then become a plasma cell, capable of producing antibodies.*

No one yet knows how the thymus knows which immunocytes to release to the general circulation and which to destroy, or why the T and B-cells react on the surface of the macrophage. Although these answers and many more are still unknown, there is enough knowledge to understand what happens when the immune system is impaired. An incompetent immune system gives every microbe the opportunity to become a pathogen, while it permits the usual pathogens to become more virulent. The incidence of cancer is much greater in the immunologically depressed person than in the general population.

CAUSES OF IMMUNOLOGIC DEPRESSION

Since immunologic depression can lead to an increased infection and cancer occurrence rate, it would be helpful to identify the conditions that predispose to immunologic depression. These conditions can be classified into six major groups: age-related defects, congenital abnormalities, malnourished states, disease conditions, iatrogenic causes, and/or autogenic causes, such as surgery, chemotherapy, alcoholism, and drug abuse.

Age-Related Defects

Persons in the extremities of life have a greater potential for immunologic depression than do those in the middle years. The premature infant is incapable of an adequate response to inflammation, and there is a decreased capacity for intracellular killing of bacteria. Children have not yet developed the capacity for production of their own antibodies and must depend on passive immunity as received from maternal antibodies. Older infants do not seem especially susceptible to infections unless they are deficient in gamma globulin.[1] The frequency of

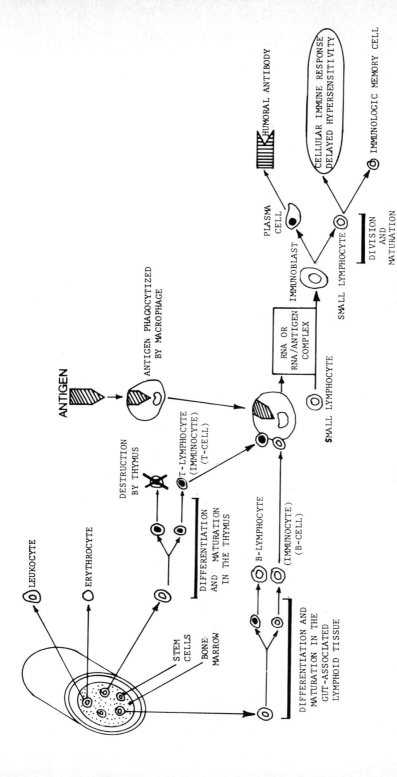

Figure 17-2 The immune response.

infection in children under the age of 5 can be attributed to the fact that active immunity does not appear spontaneously, but must be built up gradually. This can happen only after exposure to an antigen has occurred.

In the geriatric patient, cells begin to err in the copying mechanisms of DNA and RNA, and somatic mutations appear. The body loses its ability to differentiate between self and nonself, and autoantibodies are produced to destroy the body's own tissues. Thus, autoimmune connective tissue diseases may appear. The surveillance mechanism for destroying nonself tissues is impaired, and the ability to respond to the challenge of invading bacteria, viruses, and fungi is decreased. As somatic mutations increase, the immune system can no longer recognize its errors, the transformed cell is allowed to proliferate, and cancer is the result.[2] In addition, the very young and the very old usually have an interruption in nutrition and may not get all the essential nutrients in the proper amounts to allow antibodies to be produced in response to the disease.

Congenital Abnormalities

Congenital abnormalities include absence of the thymus gland, the stem cell, or the gamma globulin, that portion of the serum which stores antibodies. A deficiency of gamma globulin, or hypogammaglobulinemia, also results in impaired immunity, for antibodies cannot be stored in sufficient quantities for complete immunologic protection. Siblings who have identical immune defects may develop histologically identical cancers that are very different from the usual cancers of childhood. These cancers arise from the lymphoreticular system and include lymphocytic and histiocytic lymphomas, epithelial cancers, leukemias that differ from the usual subacute lymphatic leukemia seen in childhood, mesenchymal, and primary central nervous system tumors. This finding leads to the hypothesis that the inability to recognize and destroy transformed cells accompanies immunologic deficiency syndromes, and it points to the necessity for an intact immune system in the protection against cancer.[3]

Malnutrition

Malnutrition, whether due to poor intake and/or to poor absorption of essential nutrients, leads to an immune deficiency. The deficiency may take the form of decreased ability of the phagocyte to engulf and kill the bacteria, difficulty in the processing and recognition of the antigen, or decreased ability to produce antibody in response to some bacterial and viral antigens.

The essential nutrients referred to may be (1) vitamins, specifically pyridoxine (B_6), pantothenic acid, folic acid, A, B_{12}, and C; (2) amino acids such as phenylalanine and tryptophan; or (3) minerals such as iron, phosphate, and magnesium. Some sources implicate zinc and selenium as two more minerals that may be associated with immune deficiency. If these factors are not present in sufficient quantities, there is a derangement in the structure and/or function of the antibody-producing plasma cell. Amino acids, too, must be present in balanced quantities, or the antibodies will be produced in insufficient quantities and be of poor quality.

To illustrate the complexity of the interaction of nutrition and the immune system, a summary of the interaction of iron and the immune system is presented below.

Iron   Iron's role in immunity is not clearly understood. The onset of an infectious disease is often accompanied by a transient anemia that improves once the infection is treated. Normally, serum iron is bound primarily to a substance called transferrin and secondarily to one called lactoferrin. Free serum iron occurs when more iron is present than can be bound by transferrin or lactoferrin. Patients who have high levels of free serum iron, whether due to a hemolytic disease or to repeated blood transfusions, have a concurrent rise in infections, while free blood in the peritoneal cavity leads to increased mortality from peritonitis. "Autosequestration" is the body's ability to withhold a substance from systemic circulation. This property is used to withhold iron, phosphates, and sometimes zinc from the general circulation once an infectious process begins, to keep the causative organisms from using the minerals for their own growth. Elevation of the body temperature aids in the autosequestric process. Once supplemental iron therapy is begun in the autosequestric patient, a smoldering infection may become rampant, resulting in the patient's death.

Anemia frequently accompanies the terminal phase of cancer. It is not known if it is related to or caused by the process of autosequesteration, if it is due to the tumor's uptake of iron for its own growth, or if it is a true dietary deficiency condition. In addition, it is not known if supplemental iron therapy has a beneficial or a detrimental effect on cancer growth.

Iron deficiencies inhibit antibody synthesis, since iron is an essential constituent for adenosine triphosphate (ATP) production. Adenosine triphosphate is the energy compound of the cell and is needed for construction of the proteins which compose antibodies.

High urinary zinc levels are positively correlated with the frequent urogenital fungal infections seen in diabetics, while the onset of an infection caused by a gram-negative, rather than a gram-positive, organism is accompanied by hypophosphatemia. The phosphates fall to low enough levels to create conditions that are less than optimal for bacterial growth.

Disease Conditions

While many disease conditions contribute to the development of immunologic depression, space does not permit a comprehensive discussion of them all. Therefore, only cancer and potential or actual infectious states will be discussed briefly.

Cancer   Immunosuppression contributes to the development of cancer, but cancer is in itself immunosuppressive. Theories are now prevalent that we all constantly develop cancer cells, but our immune systems recognize them as non-self and destroy them. The body can destroy up to ten million cancer cells. When the mass of cells reaches the 100 million level, the immune system can no longer destroy these transformed cells. When clinically apparent, a cancer which measures one centimeter in diameter contains more than ten billion cells. After the cancer mass reaches this size, the cells begin to secrete antigen into the bloodstream. The immune system is depressed still further by the antigen. The question is, if the body can normally recognize and destroy cancer cells, how can cancer ever develop in the first place? The answer is, of course, that prolonged immunosuppression has occurred, or that the immune system has been overwhelmed. Carcinogens are in themselves immunosuppressive. Normally, the transformed cell is recognized and destroyed but the local concentration of carcinogens suppresses the recognition as well as the destruction of this cell. The transformed cell can then proliferate. The steady leak of antigen from a large carcinoma combines with any available antibody and prevents it from attacking the cancer cells. The leak of antigen plus the persisting carcinogen can lead to more intense immunosuppression.

Another factor that may contribute to the inability of the system to destroy a cancerous cell is that blocking factors may cover the tumor cell and produce a complex that prevents access to the cell by a sensitized killer lymphocyte [see Figure 17-3]. If the tumor is to be recognized as foreign and destroyed by the immune system, it must contain material that is not found on or in host cells. This substance is called tumor-specific antigen (TSA). TSA may combine with antibodies that enhance rather than inhibit tumor growth, or the TSA may not be recognized as foreign early enough.

Infections   Another condition that may cause immunologic depression is the presence of an overwhelming systemic infection, especially one of viral origin. All available nutrients are being used to manufacture one type of antibody, and no nutrients remain to manufacture another type. The patient will be unable to respond to the challenge produced by the second invader. This is clearly illustrated by the patient who dies very rapidly from pneumonia while recovering from another infection, such as influenza.

Other Disease Conditions   When a person is burned, the first line of defense, his skin, is lost. It is thought that the infections which arise in spite of meticulous nursing care are a result of the invasion of the body by microorganisms which normally reside on the skin's surface. The mechanisms which usually prevent pathogenicity of these bacteria are gone, i.e., the intact skin, the sweat (which contains lysozymes that help destroy bacteria), and the normal beneficial flora. In addition, the serum ooze through the burned skin reduces the body's supply of gammaglobulin and therefore antibodies.*

Patients with chronic cardiac conditions are known to be deficient in folic acid, and they are therefore more susceptible to infections than are noncardiac patients. The diabetic patient is known to be deficient in vitamin B_6, as are the pregnant woman and the woman who takes contraceptive pills.

Drug-Induced Immunosuppression

Antibiotics such as chloramphenicol, immunosuppressives such as azathioprine (Imuran), antineoplastic agents such as nitrogen mustard and cytosine

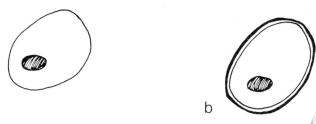

Figure 17-3 Blocking factors on the surface of a cancer cell. (*a*) Typical cancer cell. (*b*) Cancer cell with blocking factors surrounding it.

arabinoside, antipsychotics such as chlorpromazine (Thorazine), cortico-steroids, alcohol, barbiturates, heroin, and colchicine all bring about immunologic depression. The small lymphocyte (see Figure 17-2) is the most sensitive of

> all blood cells to radiation and to many of the cytotoxic drugs, including nitrogen mustard, colchicine, barbiturates, and cortisone.
>
> Interestingly enough, while small quantities of cortisol help protect the lympho-cyte from the damaging effects of these other drugs and from disease, high concentrations of cortisol cause lympholysis. Corticosteroids alter cell membranes and induce the production of various adaptive enzymes, some of which may be immunosuppressive. Steroids may either decrease or enhance antibody production, depending on the dose of the steroid and the interval between the antigenic stimulus and the time of administration*

of the steroid.

The purine antagonists azathioprine and 6-mercaptopurine, the folic acid antagonists methotrexate and aminopterin, the pyramidine antagonist cytosine arabinoside, and alkylating agents such as nitrogen mustard and cyclophosphamide all decrease antibody production. Alkylating agents are also capable of suppression of the inflammatory response and destruction of the small circulating lymphocyte; they are carcinogenic as well. Cytosine arabinoside has additional immunosuppressive qualities while also being carcinogenic. The carcinogenic ability of these drugs can be due to either the drugs' immunosuppressive quality, an irritant type of effect on the tissues, or a mutagenic effect on the cell.

The antibiotics Mitomycin C, Actinomycin D, azaserine, and chloramphenicol have a negative effect on the production of antibodies and can cause hypoplastic bone marrow as well.

Excessive alcohol consumption seems to have a direct toxic effect on the bone marrow, as evidenced by leukopenia, thrombocytopenia, and reticulocytopenia.

Iatrogenically Induced Immunosuppression

"Iatrogenically induced" immunosuppression is that which is induced by the physician. Drug therapy, which was previously discussed, radiation, surgery, and anesthesia are included in this category.

Radiation   Radiation may or may not depress a patient immunologically. Lymphoid tissue is destroyed by radiation, but the size and location of the radiated area determine the severity of the depression. Lymphoid-tissue depression ranges from complete destruction of all lymphoid tissue, when total body radiation is done before bone marrow transplantations, to very little, if any, detrimental effect when only a small area is radiated.

Surgery and Anesthesia   Surgery decreases immunologic competence in many patients undergoing major surgical procedures. There have been many advances in the areas of pharmacology, microbiology, immunology, surgical skills and techniques, cardiovascular dynamics, and others. In spite of these advances, however, there is still a higher rate of gram-negative, viral, and mycotic infections than is thought desirable by the medical and nursing professions, and dissemination of cancer still occurs. The immunosuppression seems to come from several sources that have an additive effect. The mechanical stress of surgery stimulates the adrenal cortex, which releases cortisol. As discussed previously, small amounts of cortisol help prevent infection by protecting cells from the damaging effects of drugs and microbes, while larger amounts are lympholytic. Psychologic stress also accompanies surgery and also stimulates the adrenal cortex. Thus, the adrenal cortex receives stimulation from two sources, and the amount of cortisol released by the cortex is greater than if it were stimulated by one source alone.

Another source of immunosuppression is the interruption of nutrition that accompanies major surgery. Healing tissues require a dietary source of essential nutrients. If the supply is inadequate or if the amino acids are not in proper balance, both healing and antibody production will suffer. The anesthesia itself may cause immunosuppression, as anesthesia tends to decrease the body's ability to produce adenosine triphosphate, ATP, the source of energy for the production of antibodies and for the immune response.[4]

Emotions and Immunity

Very little has been done to determine the effects of emotions on immunity in human beings. Laboratory animal research has demonstrated decreased antibody production in response to environmental stress while also finding increased adrenocortical function, leukopenia, and a higher adrenal weight resulting from social isolation or sensory deprivation.[5,6] It has been found that mild stress enhances the resistance to a disease or to postoperative complications, while high stress increases the occurrence of a disease or of postoperative complications. This finding is in keeping with the biologic effect of cortisol, as previously discussed.

Summary

Regardless of the cause, the symptoms of immunologic suppression are increased susceptibility to infection and to cancer. Organisms not normally pathogenic to humans, such as protozoa, pneumocystis carinii, cytomegalic inclusion virus, herpes zoster, *Candida,* and *Aspergillus* may overwhelm the weakened host and cause death. With a suppressed inflammatory response, a relatively insignificant infection can spread rapidly throughout the body and cause death.

Cancer is a real danger for those who are immunologically suppressed, since the risk that these people will develop cancer is many times greater than for the general population. Once established, cancer can grow very rapidly in the immunologically depressed, so early diagnosis and treatment is essential.

IDENTIFICATION OF IMMUNOLOGIC DEPRESSION

Immunologic depression may be identified by quantitative or qualitative tests. Quantitative tests include peripheral-blood counts, bone marrow examination, and immunoglobulin assays. Qualitative tests, done in vivo or in vitro, determine the quality of antibody produced and its ability to respond to an antigenic stimulus.

Quantitative Examinations

Quantitative examinations of the peripheral blood will show a leukopenia and/or a lymphopenia. The normal leukocyte count ranges from 5,000 to 10,000 cells per ml^3 of blood. In leukopenia, the count drops to below 3,500 per ml^3. If the count has been relatively stable at 8,000 to 9,000 and suddenly drops to 4,000, a relative leukopenia exists and precautions against infections should be instituted.

The normal range of lymphocytes is 1,000 to 3,000 cells per ml^3 of blood. If the lymphocyte count drops below 1,000, the patient is usually prone to infections.

Pancytopenia, a decrease in all blood cells, is a sign that the bone marrow is underpopulated. It cannot be determined from the peripheral blood alone whether the bone marrow is hypoplastic or aplastic or if this condition is temporary or permanent decrease, and a bone marrow examination must be done. Hypoplasia may affect only one particular type of cell, or all may be affected to some degree. When the white cell line is affected, all defense mechanisms will be affected. If there is trauma to the bone marrow, such as that brought about by a chemotherapeutic drug, the peripheral-blood count may not show a decreased white count for several days, depending on the marrow reserves. Normally the life span of a leukocyte is 7 to 8 hours, but the marrow contains enough reserves to last for another 8 days. If the marrow is compromised, it is unable to replace the circulating white blood cells as they die.

Qualitative Examinations

The qualitative changes in antibodies and antibody production may be assayed by in vitro methods such as phytohemagglutinin (PHA), varidase, pokeweed mitogen, and streptolysin-0. When these substances are combined with normal lymphocytes, the anticipated reaction is for the lymphocytes to undergo mitosis and form blast cells (blastogenesis). These procedures are done as screening tests before a patient is started on immunotherapy and may be done at intervals throughout the immunotherapy administration.

In Vivo Tests   Some of the in vivo tests used are the dinitrochlorobenzine (DNCB) skin test, the skin window, and the use of antigens in skin tests. The antigens used include *Candida,* mumps, varidase, intermediate PPD, and others. A patient unable to respond to these antigens is said to be "anergic," or incapable of responding immunologically to an antigenic stimulus. The anergic patient with cancer will probably have a poor prognosis with a rapidly growing cancer, and this person will be unable to benefit from immunotherapy.

   DNCB   Dinitrochlorobenzine is a chemical antigen. It is applied topically. In the immunologically responsive patient, a delayed hypersensitivity reaction will occur (see Figure 17-4).

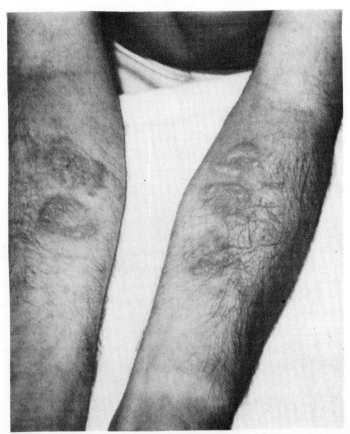

Figure 17-4   Delayed hypersensitivity reaction to DNCB skin testing. *(Photo by Diana L. Donley.)*

Skin Window The purpose of the skin window is to assay the ability of the lymphocytes to recognize an antigen and to produce migratory inhibition factor (MIH), which prevents the macrophage from leaving the area stimulated by the antigen. A sharp blade is used to carefully scrape away the upper layers of skin until the dermis is exposed but the area is not actively bleeding. A drop of antigen is then applied to the denuded area, and a glass cover slip is applied aseptically. The cover slips are changed periodically for 24 hours (see Figures 17-5 through 17-7). A bandage is then applied, and the wound heals without incident. The cover slips are fixed and examined microscopically as a means of determining the number of macrophages entering the area in a given time period.

Intradermal Skin Tests In other skin tests, substances are injected intradermally. A positive response will result in erythema and an indurated area. These tests will be done before the onset of immunotherapy and may also be

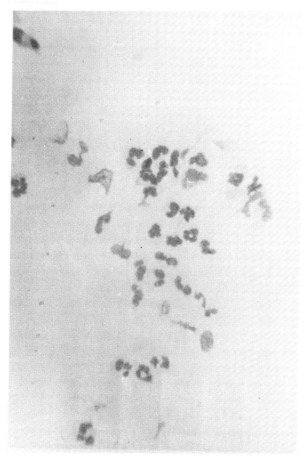

Figure 17-5 Skin window at 3 hours. High dry magnification. *(Courtesy Dr. Noboru, Oishi, Honolulu.$*

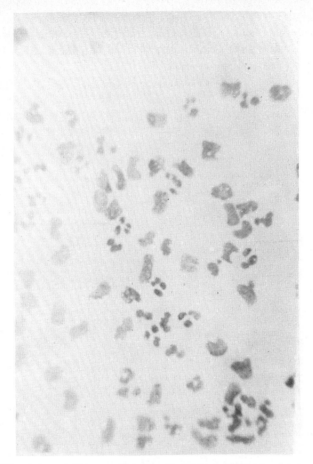

Figure 17-6   Skin window at 12 hours. *(Courtesy Dr. Noboru Oishi, Honolulu.)*

done at intervals throughout the treatment process. When performed on an anergic patient, little or no reaction will occur.

IMMUNOTHERAPY

Alteration of the depressed immune system may be accomplished by four different methods and combinations of these methods.

Active Specific Immunization

In active specific immunization, the bacterial or tumor cell and its products or antigens are reinjected into the original host. This procedure stimulates the host to produce antibodies. Antibodies may not have been produced before because of an inability to recognize the antigen due to blocking agents on the surface of

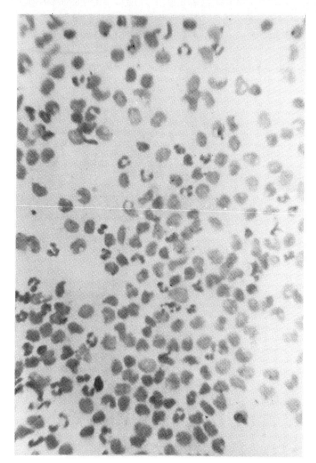

Figure 17-7 Skin window at 18 hours. *(Courtesy Dr. Noboru Oishi, Honolulu.)*

the baterial or tumor cell. The bacterial or tumor cells are usually attenuated before the reinjection is attempted, so that development of a secondary site of infection or tumor growth can be prevented.

Active Nonspecific Immunization

Antigens such as bacillus Calmette-Guerin (BCG) are used to stimulate the immune system to be more active. It is not known exactly how BCG stimulates the immune system. A leukocytosis does occur after BCG has been adminis-tered, and the patient's life span seems to increase. Small amounts of the antigen are injected intradermally or applied via the scarification technique (see Figure 17-8). BCG is never given to an anergic patient, or granulomatous hepatitis may develop. If it is given to a patient who has had tuberculosis, the tuberculosis may be activated and will rapidly disseminate. Skin tests including the intermediate

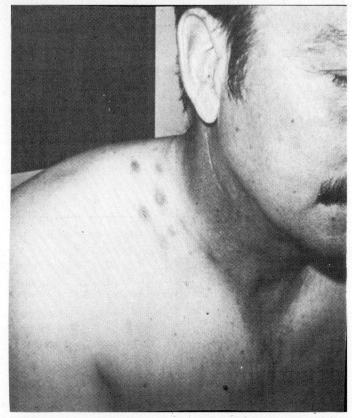

Figure 17-8   Delayed hypersensitivity reaction to DNCB skin testing. *(Photo by Diana L. Donley.)*

PPD are done before BCG is administered. If the PPD is positive but the patient has not had tuberculosis previously, and if all other tests for tuberculosis are negative, the amount of BCG given is reduced by one-half.

Other antigens in this category include methanol extracted residue of BCG (MER); thymosin, which is an extract of the thymus gland; and cornebacterium parvum.

Passive Immunization

''Passive immunization'' is the term used when the lymphocytes from a patient who has been cured of a disease are given to another patient with the same disease. The donor and recipient should be histologically identical to prevent a sensitivity reaction. The lymphocytes help the patient resist the disease.

Passive Adoptive Immunization

Lymphocytes are also used to immunize the patient in the passive adoptive method, but they are lysed by a freezing-thawing process, and a substance called transfer factor (TF) is obtained. The transfer factor need not only be given to those who are histologically identical to the donor.

Bone Marrow Transplantation

Bone marrow transplantation may be done for a patient who is totally incompetent immunologically or for a patient who has widespread bone marrow involvement with a neoplastic disease such as leukemia. It is often used in the leukemic patient who has become unresponsive to chemotherapeutic agents and who has a healthy identical twin. The skin and hair of the patient are cleansed with antiseptic agents, and the patient's gastrointestinal tract is sterilized with antibiotics, for even the normal beneficial flora can be pathogenic to the immunologically depressed patient. The patient is maintained in a germ-free environment such as a laminar airflow room or reverse isolation. He or she is given only sterilized food and has no skin-to-skin contact with another human until the transplant is functioning normally, usually 2 to 3 weeks after the transplant. The recipient receives large doses of cyclophosphamide and/or total body radiation to destroy all stem cells and lymphoid tissue in the body. Bone marrow is obtained from an histologically identical individual, usually a sibling and preferably an identical twin, by means of repeated bone marrow aspirations. The marrow is then transfused intravenously into the patient through a filter, and the stem cells migrate to the bone marrow cavities and begin to grow.

Fulgeration of Tumors

In vivo fulgeration of tumors seems to act as an active specific method of immunization. The protein of the tumor cell is liberated into the body as fulgeration occurs. The liberated protein can then be recognized as foreign and can act as an antigen, with antibodies being produced against it. This situation enhances the body's ability to destroy the remaining tumor.

Immunotherapy in a Combined Approach

Since immunotherapy is most effective when the tumor load is small, other types of cancer destruction therapy are often employed to reduce the tumor burden before immunotherapy is begun. Surgeons may remove or attempt to remove the bulk of the tumor before either chemotherapy or immunotherapy is begun. Radiotherapy may be employed for the same purpose. Chemotherapy may be initiated before immunotherapy, and the two modalities may be continued together from then on.

For treatment of some diseases, such as acute leukemia, all of the treatment modalities may be employed at various points in the treatment regime. Initially, chemotherapy is given to reduce tumor bulk. Surgery in the form of a splenectomy may be done to eliminate a potential disease reservoir. Radiation is given to the brain and spinal cord to decrease the possibility of and/or treat meningeal leukemia, and immunotherapy is employed to rid the body of the last leukemic cell.

This combined approach is not currenly used in the treatment of all cancers, but the more sophisticated way of treating this disease uses the combined approach more and more frequently.

THE NURSE'S ROLE IN IMMUNOTHERAPY

Recently, a new role for the nurse in immunotherapy has evolved: that of immunotherapy nurse. The nurse in such a position aids in the immunotherapy treatment process; educates the patient, family, and staff members as to the immunotherapy process; and supervises the nursing interventions for the patient receiving immunotherapy. He or she coordinates the patient's immunotherapy with any chemotherapy that may be given and keeps records on all the patients. The nurse is able to discuss the treatment and its rationale with the patient at the patient's level and to teach prevention of infections to all concerned.

A brief review of nursing interventions for the immunologically depressed patient will be followed by a discussion of nursing interventions for the patient receiving immunotherapy.

Nursing Implications for the Immunologically Depressed Patient

The most important nursing intervention for the care of the immunologically depressed patient is the prevention of infections.

Care of the Patient's Environment   To prevent exposure of the patient to infections, the nurse must recognize the potential reservoirs of disease. The room should be kept clean and should be damp-dusted with a disinfectant solution rather than dry-dusted, since dry dusting tends to scatter rather than remove the dust. Humidifying the air also helps to reduce microorganisms, since they become laden with moisture, drop to the floor, and die. Standing water found in bedside pitchers, denture cups, suction and respiratory equipment, and flower arrangements is an excellent medium for bacterial, fungal, or protozoal growth. Equipment should be disposable or sterilized frequently. Fomites such as blankets, sheets, newspapers, magazines, and backrub lotion should be eliminated. Individuals with colds should not tend to this patient's needs. If the day's work is planned so that these patients receive care first, bacteria are less likely to be carried to them on the nurse's uniform. Hand washing before, during, and after giving patient care should be an established routine.

Care of the Patient   The body's first lines of defense are the intact skin and mucous membranes. When the skin becomes paper thin and tears easily, as occurs with long-term steroid therapy or in advanced age, good skin care becomes essential. Even a minor injury such as a venapuncture site, insignificant as it is for most people, may become a portal of entry for a fatal infection in the immunologically depressed person.

Decubiti can be prevented by control of pressure on bony prominences, use of lamb's wool pads, alternation of pressure pads, or use of water beds, and friction burns may be prevented by lifting rather than sliding the patient and by using powder on the skin.

Dry skin can lead to cracking, which also provides a portal of entry for microbes. Dry skin can be alleviated by using emollients and by increasing humidity of the air, as well as by reducing the number of complete baths or the use of soap.

Excessive moisture on the skin may lead to maceration, and if soaks are ordered, periodic drying must be provided to prevent skin damage.

Sunburn, a potential problem for this patient, should be avoided by reducing time spent in direct sunlight or by using a commercial sunscreen. Insect bites, another potential source of infection, should be avoided.

Care of the mucous membranes includes prevention of trauma due to ill-fitting dentures and inadequately lubricated tubes and catheters. Foods that are very spicy or are high in roughage, such as bran, should be avoided, as should solutions that are very hot or chemically irritating. Prolonged or excessive irrigations, such as douches or antiseptic gargles, should be discouraged, as they will disturb the normal flora and lead to overgrowth of other organisms.

Since the immunologically depressed patient is so vulnerable to infections, he or she should be protected from visitors, staff, or other patients who have infections. If the immunosuppression is severe, with a leukopenia of less than 3,000 and/or a lymphopenia of less than 800, it is wise to place the patient in protective or reverse isolation. If the patient is totally incompetent immunologically, it may be necessary to place the person in a totally germ-free environment, such as a laminar airflow room, until some measure of immunologic competence is again developed.

Good nutrition and plenty of rest and sleep are essential for this patient, for metabolic requirements are higher when a patient is stressed immunologically. The dietitian can aid the patient to choose food that meets esthetic and ethnic preferences while still remaining within the ideal of a well-balanced diet, regardless of whether the food is prepared at home or in the institution. The patient can be assisted to obtain the goals of rest and sleep by reduction of physical discomfort; visual, auditory, and cutaneous stimuli; and intrusive thought patterns. Many patients could benefit by less use of tranquilizers or mood elevators and more opportunities to ventilate hopes and fears.

Care of the Patient in Reverse Isolation   Since physical care of the patient in reverse isolation has been discussed thoroughly by the authors of many nursing texts, only some psychosocial aspects of isolation will be discussed.

The patient can be helped to understand the necessity for isolation techniques by keeping explanations as simple and as concise as possible. Immunosuppression rarely arrives unheralded, although it may predispose to other conditions that are of rapid onset, such as a massive infection. More usually, the onset is gradual and teaching can be done as the condition evolves.

Patients may find it difficult to tolerate isolation without emotional support from the nursing staff and the family. The patient who has cancer may be very depressed simply because he or she has much uninterrupted time to think about the condition and prognosis. Visits from the hospital staff drop off rapidly once reverse isolation is begun. The patient may be kept in contact with the outside world by a disinfected television or radio, by sterilized newspapers or magazines, and by frequent visits from the nurse. The time it takes to don a gown and mask is well worth the effect visits have on the patient's mental health.

The patient continuing in reverse isolation begins to withdraw. When able to be with others once again without gown and masks interfering with normal communications, he or she must be helped to reestablish normal communications with others.

Family members, too, must be made to feel that they have a part in aiding their loved one to get well. They can be taught the principles of immunosuppression and the care of the patient as the condition evolves. Anticipatory teaching will prevent the family from fearing to visit once the patient is in reverse isolation. When the patient is discharged, the family members can be taught that prompt attention to an injury that might appear trivial to them, such as a scratch on the arm, is essential.

These interventions are only a basic outline of the areas to be considered. Undoubtedly, the reader will think of many more that are specific to his or her particular situation.

Nursing Implications for the Patient on Immunotherapy

Patients on immunotherapy are usually considered to be immunologically depressed, and therefore the previous discussion on care of the immunologically depressed patient applies to the patient receiving immunotherapy as well.

The types of immunotherapy and the substances used for alteration of the immune system differ, as do the methods of administration. Immunotherapy, unlike chemotherapy and radiotherapy, usually causes few severe side effects depending on the type of agent used. Many substances, from a vaccine prepared from the patient's own tumor (autologous vaccine), to bacillus Calmette-Guerin BCG, to bacterial products or chemical antigens, may be used in immunotherapy. Currently, however, BCG is the vaccine used more often for immunotherapy than any other type of vaccine. This is for several reasons. First, BCG has been used for many years in the prevention of tuberculosis, and many clinicians are familiar with its use. It is now used infrequently for prevention of tuberculosis because of the low incidence of tuberculosis in the United States, not because of the side effects of its use. As long as the patient is immunologically competent and has not had either active or latent tuberculosis previously, the few side effects of BCG therapy are transient and comparatively mild. Another reason for the use of BCG is that it is widely available through established commercial laboratories, and thus the quality, strength, and purity of the vaccine are assured.

The best reasons for using BCG, or any type of immunotherapy, are that is is specifically cancericidal, that normal tissues and cells are unaffected by the therapy, and that it works. The exact mechanisms by which BCG stimulates the immune system are still being researched and are not well understood at this time. The amount of tumor-specific antigen (TSA) is increased during successful BCG therapy, as are the number of circulating lymphocytes. These lymphocytes seem to be sensitized to fight the cancer more readily.

Since BCG is the method of immunotherapy most often used, most of the following discussion will be focused on use of this vaccine, with other vaccines being mentioned where appropriate. Nursing interventions vary somewhat with the method of administration used, and so will be presented in this fashion.

Methods of Administration   The vaccines used in immunotherapy may be administered by intravenous injection into a tumor nodule or adjacent area, intradermally, via the scarification technique, or by multiple puncture injections. Few vaccines are given intravenously because most are more easily accepted by the body when given into the tissues. Some vaccines do work better this way, however. Side effects depend on the specific vaccine used.

The intralesional method allows for injection of the antigen into obvious subcutaneous nodules or adjacent areas. This technique has been used for cutaneous metastases from breast and colon carcinoma and for malignant melanoma. BCG injected into these nodules causes regression in a percentage of patients but not in all of them. An obvious obstacle to the success of this type of therapy is the absence of any cutaneous lesions. Noninjected nodules do not always regress, and the visceral tumors are usually untouched. There is the potential for stimulating the growth of the injected nodules. This technique therefore is not as widely used since the development of the scarification technique. When nodules are injected, the possible reactions are erythema, induration, and possibly ulceration with drainage, leading to potential infection. Transient ipsilateral lymph node enlargement is also seen.

The intradermal method of administration was frequently used for BCG therapy until the advent of scarification. It is used less often now with BCG, because the side effects the patient experiences are less intense when BCG is given by scarification than when given intradermally. It is still used with other types of vaccines, such as autologous vaccine. Reactions may be the same as with intralesional injections, i.e., erythema, induration, ulceration with tissue sloughing, and a potential portal for infection.

The Scarification Technique   The scarification technique makes use of multiple scratches etched on the arm or thigh with the beveled cutting edge, rather than the point, of a needle. An area 5 cm² is described on the previously sterilized skin, and 8 additional horizontal and vertical lines are etched approximately every ½ cm inside the square to form a grid. The scratches are deep enough to cause oozing but not frank bleeding. The BCG or BCG and mixed vaccine are then applied drop by drop on the scarified area and massaged in with the flat of the needle. A hair dryer set on cool—as heat destroys BCG—may aid in the drying process. The site will not be sticky, and a glaze will form. A small petri dish, small plastic Frisbee, or similar object is set over the scarified areas, and the area is left untouched for 24 to 48 hours. The protective dressing may then be removed. After 48 hours, the area may be washed with soap and water twice a day until healing is complete. The area should not be scratched. If it becomes dry or itchy, a small amount of nonperfumed lotion may be massaged into the area. Alcohol should not be used as it can cause further drying.

The sites for scarification may be the arms and thighs, and the sites are altered. BCG will be given at weekly or longer intervals depending on the protocol used.

Each previous treatment site may again become active when a new scarification is performed. The side effects of the scarification itself, i.e., ulceration, induration, and drainage, are less frequently observed than when BCG is given by other routes. The systemic reactions may be a flulike syndrome with malaise, chills, fever, and myalgia. The fever may appear within 6 hours and may be controlled with acetominophen (Tylenol). Reactions are dependent on the number of previous injections, the route of administration, and possibly the number of BCG organisms used.

BCG and Cultured Cell Vaccines   BCG can be mixed with cells cultured from a patient and given intradermally. Reactions tend to become greater with each immunization and include transient ipsilateral lymph node enlargement, induration, and sometimes ulceration of the vaccination site, malaise, headache, myalgia, chills, and fever. The reactions may be lessened by administration of acetominophen. Reactions usually subside in a day or two, but may last as long as 4 days.

SUMMARY

Immunology and immunotherapy are new fields whose limits continue to be defined daily. Immunotherapy as a treatment for cancer is becoming more sophisticated and is used in combination with surgery, radiotherapy, and chemotherapy to help achieve long-lasting remissions in some cancers. The role of the nurse in immunotherapy or in immunology is not yet clearly defined. Nurses who now occupy such positions are pioneers in these fields. As they continue to define their roles, the rest of the nursing profession will look to them for guidance in caring for the patient receiving this newest method of cancer therapy.

REFERENCES

1   J. Alexander and R. Good. *Immunobiology for Surgeons.* W. B. Saunders, Philadelphia, 1970.
2   L. Robert and B. Robert. "Immunology and aging." *Gerontologia,* **19,** 1973, pp. 330–350.
3   J. Kersey, B. Spector, and R. Good. "Primary immunodeficiencies and cancer: the immunodeficiency—cancer registry." *International Journal of Cancer,* **12,** 1973, pp. 333–347.

4 T. Park et al. "Immunosuppressive effect of surgery." *Lancet*, **1**, 1971, pp. 330–350.
5 W. B. Gross and P. B. Seigal. "Effect of social stress and steroids on antibody production." *Avian Diseases*, **17**, October–December 1973, pp. 807–815.
6 H. Baer. "Long-term stress and its effects on drug response in rodents." *Laboratory Animals in Science*, **21**(3), June 1971, pp. 341–349.

BIBLIOGRAPHY

Alexander, J. and R. Good: *Immunobiology for Surgeons*, W. B. Saunders, Philadelphia, 1970.

Baer, H.: "Long-term stress and its effects on drug response in rodents," *Laboratory Animals in Science*, **21**, (3), June 1971, pp. 341–349.

Bast, R. C., et al.: "BCG and cancer," *New England Journal of Medicine*, **290**, (25), June 20, 1974, pp. 1413–1420.

———: "BCG and cancer (second of two parts)," *New England Journal of Medicine*, **290**, (26), June 27, 1974, pp. 1458–1469.

Beeson, P. and W. McDermott: *Textbook of Medicine*, W. B. Saunders, Philadelphia, 1975.

Beland, I.: *Clinical Nursing: Pathophysiological and Psychological Approaches*, Macmillan, New York, 1970.

Berenyi, M., B. Straus, and D. Cruz: "In vitro and in vivo studies of cellular immunity in the alcoholic," *American Journal of Digestive Diseases*, **19**, March 1974, pp. 199–204.

Bodey, G. O.: "Isolation for the compromised host," *Journal of the American Medical Association*, **233**, August 11, 1975, pp. 543–545.

Boyd, W.: *Fundamentals of Immunology*, Interscience, New York, 1966.

Brown, S. M., et al.: "Immunologic dysfunction in heroin addicts," *Archives of Internal Medicine*, **134**, Dec. 1974, pp. 1001–1006.

Burnet, M. *Cellular Immunology*, Cambridge University Press, London, 1969.

Clement, C. and D. Kramer: "Effects of radiotherapy on immunity," *Cancer*, **34**, July 1974, pp. 193–196.

Craddock, P. R., et al.: "Acquired phagocyte dysfunction: a complication of the hypophosphatemia of parenteral hyperalimentation," *New England Journal of Medicine*, **290**, (25), June 20, 1974, pp. 1403–1407.

Day, D.: *The Immunochemistry of Cancer*, Charles C Thomas, Springfield, Ill., 1965.

Donley, D.: "Nursing the patient who is immunosuppressed," *American Journal of Nursing*, **76**(10), October 1976.

Faulk, M., et al.: "Some effects of malnutrition on the immune response in man," *American Journal of Clinical Nutrition*, **27**, June 1974, pp. 638–646.

Fefer, A.: "Bone marrow transplantation for hematologic neoplasia in 16 patients with identical twins," *New England Journal of Medicine*, **290**(25), June 20, 1974, pp. 1389–1393.

Fiennes, R. N. and A. J. Riopele: "Using primates in medical research: hazards for man and models for research," *Primates in Medicine*, **3**, 1969, pp. 93–103.

Goodhart, P. and M. Shils: *Modern Nutrition in Health and Disease*, Lea and Febiger, Philadelphia, 1973.

Gross, W. B. and P. B. Seigal: "Effect of social stress and steroids on antibody production," *Avian Diseases*, **17**, October–December 1973, pp. 807–815.

Holmes, E. C., F. Eilber, and D. Morton: "Immunotherapy and Malignancy in Human," *Journal of the American Medical Association,* **232**(10), June 9, 1975, pp. 1052–1055.

Hontela, S.: "Iron deficiency and infection," *Lancet,* March 22, 1975, p. 685.

Isler, C.: "Newest treatment for cancer: immunotherapy," *RN,* **39**(5), May 1976, pp. 29–31.

Kersey, J., B. Spector, and R. Good: "Primary immunodeficiencies and cancer: the immunodeficiency-cancer registry," *International Journal of Cancer,* **12,** 1973, pp. 333–347.

Leveen, H. H., et al.: "Tumor eradication by radiofrequency therapy," *Journal of the American Medical Association,* **235**(20), May 17, 1976, pp. 2198–2200.

Masawe, A., J. Muindi, and G. Swai: "Infections in iron deficiency and other types of anaemia in the tropics," *Lancet,* August 10, 1974, pp. 314–317.

Nordmark, M. T. and A. W. Rohweder: *Scientific Foundations of Nursing,* J. B. Lippincott, Philadelphia, 1967.

Notkins, A. B.: "How the immune response to a virus can cause disease," *Scientific American,* **228,** January 1973, pp. 22–31.

Park, T., et al.: "Immunosuppressive effect of surgery," *Lancet,* **1,** 1971, pp. 330–350.

Robert, L. and B. Robert: "Immunology and aging," *Gerontologia,* **19,** 1973, pp. 330–350.

Rodman, M. and Smith, D.: *Pharmacology and Drug Therapy in Nursing,* J. B. Lippincott, Philadelphia, 1968.

Sbarra, R., et al.: "Bactericidal activities of phagocytes in health and disease," *American Journal of Clinical Nutrition,* June 1974, pp. 629–633.

Schlesinger, M. G. and A. Stekel: "Impaired cellular immunity in marasmic infants," *American Journal of Clinical Nutrition,* June 1974, pp. 615–620.

Silverstein, M. J. and D. L. Morton: "Cancer immunotherapy," *American Journal of Nursing,* **73**(7), July 1975, pp. 1178–81.

Sokal, J., C. W. Aungst, and T. Han: "Use of bacillus calmette-guerin as adjuvant in human cell vaccines," *Cancer Research,* **32,** July 1972, pp. 1584–1589.

Strauss, A. A.: *Immunologic Resistance to Carcinoma Produced by Electrocoagulation: Based on 57 years of Experimental and Clinical Results,* Charles C Thomas, Springfield, Ill., 1969.

Weinbert, E.: "Nutritional immunity: the host's attempt to withhold iron from microbial invaders," *Journal of the American Medical Association,* **231**(1), January 6, 1975, pp. 39–41.

Wu, A., I. Chanarin, and A. Levi: "Macrocytosis of chronic alcoholism," *New England Journal of Medicine,* **291**(18), May 4, 1974, pp. 829–835.

Chapter 18

Development of an Oncology Unit

Diana L. Donley

An oncology unit, like the disease that is its focus, does not start on a Monday morning. Instead, the formation is a gradual one brought about by a gradual realization of the necessity of and research into the feasibility of such a unit and the development of an underlying philosophy and a period of planning for such a change. The physical design and location of an oncology unit is of less importance than the philosophical and emotional climate created by the nurses, physicians, patients, families, administration, and supporting services of the institution. This climate takes time to achieve. Although a unit may open in January, the change in focus from technical, task-oriented nursing to psychosocial, process-oriented nursing may not occur in less than a year.

This chapter is designed to give some of the reasons for an oncology unit and to define those situations in which an oncology unit would not be feasible. Assuming the decision has been made to develop an oncology unit, one measure of the potential success of the unit is the type of support system available and the extent to which it is used by nurses and patients alike. The support system is composed of many types of services, some of which, such as social, nutritional, and religious services, are well known and utilized now. Other areas, such as music therapy, bibliotherapy, and art therapy, are now being developed and tried

381

in various institutions throughout the country. The support system, its importance, and its function will be discussed.

IS AN ONCOLOGY UNIT FEASIBLE?

When one explores the possibility of an oncology unit, one must first consider if there is a need for the unit. The following points can be evaluated.

Patient Census

Does the percentage of cancer patients in proportion to the total hospital population indicate that there are sufficient numbers of cancer patients to keep the unit filled to 80 percent capacity at all times? An 80 percent occupancy rate is the figure frequently used by hospital administrators to justify the existence of any unit. Less occupancy results in increased cost to the institution for nursing service, dietary service, and other types of support services needed to keep a unit open.

If there are adequate numbers of patients who have the diagnosis of cancer, but their physicians are unwilling to admit them to such a unit, then again the feasibility of the unit must be questioned.

Physician Support

Are there adequate numbers of physicians interested in assisting the development of the unit? These can be physicians specializing in hematology, oncology, gastroenterology, proctology, genitourinology, obstetrics, or gynecology; or they can be practicing in family medicine, in general practice, or in any other area of medicine, surgery, or psychiatry. Although they do not have to be specialists in oncology, they should be committed to the concept of holistic cancer care. They should be willing to support the unit with patient admissions, allowing their patients to receive the full benefit of the support system of the unit. Their willingness to contribute to the educational interchange will allow for full professional and personal growth potential of the staff members, resulting in increased benefits to the individual patient.

Administrative Support

The priority of an oncology unit as compared with that of other types of specialty units will be considered by the institution's administrative personnel and board of directors. If the institution's primary reason for existence is to serve a certain segment of the community, such as women with obstetrical or gynecological problems, this intent may or may not be further served by the inclusion of an oncology unit. Even though the institution may not be focused on a particular health problem, if other nearby institutions already have large oncology units, the board of directors and administration may feel that development of a different specialty unit, such as one in cardiology or orthopedics, might better serve the needs of the community and avoid interagency competition as well.

The board of directors and administration must be willing to set up policies to make the operation of the oncology unit possible. For example, if psychological counseling has been available only on a limited basis, they will want to consider its expansion so that all patients on the unit could benefit from the service. Because doing this could involve the hiring of additional personnel, the board and administration must be willing to support the unit financially as well as through policy-making procedures.

Nurse Support

There must be sufficient numbers of nurses to adequately staff the unit. Ideally, these nurses should be volunteers to the unit staff and should be willing to help develop the emotional as well as physical climate of the unit. They therefore should be open to change. Many institutions are concerned about staffing, for they feel that nurses might not be available to assure continued coverage of the unit once it was in existence. This concern is due in part to the general belief that a cancer unit is a depressing place to work. This "truism" need not be true. An oncology unit is only as depressing as the combined approach to patient care makes it. It can be an extremely rewarding place to work, depending on the attitudes of the physicians and staff nurses, the support systems available to patients and staff alike, and the tone set by the head nurse and/or supervisor. It is a place in which the nurse can practice patient care as it was taught—that is, care of the person as a unified whole and where every facet of nursing service, from orthopedics to cardiology, can be used.

Policy-Making Committee's Support

The policy-making committee is composed of representatives from medicine, surgery, nursing, administration, social services, and others. This group must be able to reach agreement on several issues.

Admission Policies   Will medical and surgical patients be placed on the same unit? Will newly diagnosed patients be admitted along with the terminally ill? Will the nursing staff or the admissions office control placement of the patients, to avoid interpatient conflict? Will a newly diagnosed patient be placed next to a patient who is in the terminal phase and who has the same diagnosis? Are patients admitted to other units to be transferred to the oncology unit once the diagnosis of cancer has been made? Will patients accustomed to the unit be transferred off once they reach the terminal phase, to avoid depression in other patients? If so, what about the dying patient and family? Will they be able to keep in contact with the nursing staff they have grown to know and trust to help them through the dying process?

Support Services   Will the nurses as well as the patients be given support to prevent staff morale from deteriorating? Will nurses be able to ask for and receive temporary reassignment to another unit should they feel the need? Will the support service concept be supported by administration so that the unit can be adequately staffed while in-service programs or "screaming sessions" designed to handle nurses' feelings are conducted?

Staff Rotation   If an oncology outpatient clinic is also in existence or is planned in the institution, would the nurses be rotated to that area? This plan would not only increase continuity of care, but would also help the nurses see a more positive aspect of care in which patients are able to continue daily living in spite of a diagnosis of or treatment for cancer. If a hospice is nearby, will the staff be able to rotate to that institution so that fresh ideas about caring for the terminally ill might be generated? In the absence of a home care system, will the staff nurse be able to perform a home visit for discharge planning or for follow-up as he or she feels is necessary?

Other Policies   Other policies to be decided upon include the type of support systems to be made available to both nurses and patients, the issue of a higher wage scale for nurses on the unit due to its specialty nature, and the availability of other staff nurses to float in as needed.

PHILOSOPHY

The purpose of the philosophy is to provide the individual caregiver with a point of view on which to base the rationale for the type of care given. It also provides all caregivers in a certain setting with a similar point of view, so that the care given by each may be complementary to others' work and there may be a unified approach to care. For example, one philosophy, regarded by nearly all health professionals as being outmoded, viewed human beings as entities with needs in *either* the biologic *or* the psychologic realm and viewed nursing as being that care given to human beings which would help to prevent complications once a disease process was established. Now, however, the majority of institutions and schools of nursing, whether hospital-, college-, or university-based, utilize a philosophy that resembles that which follows:

> *The human being:* The human being is a unique being who has intrinsic value and whose life is therefore worthwhile. The human being is a holistic being whose needs in one facet of life are dependent upon and interact with the needs felt in every other facet of life. The human being is a thinking, feeling, and behaving individual who has inherent internal goals of growth, ever moving toward increasing complexity of function. (See Figure 18-1.)

> *Nursing:* Nursing is a process by which an individual, group of individuals, or community is assisted to move toward and to maintain optimal health. Health is seen as being on a continuum, with optimal health being that which is required for maximal utilization of thoughts, feelings, and actions. Nursing is so designed as to assist the individual to perform those tasks that he or she would normally do for himself, or herself but is now unable to do. Nursing is planned so that the assistance given to the individual diminishes as the individual's ability to function independently increases. (See Figure 18-2).

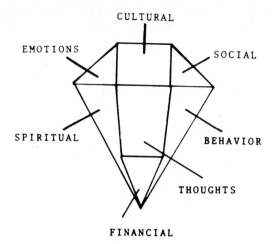

Figure 18-1 Facets of person: the forces acting upon and within each individual.

Regardless of what type of philosophy is designed and/or adopted, it is useless unless the policies of the unit reflect the philosophy in their design and operationalization.

POLICIES OF AN ONCOLOGY UNIT

The oncology unit is almost always a department that is responsible to nursing service rather than to administration. Therefore, many of the policies of the unit

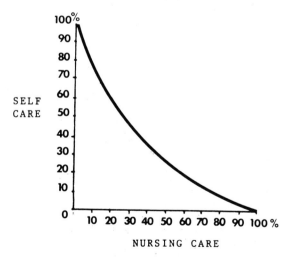

Figure 18-2 Self-care in relation to nursing care. The percentage of nursing care increases as the amount of self-care decreases.

will be dictated by those policies already in existence throughout the institution. Some policies, however, can be devised or revised so as to be unique to the oncology unit. Although each group of nurses can undoubtedly think of many policies they would like to see in operation on their units, some commonalities can be seen in the general types of policies used in many institutional settings.

Policies on Patient Activity

One policy in this category is the amount of freedom the individual patient will have to guide and participate in his or her own care. Will the patient be given the freedom to decide, within the constraints of time and individual ability and when guided by the nurse, the type and timing of care and/or procedures he or she is to receive? Will the patient be encouraged to assume partial responsibility for administration of medications, or will this function be assumed entirely by the professional staff? Giving the patient some degree of control in these areas helps to prevent or alleviate some of the inevitable loss of self-esteem that accompanies admission to the hospital and assumption of a "dependent patient" role.

Another policy considers structuring of patients' time. If the programs for patients emphasized group interaction as a means of obtaining peer support for the individual, will policies of the unit support this? Some possible methods of meeting this goal include provision of a coffee hour for patient interaction, setting aside of a portion of time each day for the patient to visit a solarium or dayroom for interaction, or a similar type of policy. Will each patient have some free time each day to fill as desired? Will adequate time for patient education in the areas of physical needs, psychosocial needs, or knowledge of the disease and its process be provided as the patient needs or desires?

Will patients be provided a mechanism for feedback into the system, a method by which patients can have some voice in the policies of the unit? One method to fulfill this goal is to have a patient or former patient be a full- or part-time member of the policy-making committee. Another method is to ask the patients for written or verbal suggestions, and a third method would utilize the nurses' observations of the effectiveness of the current policies in meeting patient needs.

Policies on Family Support and Participation

The policies of the unit should reflect a realistic picture of the amount the patient's family may participate in patient care or the amount of staff support the family may expect. Will the patient's family be allowed to visit at any time, or at designated hours only? What about the visitation of a patient by young children? Will an area be provided in the patient's room, in the institution, or in a nearby hotel or motel should the family feel the need or desire to be near the patient? Many institutions make arrangements with nearby hotels so that rooms may be provided at a reduced rate should the family desire it. The patient is a member of a family unit and, as such, not only receives but also gives support to the other family members. The nearness of the family may meet the needs of the family as much as it meets the patient's needs. Many institutions, especially those involved with the care of children, provide space in or near the patient's room for the family. Thus the intrafamily support system is disrupted as little as possible.

Are families expected or allowed to participate in the care of the patient? If they are expected to do so, as in the care of a child or very dependent adult, will the nurse spend some time with the care-giving family member(s) to devise a rational plan for a combined approach to patient care? Who is to give the physical care, and how much and when is he or she expected to perform these tasks? Once the decisions are reached jointly by the patient, family, and staff, friction between the staff and family can be minimized and the potential for maximal cooperation in attaining patient care goals can be reached.

Can the family expect a planned type of counseling from the staff, or will counseling occur on a "need felt–help given" prn basis? Will the family's needs be considered as secondary, and important to the staff only to the extent that they affect the patient? Or will these needs be met as much as possible to prevent further trauma and family disruption? Will the nurses recognize that the needs of the family dictate that the family also be recognized as a "patient"? Intervention by the nurse or other members of the support team will help the family maximize its potential for normal functioning in the present or the future.

Policies on Staffing

The type of nursing assignment most effective on an oncology unit is now under study, with both team and primary nursing being evaluated. Both methods have advantages as well as disadvantages. With primary nursing, the staff nurse has both the responsibility and the accountability for a small group of patients (usually four to six) from the time of their admission to the time of discharge. All patient care is planned with input from the patient, and a very close nurse-patient relationship results. The continued contact between nurse and patient encourages the patient to air feelings with increasing comfort and confidence in his or her nurse. The major disadvantage of primary nursing in the oncology setting is that patients may be on the unit for extended periods, perhaps as long as several months. The continued responsibility may leave the primary nurse feeling drained not only emotionally but also in terms of creative approaches to nursing interventions. This situation can be avoided if the problem is discussed with the patient and/or family and an arrangement is made for another nurse to assume the primary nurse role, with the first nurse acting as consultant to the second.

Most hospitals currently use the team approach to patient care assignment. The major advantage in maintaining this type of approach is that staff on the unit will have fewer changes to adjust to when the unit is first opened. Primary nursing can be explored as a new method later, when the staff is more used to functioning in this setting. One major disadvantage of team nursing is the more distant relationship that exists between the patient and nursing staff. A second disadvantage is the higher cost of team nursing in comparison with primary nursing. Proponents of primary nursing have also found a lower turnover rate and a higher rate of job satisfaction than is seen with the team concept.

The primary nursing concept suggests the use of an oncology clinical specialist or nurse of similar education and training as the head nurse, or, as she is sometimes called, the "unit coordinator." This nurse can then serve as a role model for the other nurses on the unit.

Regardless of the method of patient care assignment, it is ideal that the head nurse have the prerogative to interview prospective members of the nursing staff and that her suggestions regarding hiring, firing, or transfers be followed by the nursing or personnel office.

PHYSICAL FEATURES OF THE UNIT

It has been noted that the philosophical and emotional climates of an oncology unit are more important than the physical features. Yet the physical features are of considerable importance to the comfort of patients, their families, and the staff. They therefore can influence the amount and type of patient-patient, patient-family, and patient-nurse interactions that occur.

The rooms may be furnished in accordance with the philosophy and focus of the unit. If patient-patient interactions are to be encouraged, then one should consider eliminating televisions from the room of ambulatory patients and placing a television in a solarium or dayroom. If one goal is family participation in patient care, location of supplies, for example, can be decentralized so that they are readily available to the family. If nurse-patient or nurse-family interactions are the goal, areas should be provided in or near rooms to ensure privacy for those interactions. Patient interaction can be encouraged or discouraged by use of furnishings in the patients' rooms and in the solarium and associated rooms (see Figures 18-3 through 18-5).

About one-third of the rooms on a 20- or 30-bed unit should be private. This arrangement allows for greater privacy for patients who desire it and will enable the private rooms to be converted into isolation rooms as needed. Some institutions provide a dressing or treatment room in which to carry out painful or uncomfortable procedures. Of the institutions that care for children, some provide a solarium or dayroom to be known as a "no-hurt" room. No painful procedures, regardless of their brevity, may be carried out there.

Other physical features that add to the comfort of the patients and families are a nearby nondenominational chapel and a quiet room, also known as a "screaming room," for the families to escape the ever-present reality they must face in the patients' rooms. Patients' and families' use of kitchen facilities to make coffee or sandwiches or to heat meals from home helps to make the hospital routine less regimented and can give the patients and families some control of their daily routine.

While these additional features, e.g., the kitchen, the quiet or screaming room, or possibly a library or counseling room, are not essential, they do help both patients and families get the message that their needs are considered and are felt to be important.

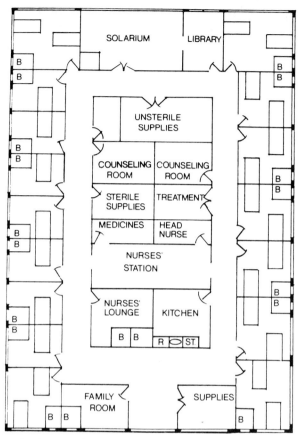

Figure 18-3 Example of an oncology unit arrangement.

STAFFING

Some oncology units have been opened with a hand-picked staff of all volunteers, while others have opened with staff already assigned to the unit. As long as there is adequate psychological support, either method seems to work well. Usually the turnover rate is not greater on an oncology unit than on another type of unit. It may even be less because of the extra attention and the support system available to staff members.

The staff should be open to change and committed to the concept of holistic patient care. The nurses should have a strong sense of personal identity and be able to ask for and accept assistance when it is needed. They should be able to share themselves with others—not only with patients and their families but also with other staff members. The nurses should have a strong sense of responsibility and be willing to be held accountable for their actions. Many nurses find an

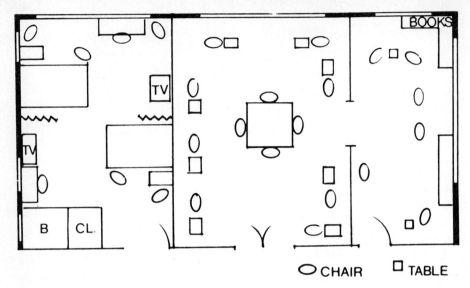

Figure 18-4 Sociofugal setting for interaction. A "sociofugal" setting is one that discourages social interaction. In this setting, patients will be less likely to leave their rooms or to converse in the solarium or library.

oncology unit to be a dynamic, intellectually stimulating, and personally fulfilling setting in which to practice their profession.

The burden of paperwork can be greatly reduced by the use of a computerized system of record keeping if it is feasible in the institution. The use of

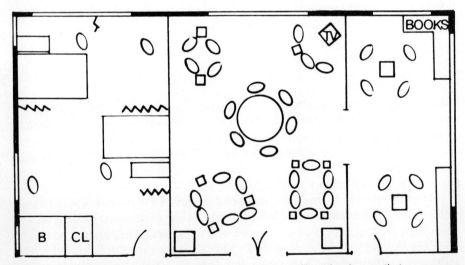

Figure 18-5 Sociopetal setting for interaction. A "sociopetal" setting is one that encourages patient interaction. Patients' rooms are sparsely furnished while the solarium and library are more elaborately furnished.

the "acuity system" will help to provide adequate staffing from shift to shift. Basically, the acuity system involves an assessment of each individual patient on the unit according to the level of nursing intervention needed (whether physiologic or psychologic). The total hours and the quality of nursing care needed on the unit for the following 8-hour shift are then used to accurately calculate how many R.N.s, L.P.N.s, and nurses' aides are needed to meet patient needs. This type of system cuts the expense of overstaffing and prevents excessive patient care loads for nurses which reduce the quality of patient care that can be given on days when patient needs are at their peak.

Physicians who use the services of the oncology unit for their patients are usually encouraged by the atmosphere of the unit to be open and honest with the patient and family. The nurse may view as overwhelming the prospect of caring for one oncology patient for several months, since some of these patients may be hospitalized that long or longer. The physician may also feel this to be an overwhelming task, especially when progress is not evident in the patient's condition. The atmosphere of an oncology unit may be as supportive to the physician as to the nurse, patient, or family. Physicians may come to rely on the nursing staff or other support services to meet the psychosocial needs of their patients, leaving themselves free to concentrate on treating the physical conditions. Thus, a multidisciplinary approach to patient care can be fostered on an oncology unit.

Physicians are taught from medical school on to view death as the enemy— the final defeat, the ultimate failure. Over a period of years, the death of many patients takes its toll on physicians. If physicians can be encouraged to attend sessions that focus on dealing with the feelings aroused by caring for cancer patients, or if the nurse can understand that these feelings are operant in nearly all physicians, interdisciplinary understanding and mutual support can result.

SUPPORT SERVICE SYSTEM

The purposes of a system of support services are threefold.

1   A wider range of services offered by experts in each area are available to every patient.
2   The nurse is freed of many concerns for the welfare of the patient and family and can concentrate on planning and delivering effective high-quality patient care.
3   The staff benefits from increased support for personal reactions to caring for these patients. The staff may find the employment experience to be one that fosters personal and professional growth.

The areas in which support is considered essential are social services, nutritional counseling, religious support, psychological counseling, oncology clinical specialists, rehabilitation, family support, educational support, and housekeeping.

Social Services

Typically, nurses have thought of social service as offering only financial counseling to patients. This tended to be the role of social service in areas where social workers were employed only by federal or state welfare agencies. In the institutional setting, there often was only one social worker for the entire institution, and it was physically impossible for one person to attempt more than just meeting the basic referrals for financial counseling that were sent to him or her.

Because social workers of the past were often representatives of a welfare agency, many hospital administrators, patients, doctors, and nurses have regarded the use of their services in a negative light. The social worker of today is as likely to run group therapy sessions or do individual patient counseling as to handle financial problems. The negative connotation of the social worker is being replaced by the more enlightened and realistic picture evolving today. Although there is still a nationwide shortage of social workers, most institutions employ at least one and more often several to offer a wide variety of services.

Financial Counseling   Having cancer is costly unless one is either very wealthy or very poor. The wealthy can afford to pay the bills, while the poor rely on governmental support to pay. The burden falls on those who are in between these two groups. Nearly all insurance companies set limits as to the amount they will pay for a single illness. Patients just beginning this illness need advice on how to manage their finances so that the drain on the family will be as little as possible. Social workers can either offer this help themselves or refer the patient to a financial adviser.

Community Agency Liaison   Social workers often have more awareness of the help available to the patient than anyone else does. They assess the patient, the person's needs, and his or her areas of personal, social, financial, and family support and then refer the patient to the agency most likely to be able to help.

Counseling   Most social workers conduct individual or group therapy or counseling sessions, although each individual has his or her own areas of interest and expertise. When a nurse encounters a patient who resists help, the nurse can refer the patient to a social worker. Persons who have a master's degree in social work have learned counseling skills and may suggest to the patient's physician that the patient be referred to a psychiatrist or psychologist if the patient also resists the social worker's efforts to help. Social workers counsel patients, families, or staff. They work with doctors and nursing staff to help the patient make the transitions from hospital to home or to an extended-care facility.

Nutritional Services

Many patients experience difficulties in their dietary regimes while undergoing cancer therapy. A dietician can help the patient or family plan nutritionally sound meals that are ethnically and esthetically pleasing to the patient. Since many of the gastrointestinal reactions to surgery, chemotherapy, immunotherapy, or radiation therapy can be anticipated, the dietician can advise the patient on a pretreatment and during-treatment diet. These diets, usually high in proteins, vitamins, and minerals, will help the patient withstand the rigors of therapy.

Religious Support System

A chapel or quiet room that can be converted to this purpose should be easily accessible to the cancer patient and family. Religious services can be conducted there as the patients and religious leaders desire.

Many institutions find that their patients benefit from the use of clergy on a full- or part-time basis. The ministerial services may be rotated to provide a wide variety of denominational approaches. Regardless of the denomination, the clergy should have two things in common. The first is a sensitivity to the needs of cancer patients, and the second is an ability to communicate an atmosphere of love and acceptance rather than rejection and damnation.

Psychological Services

Psychological services may be divided into two general categories: patient-oriented and staff-oriented. Persons who conduct the counseling sessions may vary: Nearly all nurses have the ability to counsel patients individually, but nurses may not feel qualified to counsel family groups or groups of patients. The psychiatric nurse clinician, a clinical specialist, a psychologist, or a well-trained religious leader or social worker may be the ideal person to lead such a group. Regardless of who leads the group, the person chosen should have some basic understanding of the biologic and psychologic effects of cancer and its treatment.

Patient Programs   These programs are designed to help the individual work with and through the feelings associated with having cancer. Individual counseling was the first method used and is still the one most frequently seen. Group counseling may be held with the family alone, the family and the patient, or a group of patients. Individual counseling may be done formally or informally. Group counseling is nearly always done formally in that a definite appointment time is scheduled, there is a designated leader, and the experience may be more or less structured.

Previously, approaches to counseling involved mainly verbal communication. With the numerous recent advances in the social sciences, however, many new approaches are currently being seen.

The patients' coffee hour is an informal gathering of patients designed to allow patient interaction and peer group support. Patients may express feelings about treatments and about the disease process itself. Usually, the presence of staff in these coffee hours is not needed, although the staff may be nearby to answer questions if they arise. The patients may even enjoy being "on their own" for a while.

Recently, some novel experimental techniques have been devised to aid patients in expression of emotions. *Bibliotherapy* is one of these approaches. The group leader or a group member reads a selection of prose or poetry to the group. Group members then discuss their reactions to the reading. The readings are carefully selected by the leader to explore a particular topic and to be at the proper level of understanding for the group as a whole. For example, if the topic that needed to be dealt with was fear, the selection could be one focusing on the arousal of fear, its effects on the person, or the resolution of fear. However, some people are more oriented towards expression of emotion through language and others are more oriented toward expression through physical measures. Theoretically all patients would benefit from bibliotherapy, but some might benefit to a lesser degree than others.

Music therapy is another new approach. A selection of music is carefully chosen by the leader for its potential effect on the listeners. To assist the listeners in expression of anger, for example, one might choose a passage that at first sounded light and pleasing, enabling the patient to relax. The tone would then become more ominous and foreboding. This change could arouse feelings of anger in the patient, as it did in the author. If patients have a great deal of unexpressed anger of which they may or may not be aware, this is an excellent technique to uncover and release those feelings.

There seems to be a physiologic basis for this response to music. Electroencephalographs show a slowing of brain waves in response to a slow, soothing type of music and an increase in wave activity when faster, more exciting music is played. Many mothers make use of this principle in singing lullabyes to their children.

This technique is potentially more useful than bibliotherapy or art therapy since the response to music seems to be more universal than the response to the printed or spoken word or to art.

Art therapy is another useful technique to help patients express deeply felt emotions. The stimulus may be a picture or a piece of sculpture, that is discussed by the group, or it may be drawing or sculpting by the patient. One can observe much about a patient's inner emotional state by simply observing the way the patient uses his or her hands and the finished product. This technique is limited by the space available to work on and to store the projects until they are completed. Limitations may also be seen when patients feel that they have no artistic ability and so are unwilling to participate in the therapy. This method seems to be an outgrowth of occupational therapy, to be discussed later.

It should be remembered that each culture has different responses to the same stimulus. Thus, a poetic selection or musical passage that elicits a fearful reaction in the American culture may have a different effect on the person of Hispanic or Japanese origin.

Staff Programs   Working with cancer patients engenders many conflicting feelings within each staff member. If these feelings are not dealt with, the individual may be unable to continue working on the unit and may be left with more intense reactions to illness, pain, or death than the person had previously. Nurses frequently go through a process of grieving for the patient as well as with the patient. Patients usually resolve this process before they die, but the nurse cannot do this without withdrawing from the patient. Nurses need help before, during, and after the terminal phases, which on an oncology unit means nearly continuously. Group sessions held once a week by someone other than a staff member may be used for griping, crying, or just plain screaming. The group leader should be trained to help staff members express their emotions constructively. Bibliotherapy or music therapy could also be used on occasion to aid in expression of emotion.

A clinical specialist or other trained person could be on call to counsel the individual staff member as feelings arise. Nurses will increase in self-knowledge and in the comfort they feel and are able to give to the patients as they become more comfortable with how they as individuals feel about death.

Thanatology Teams   Some institutions now have a team or a core group of people interested in discussing death with others. This team may include psychologists, clinical specialists, physicians, staff nurses, clergy, and social workers. These people may be on call to lead group discussions throughout the institution and to offer advice and guidance on how to handle problems associated with death or dying.

These programs, although discussed in terms of patient or staff participation, also extend to the counseling of families. This counseling may be done formally or informally and may be conducted with individual family members, the family as a unit, or a group of families.

Nurse Specialists

Nurse specialists comprise a core of people with expertise in various nursing fields. The oncology clinical specialist has educational preparation at the master's level and has specialized in oncology. This person can advise on topics ranging from physical to psychological problems. He or she may fill a head nurse position or may be a consultant to the staff.

The clinical care coordinator may be a nurse of varying educational preparation, but is well experienced with cancer patient care. This person may act as a liaison agent with the home, hospital, outpatient clinic, or extended-care facility to improve the continuity of care. He or she also functions as a resource person for the oncology unit staff and may assist in inservice education of the staff.

Chemotherapy nurses are those who are specially trained in the handling, administration, and management of toxicity of chemotherapeutic agents. They usually provide counseling to the patients and the staff, especially on the drug effects. It is frequently advisable to train staff nurses to give these drugs. The chemotherapy nurse, who is usually institution-based rather than unit-based, is then freed to act as a consultant for the administration of drugs and the observation of toxic reactions. In addition, the chemotherapy nurse will give drugs to any patient in the institution who is not on the unit and may administer the drugs in the outpatient clinic as well.

Immunotherapy nurses administer immunotherapy and observe the patient after therapy. They counsel patients, family, and staff on the type of agent used and the expected results, both positive and negative.

Radiation therapy nurses are usually located in the radiation therapy department of the institution. They counsel patients before, during and after therapy to minimize unpleasant side effects.

Infection control nurses, or epidemiology nurses, advise the staff on measures of infection control. They can describe the usual course of an infectious disease and can advise if and when isolation precautions are needed for a specific type of infection.

The participation of all these types of nurses has the potential for fragmentation of patient care, with resultant decreased quality of care and increased patient isolation. The patient may have no one specific nurse to relate to and may feel "lost in the shuffle." If one nurse can coordinate the contributions made by all these people, the process can be made meaningful and perhaps even organized for the patient. (See Chapter 19, "The Oncology Nurse Coordinator— An Expanded Role.")

Rehabilitation Team

Physical Therapy   The patient who has undergone mutilating but potentially life-saving surgery needs to learn how to use the rest of his or her body to compensate for the missing part(s). For example, after a radical mastectomy, the patient needs to learn how to use other muscles to raise her arm. The patient who has had an amputation needs to learn how to compensate for the lost limb. Other patients may lose the function of a body part, such as in paralysis of an extremity, and compensatory functions of other extremities must be learned. As the patient regains control of his or her body, the person's self-esteem will begin to rise correspondingly. Emotional counseling is therefore a useful adjunct to physical therapy.

Occupational Therapy   Occupational therapy aids the patient to adjust to the changed body and body image. A person who has recently become partially paralyzed may feel incompetent and therefore useless because the family's needs can no longer be met. This person can be helped to learn new ways of functioning to meet some of the family's needs, such as cooking from a wheelchair, and may require occupational advising. A woman patient may need assistance in revising her expectations of the womanly role, and a man may need help in adjusting to his altered male image. The person may find more time to talk to the family since time is no longer filled with the role of housekeeper or breadwinner. Body image will change, and the person, although limited in what can be done, may find that new skills can be developed, with the change in body image not necessarily negative.

Teaching Teams   The teaching team may consist of an enterostomal therapist, nurses skilled in teaching patients postoperative care of radical head and neck operations, persons to teach mastectomy patients postoperative care and exercises, persons to give diabetic teaching, etc. These people supplement but do not replace the teaching done by staff nurses.

Home Care   The nurses from a home care agency visit patients prior to discharge and also evaluate the home setting to be sure the patient can be adequately cared for at home. They may obtain the needed equipment and aid in its placement in the home. They follow the patient's progress at home. Should the patient need readmission, these nurses will aid in the transition from home to hospital, thereby maintaining continuity of care as much as possible.

Family Support

Family support services, as discussed earlier in this chapter, include visiting policies, ability of the family to become involved in patient care, counseling of family members, and use of a quiet or screaming room, as the need may be. These services are important not only for the well-being of the patient but also for prevention of future pathology in the family. (See Chapter 11, ''The Psychosocial Aspects of Cancer.'')

For patients hospitalized for any length of time, inhibition versus expression of sexuality becomes a problem. To touch and be touched is a basic human need that is often frustrated in the hospital setting. Patients often feel isolated and need the comfort of their spouses. Some time may be set aside for patients and their spouses to be alone together, and the policy of always knocking on a closed door before entering should be strictly observed by all. This topic is more fully discussed in Chapter 13, ''Sexuality and the Oncology Patient.''

Educational Support of the Staff

Staff nurses working on an oncology unit need educational support. One frequently observed request is for information about how to improve one's communication and counseling skills, especially in regards to the terminally ill and their families.

Physical care of the oncology patient may differ somewhat from care of other patients in the amount and depth of assessment. Care planning has somewhat different goals than those set for care planning with patients with noncancerous conditions in the amount and type of psychologic intervention needed. Education as to new drugs and new types of therapy can be done on a regular basis, since new data about these topics becomes known frequently.

Having a staff nurse function part time as a unit in-service instructor helps to meet the needs of the staff on the unit and also tends to gear information given to the information needed and/or desired by the staff.

Housekeeping Support

The ability of the housekeeping team to function as a part of the patient care team is a frequently underestimated resource. Some patients, whether because of socioeconomic status or personal feelings about the professional staff, may find it more comfortable to communicate with members of the housekeeping staff. Should this situation arise, the nurse assigned to the patient may let the process continue for as long as needed. In the interim, the nurse can guide the housekeeper as to how to proceed while trying to establish good rapport with the patient. This can be done by helping the housekeeper guide the patient to the nurse or by the nurse trying variations in approach in an attempt to gain the patient's confidence.

When a patient has a behavior problem, becomes critically ill, or dies, the nursing staff should not neglect to include the housekeeping staff in a grieving session. Although these people do not usually develop close rapport with patients, they, too, are involved with the patients' care and feel grief along with the rest of the staff. Thus, working on the oncology unit can be a means for personal growth for all concerned.

SUMMARY

This chapter has dealt with the reasons for establishing an oncology unit and some of the points and policies to consider in planning and operating such a unit. It is expected that each institution's needs will be different, as will its means for meeting these needs. Thus, this chapter has offered a general guideline rather than definitive solutions in each area.

An oncology unit can be a rewarding setting for the personal and professional growth of each staff member. An oncology unit with the proper philosophical and emotional climate will also help patients learn to live or to die without fear.

BIBLIOGRAPHY

Association of Hospitals and Institutional Libraries: Committee on Bibliotherapy: *Bibliotherapy: Materials and Methods,* Chicago, American Library Association, 1971.

Bonny, Helen: *Music and Your Mind: Listening with a New Consciousness (Suggested Recordings for Altered States of Consciousness),* New York, Harper and Row, 1973.

Bright, R.: *Music in Geriatric Care,* New York, St. Martin's, 1973.

Capurso, A., et al.: *Music and Your Emotions: A Practical Guide to Music Selections Associated with Desired Emotional Responses,* New York, Liveright, 1970.

Charnock, J.: "Leadership and the search for excellence in hospitals," *Health Social Service Journal,* **84,** March 16, 1974, pp. 604–605.

Ciske, K.: "Primary nursing: an organization that promotes professional practice," *Journal of Nursing Administration,* **4,** January–February 1974, pp. 28–31.

Daeffler, L.: "Patients' perception of care under team and primary nursing," *Journal of Nursing Administration,* **5,** March–April 1975, pp. 20–26.

Dunn, A.: "Hospitals should be coloured optomistic," *Nursing Times,* **71,** September 4, 1975, pp. 1398–1399.

Durrant, J.: "Library service to geriatric patients in the hospital," *Health Welfare Library Quarterly,* **1,** December 1974, pp. 87–89.

Gaston, E. T.: *Music in Therapy,* New York, Macmillan, 1968.

Grace, M. J.: "The psychiatric nurse specialist and medical-surgical patients," *American Journal of Nursing,* **74**(3), March 1974, pp. 481–483.

Greenberg, I.: *Psychodrama: Theory and Therapy,* New York, Behavioral Publications, 1974.

Grof, S.: *Realms of the Human Unconscious: Observations from LSD Research,* New York, Dutton, 1976.

Hogan, R.: "Development of an empathy scale," *Journal of Consulting and Clinical Psychology,* **33,** 1969, pp. 307–316.

Horne, E. M.: "A look at bibliotherapy," *Special Libraries,* **66,** January 1975, pp. 27–31.

Howell, D., and W. Boxx: "Motivating workers on routine jobs," *Supervisor Nurse,* **4,** May 1973, pp. 44–53.

Kravitz, S., et al.: "Consciousness-raising groups," *Supervisor Nurse,* **6,** October 1975, pp. 26–27.

Lerner, A.: "Poetry therapy," *American Journal of Nursing,* **73**(8), August 1973, pp. 1336–1338.

Luber, R. F.: "Poetry therapy helps patients express feelings," *Hospital Community Psychology,* **25,** June 1973, p. 387.

Lyddiatt, E. M.: *Spontaneous Painting and Modelling: A Practical Approach in Therapy,* London, Constable Press, 1971.

Manthey, M.: "Primary nursing," *Nursing Forum,* **9**(1), 1970, pp. 65–84.

———: "Primary nursing," *Nursing Forum,* **9**(4), 1970, pp. 356–379.

Marram, G., K. Flynn, W. Abaravich, and S. Clarey: *Cost Effectiveness of Primary and Team Nursing,* Wakefield, Mass., Contemporary Publishing, Inc., 1976.

———: M. Schlegel, and E. O. Bevis: *Primary Nursing: A Model for Individualized Care,* St. Louis, C. V. Mosby, 1974.

Pienschke, D., Sr.: "Guardedness or openness on a cancer unit," *Nursing Research,* November–December, 1973, p. 204ff.

Podolsky, E.: *Music Therapy,* New York, *Philosophical Library,* 1954.

Riehl, J., and C. Roy: *Conceptual Models for Nursing Practice,* New York, Appleton-Century-Crofts, 1974.

Rogers, M.: *An Introduction to the Theoretical Basis of Nursing,* Philadelphia, F. A. Davis, 1970.

Ryan, T., et al.: "System for determining appropriate nurse staffing," *Journal of Nursing Administration,* **5,** June 1975, pp. 30–38.

Small, J. E.: "Why consider unit management?" *Hospital Progress,* **55,** April 1974, pp. 74–78.

Stopera, V., and D. Scully: "A staff development model," *Nursing Outlook,* **22,** June, 1974, pp. 390–393.

Van de Wall, W.: *Music in Hospitals,* New York, Russell Sage Foundation, 1946.

Waddicor, J.: "Library service to nursing homes: a regional study," *Library Journal,* **100,** October 15, 1975, pp. 1892–1895.

Washington (State) Library: *Music the Healer: A Bibliography,* Olympia, Wash., Institutional Library Services Division, 1970.

Watzlawick, P., J. Weakland, and R. Fisch: *Change: Principles of Problem Formation and Problem Resolution,* New York, Norton, 1974.

Wethered, A.: *Movement and Drama in Therapy: The Therapeutic Use of Movement, Drama, and Music,* Boston, Plays, Inc., 1973.

Chapter 19

The Oncology Nurse Coordinator—An Expanded Role

Luana Venard

THE ONCOLOGY NURSE COORDINATOR

Today in America it appears, professional nurses are searching for expanded roles. Oncology offers a wide variety of opportunities for expansion. In different parts of the country, there are clinical specialists in oncology, chemotherapy, radiotherapy, and immunotherapy; research nurses; out-patient oncology nurses; in-service oncology nurses; leukemia nurses; pediatric oncology nurses; and a myriad of other roles. It is hoped that each is effectively and efficiently meeting the needs of the patients.

The present chapter will describe a comprehensive nursing role, one that was recently conceived, is now in the implementation phase, and is desperately needed. The role is a result of a contract between The Queen's Medical Center, Honolulu, Hawaii, and the National Cancer Institute, Division of Cancer Control and Rehabilitation.* The project has been renamed the Comprehensive Cancer Care Project and employs oncology nurse coordinators.

The oncology nurse coordinator is a knowledgeable, consistently present, major resource person for a caseload of cancer patients. The coordinator is the

*Funded by Contract NO1-CN-65197, "Development and Implementation of Cancer Care Coordinating Teams." The Principal Investigator is Noboru Oishi, M.D.

health professional consistently available to the patient and family throughout the illness, rehabilitation, and continuing-care phases of the disease. This person fills the gaps in the present health care system with knowledge, understanding, experience, and results. The coordinator is trained extensively in the aspects of cancer from initial screening to vocational rehabilitation, in the psychosocial impact of the disease and the nursing interventions to assist in coping, and in the utilization of existing community resources. Thus, the oncology nurse coordinator is responsible for coordinating all phases of health care for the cancer patient.

DEVELOPMENT OF THE ROLE

After caring exclusively for cancer patients for a number of years, the writer felt that she had heard every possible complaint from every possible source. The complaints went something like this: "Not enough staff for conferences." "But the doctor won't tell him the diagnosis; what can I do?" "Who can I call when. . . ?" "No one really cares what happens after I leave this hospital." "There's not enough in-service; if the nurses only knew what they were doing!" Sound familiar?

One specific patient experience motivated this nurse to take action. The patient was a 45-year-old woman who had experienced complete remission from her lymphoma for about 2 years. She was divorced and was attempting to rear two teen-age boys whom she considered "wayward." She was unemployed. She had had a minimum of formal education but was well experienced as a legal secretary. She was on maintenance chemotherapy that required no hospitalization but did require some outpatient visits. She had been taught subcutaneous injection for some administering of her own drugs. After having had contact with so many less fortunte cancer patients, this nurse felt that she was one of the lucky ones who had many productive years ahead. Many hours were spent in discussing her semirelated social, sexual, and vocational problems. Many hours were spent in seeking assistance. And then one day she committed suicide. Guilt hung heavy, followed by rationalization about personal limitations; then came motivation. I, we, the health care system had failed in this case. However, with that failure came the knowledge that there was a better way to utilize the existing system, to strengthen the weak areas, and to fill in the gaps to avoid similar tragedies in the future.

The first step in the nursing process is to define the problem and then gather a data base from which to work. The problem here appeared simply to be a lack of resources for cancer patients in this facility and in this community. In gathering data, however, we found the assumption to be incorrect. Through careful analysis, the problem was identified as poor utilization of existing resources by ill-prepared but highly motivated health professionals.

It should be pointed out here that each nurse has his or her own "problem" patients, ideals of care, and ever-changing health/illness environment. Although each health professional tends to view these problems as unique, it is reasonable to assume that similar barriers to quality care are shared by all nurses. As a consequence, it is the rare patient anywhere in America who enjoys consistent excellence in quality of care and total continuity throughout his or her illness.

All nurses at one time or another have been presented with a diagram of ideal patient-centered care. The patient is located at the center of the diagram and is surrounded by any number of eager health professionals. With family cooperation, excellence in patient care is the anticipated result. At the same time, our health care system and innumerable scientific advances have demanded specialization among those same health professionals who care for the patient. These medical advances and specialties, promoted in the interest of patient care, have resulted in the "lost patient" syndrome. The lost patient syndrome is not solely a product of small hospitals, but is perhaps more evident in large, highly specialized facilities. Our progressive system has made so many "advances" that one patient may come in contact with 20 or 30 "outsiders" during an illness and recovery or death. As a consequence, we have created an unwieldy system that professionals have difficulty dealing with and that may leave the patient stranded. A recent visit with a patient included the following monologue:

> I have seven doctors. Three have beards so they must be students. I really don't know who actually cut on me. There's the nurse with the needles [the chemo-therapy nurse], the one who changes the yellow bags [total parenteral nutrition], the cute one in the outpatient department, the starched one who told me when I'd be discharged [utilization review], the one who exercises that dead leg of mine [the physical therapist], and some lady with glasses who always wants to know how I *feel* about my disease. I don't know who you are, but tell me, do you really think I'd get sicker if I had a cold beer?

Although this may be an exaggerated case, the question remains, How many of the thousands of cancer patients present in America today feel similar frustrations? Has the ideal circular patient-centered system collapsed before the health professionals' very technological eyes?

The more this writer looked around, the clearer it became: The patients do not suffer from a lack of resources; they suffer from an inability to use the resources appropriately. One solution to this dilemma is to add the oncology nurse coordinator to the health delivery system. The role of this nurse is to take the patient out of the circle (circus?), raise him or her and the family above it, and then help the patient to effectively use the services of the system throughout the health-illness continuum.

THE PRACTICALITIES

Effecting any change is difficult in terms of emotional response as well as dollars and cents. This project has the benefit of federal funds to alleviate half the problem temporarily. Any reader recognizing the problems cited above and wanting to alleviate them will want to know the specifics of this program.

Project Philosophy

In spite of the sophistication of modern medical and nursing technology, there is a lack of satisfaction in the lives of many cancer patients. Too many patients and families feel lost in their struggle for survival and their struggle for health and respect. Though surrounded by experts, many patients have no idea from whom they should seek certain information or counseling. Although many excellent services exist in a facility or community, there is a lack of integration of these services and a lack of continuity in care.

The stress of illness weakens the patient, often precipitating feelings of anxiety, fear, dread, confusion and grief. The goal of the oncology nurse coordinator is to return each patient to the person's preillness level of physical, emotional, and social health. Optimal nursing care endeavors to help meet a wide range of patient needs, including basic physiologic requirements for life; the need to feel safe; the need to love and be loved; the need to respect self and others; and the needs to learn, achieve, and create.

Quality nursing care is a commitment to personalized care. It requires conscientious observation, communication, validation, and intuition, not just mechanical implementation of medical and nursing orders. Optimal care of the cancer patient challenges the skills of health professionals and demands their educated hearts, hands, and minds.

The emphasis of the project is on assisting cancer patients to live with their disease. The focus is on life, not death; on continuity, not fragmentation; on the whole individual, his or her family, and the environment, not pieces of the whole.

Project Goals

The overall goals of the Comprehensive Cancer Care Project are to:

    1 Improve the adequacy, continuity, and general quality of care of the cancer patient and family
    2 Improve the appropriate utilization of existing community and hospital resources, services, facilities, and personnel
    3 Minimize the number of physician hours devoted to nonmedical tasks

Approach

The goals will be met and the philosophy realized by the introduction of the oncology nurse coordinator into the patient's health-illness experience. The model remains patient-centered but elevates the patient to a rightful position above health professionals. The result is a three-dimensional patient care structure (Figure 19-1) with a central figure (the oncology nurse coordinator) *coordinating* the efforts of the health care team.

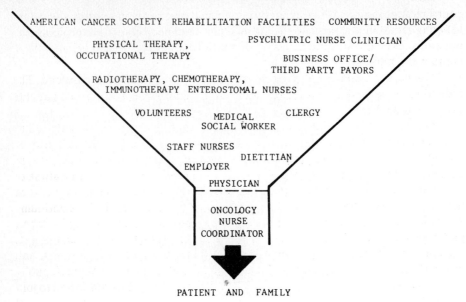

AMERICAN CANCER SOCIETY REHABILITATION FACILITIES   COMMUNITY RESOURCES

PHYSICAL THERAPY,   PSYCHIATRIC NURSE CLINICIAN
OCCUPATIONAL THERAPY
                                           BUSINESS OFFICE/
                                           THIRD PARTY PAYORS
RADIOTHERAPY, CHEMOTHERAPY,
  IMMUNOTHERAPY ENTEROSTOMAL NURSES

    VOLUNTEERS   CLERGY
                     MEDICAL
                  SOCIAL WORKER

      STAFF NURSES
                        DIETITIAN
         EMPLOYER

           PHYSICIAN

           ONCOLOGY
            NURSE
          COORDINATOR

        PATIENT AND FAMILY

Figure 19-1 Patient care structure.

  It is most important for that central figure to recognize the benefits of the team approach, the skills and talents of each member, and the fact that she or he coordinates the efforts of others and does not attempt to become a team member. The coordinator becomes the primary resource for the patient in the patient's seeking of care and the primary resource for the other team members in their provision of care. The coordinator becomes the link to the community, the catalyst in helping the patient to seek ways of meeting needs.

  When the patient is referred to the project, the oncology nurse coordinator interviews the patient and family and does a complete physical and emotional health assessment. He or she seeks contact with all other professionals and significant people in the patient's environment. After consulting with the patient, family, physicians, and significant others, the nurse develops an individual patient care plan to supplement the standard care plan previously devised. It may be advantageous to bring the patient to the attention of the project multidisciplinary support team for advice in care planning and implementation. It is the nurse's responsibility to coordinate team members' activities in designing the care plan, adhering to the timetables, attaining the goals, and evaluating the care. The nurse consistently reevaluates changing patient problems, assesses who can best solve identified problems, and personally communicates with any new team member. The oncology nurse coordinator plans and helps to implement quality care while the patient is in the acute care setting and always anticipates potential discharge needs. He or she makes at least one home visit after discharge to reevaluate progress in the patient's response to the home environment and the family's response to the caretaker role. The nurse's task of planning, referring, coordinating, and reevaluating continues until the patient meets mutually established rehabilitation goals or dies. Upon death or the attainment of the goals, the patient is taken off the active caseload, but the patient and/or family can always contact the nurse at any later date.

The nurse begins by carrying not more than 20 patients on the caseload. The individual nurse and the project director jointly determine if additional patients can be handled safely, efficiently, and effectively.

The nurse has available the 10-member multidisciplinary support team. This team consists of people who have functioned as a team for 6 months prior to the implementation of the project. They have each had an 8-hour overview of cancer, the team approach, rehabilitation, and project philosphy. An outline of the team's curriculum appears as Appendix One. This team meets once a week for patient care planning with the nurses and twice a month for continuing education. The team consists of the following personnel: medical social worker, psychiatric nurse clinician, chemotherapy nurse, radiotherapy technologist, dietitian, two clergy, enterostomal therapy nurse, occupational therapist, and physical therapist. Other members, such as the patient, family members, public health nurse, staff nurse, pharmacist, speech therapist, etc., will be asked to join particular patient planning sessions. The nurse is, of course, in constant contact with the patient's physician to ensure mutually acceptable patient goals.

The advantages of this nurse to the patient are many. The first is the nurse's availability and knowledge of the patient over a period of time. The nurse has the ability to provide appropriate consultants because of knowledge of community and hospital resources and ability to cut red tape in providing care. An open line of communication exists between the nurse and the physician, family, and other health team members. Most importantly, the nurse cares for and about his or her patients throughout their illness. (Please refer to Appendix Two for the overall job description of the oncology nurse coordinator.)

Educational Preparation

The nurse described here has an expanded role sought by many but held by few. It takes a very special person to meet the demands of such a position. As part of this National Cancer Institute—funded project, four nurses were educated for 6 months. These nurses were chosen on the basis of a strict 16-point checklist and some intuition exercised by the project director and medical consultant. All the nurses have at least a baccalaureate degree in nursing and 2 years of medical-surgical or public health nursing, oncology, and teaching experience.

The nature of the project and the people involved provides great freedom in the 6-month curriculum. The small class size allows for individual attention to each nurse's personal growth. Each nurse determined personal objectives for education, growth, and experience. Nearly one-quarter of the time was devoted to directed reading and independent study on related topics.

The learning experience comprised lectures by various nurses, physicians, psychologists, patients, and all members of the health team with expertise in a certain area. These lectures were followed by extensive, searching discussions of how the particular information applied to cancer patients, to this project, and to the nurses individually. Nearly one-third of the time was spent in practical application of theory and concepts.

A four-week block of time was devoted to exploring community resources by actually spending several days with various health professionals and lay volunteer groups. In this way, it was possible to get a ''feel'' for their services, establish working relationships, and determine on a personal level what services they offered. One of the many positive results of this experience is the *Community Resource Manual for Cancer Patients* in this community.

Another 4-week block was devoted to getting to know the referring physicians. Each nurse spent at least 15 days with a variety of physicians who would soon have patients on the caseload. This experience served many purposes. The physicians and nurses were given an opportunity to mutually explore this new role and how it would affect their patients. The area of medical versus nonmedical tasks was discussed between individuals. Mutual respect, role distinction, and role compatibility were the outcomes of this experience.

A more tangible result of the education was a thorough annotated bibliography on a variety of aspects of cancer nursing. This bibliography serves us all as a ready reference to new problems.

An outline of the 6 months' curriculum and approximate number of weeks in each core area appears as Appendix Three. Each week the nurses and project director met for at least 2 hours to continually assess the program and developing needs. The focus of life, not death; of continuity, not fragmentation; and the holistic approach to care were discussed at length. Self-awareness grew throughout the 6 months period.

IMPLEMENTING THE SERVICES

Professional and patient information is the single most important prerequisite to delivering the service described above. If physicians and patients are not convinced of the worth of services, they will certainly not be requested.

The nurses' six months of education focused not only upon becoming prepared technically but also upon informing other health professionals about the services in a nonthreatening manner. In addition, the multidisciplinary support team was thoroughly prepared. This was accomplished via the 8 hour education program. Much groundwork must be done with heads of departments to which the individual team members report. In theory, all department heads are in support of continuing education and the team approach; however, in practicality these departments must continue to function when one member is absent for meetings or education. It must be emphasized to department heads that all the department's employees will benefit from one person's education and that eventually all patients will be the benefactors of continuing education. The time one employee spends away from his or her duties is much more palatable if the salary for that time can be absorbed by the project. This was possible with contract funds from the National Cancer Institute.

Informing Physicians

The next major challenge is informing physicians of the service and then "selling" it to them. This was accomplished by first closely determining which physicians treated the majority of the cancer patients. Letters of information from the physician principal investigator and medical consultant were sent to this group three times during the 6 month education phase as a means of preparing them for the service. As the implementation time drew close, the medical consultant and project director spoke directly to physician groups via the local medical association, hospital medical advisory committees, and announcements in American Cancer Society professional newsletters. It was important to deal directly with any hesitancy a physician might have. For instance, some physicians had very legitimate questions regarding the project goal of decreasing physician hours devoted to nonmedical tasks. But physicians in general were more than eager to relinquish tasks to nurses who were not seeking to usurp the physician role of medical practitioner. The project greatly admires the physician who expends the time and effort to investigate those providing care to his or her patients.

To inform patients of the services, brochures were placed on nursing units and in the admitting department. The local newspaper carried articles about upcoming services, and the American Cancer Society announced it through newsletters.

Identifying Patients

By design, the nurses originally carry only 20 patients at any one time. Some of these patients are acutely ill, hospitalized patients; some are on the road to rehabilitation at home. During a day's work, the nurse attempts to meet a variety of physical, psychological, and social problems with a wide spectrum of patients. Also by design, only patients referred by their physicians are accepted. This procedure ensures cooperation among health professionals in establishing treatment and rehabilitation goals.

Based on initial response from the community regarding the services, a desire to serve patients most in need, and a wish to adhere to the National Cancer Institute contract, the following criteria for patient selection were established:

I   Prerequisites
   A   Patient must be referred by a physician.
   B   Patient must have one of the following primary cancers: head and neck, lymphoma, leukemia, stomach, colorectal, lung, breast, female genital, or prostate.
   C   One of the oncology nurse coordinators must have space available on her caseload.
II   Desirable conditions
   A   Patient is referred while an inpatient.
   B   Patients have multiple (more than two) problems.
   C   Patients do not have alternative sources of support.
   D   Patients have been diagnosed within the last month.

III Caseload makeup
  A 100 percent of the caseload must meet at least one of the criteria.
  B At least 75 percent of the caseload must meet at least two of the criteria.
  C At least 25 percent of the caseload must meet at least three of the criteria.

The project receives notification of the cancer patient census through the admissions department and pathology department. If there is space on a nurse's caseload, a physician may be contacted for a patient referral. Also, the staff nurses and any member of the multidisciplinary support team may contact the project regarding a potential patient, and the project director will contact the physician.

EVALUATION

The only way to continue or expand a service is to prove that the service is beneficial. The methodology for evaluating this project is extensive, sometimes cumbersome, but will answer a variety of questions in the future. There are three major reasons for thoroughly evaluating the project. The first, of course, is to consistently improve patient services while maintaining flexibility. The second is that it is felt that the services of a nurse coordinator should be extended to hospital patients with many other diseases. Ideally, positive evaluation will encourage hospital administrators to make such a commitment. The third reason is that third-party payors will be more willing to cover the costs of oncology nurse coordinator services after federal funding has expired if long-term benefit can be demonstrated.

The methodology for evaluation has been developed by an expert consultant in measurement with the assistance of Nursing Quality Assurance within this facility. Only a brief description will be given here.

Objectively evaluating quality and continuity of care is a most difficult task. After reviewing a number of existing tools and attempting to modify them to meet project needs as well as time and financial limitations, we devised three methods. First, retrospective chart auditing will be done to determine the percentage of patients on and off the caseload who have complete nursing care plans (standard and individual) and nursing histories.

Second, chart abstracting and patient observation will determine if patient outcomes were met and established nursing interventions were actually performed for patients on and off the caseloads. Care will be taken to evaluate not only if outcomes were met but also if they were appropriately established by the nurses.

Third, inventories to determine general satisfaction will be administered to patients, physicians, and the nurses themselves. Numerical values have been assigned to responses on these inventories to provide an objective measure of satisfaction. Incidentally, the average number of patient hospital days and average cost per day will be determined for comparative patients off and on the project.

As a means of evaluating the second objective, regarding utilization of resources, a close watch is kept on the number of referrals the nurse coordinators make for their caseload. Later, patients will be interviewed to determine the appropriateness of those referrals.

Minimizing of physician hours devoted to nonmedical tasks is evaluated by observing physicians. An independent evaluator will make extensive observations of a number of physicians and record the number of tasks, time it takes to perform the task, and percentage of total patient time a physician spends on nonmedical tasks in caring for patients on the project caseload and for similar patients not on the caseload. A checklist of nonmedical tasks has been prepared by means of a poll of physicians.

CONCLUSION

The reader has been bombarded with the strength of this service. The project has one important limitation: it cannot serve all the patients who might benefit. In spite of this limitation, the oncology nurse coordinator can have a positive impact on the overall care delivered to the cancer patient.

Obviously, it is hoped that, compared with other patients, project patients will be more satisfied, they will suffer less financial drain, their physicians will be happier and less burdened, and the patients will be able to enjoy the best of a variety of services while still having a primary resource to rely on. It is firmly believed that these cancer patients will feel a sense of continuity in their health care and continuity in their lives.

APPENDIX ONE: Multidisciplinary Support Team Education

The 10 individual team members each attended 80-hours of education over the 6-months of the group's training period. Each phase consisted of 20 hours in each week.

Phase I, Cancer the Disease: Basic epidemiology and pathophysiology of cancer and basic information on each of the nine disease sites covered by the project.

Phase II, The Team Concept: Introduction to the team concept: 8 hours of experiential training in group process and development of individual role descriptions.

Phase III, Psychosocial Aspects of Cancer Care: Awareness of the psychosocial impact of cancer on the patient, family, community, and health professional. Basic communication and interviewing skills; continuing and terminal care.

Phase IV, Treatment and Project Integration: Basic information on treatment modalities and patient physical and psychosocial reactions; team conferences with oncology nurse coordinators.

APPENDIX TWO: Oncology Nurse Coordinator
Job Description

GENERAL DEFINITION

Serves as the primary resource person to a caseload of selected oncology patients, providing excellence in quality of nursing care and continuity of care in all phases of diagnosis, treatment, convalescence, rehabilitation, and follow-up.

Is responsible to the project director for purposes of supervision and direction.

TYPICAL DUTIES AND RESPONSIBILITIES

1 Assesses the physical, social, emotional, and spiritual needs of the patient and family and intervenes, utilizing appropriate resources

2. Assists patient and family in adapting and adjusting to all phases of illness, hospitalization, convalescence, and rehabilitation and/or terminal phase

3 Interprets to patients, families, and staff the medical treatment objectives in conjunction with the primary physician

4 Distinguishes nonmedical tasks and decisions with the assistance of the medical supervisor, acts on those nonmedical tasks and decisions, and refers the patient/family to the primary physician for intervention of medical tasks and decisions

5 Provides short-term or emergency counseling for patients/families

6 Keeps accurate written records on all patients, including ongoing care plans and project implementation evaluations

7 Enlists the aid of the multidisciplinary support team to meet patient goals

8 Serves as a teacher and resource person to other nurses in the hospital and in the community

9 Utilizes a wide variety of resources in the hospital and community to assist patients in meeting goals

10 Attends a variety of meetings, e.g., cancer committee meetings. Comprehenhensive Cancer Care Project staff meetings, support team meetings

11 Assists in case finding

12 Performs other duties as assigned by the project director

APPENDIX THREE: Six-Months' Education of
Oncology Nurse Coordinators

Core area I: Orientation to the medical center and the project is presented. One week.

Core area II: The community oncology nursing project core course and an overview of oncology nursing are discussed. Two weeks.

Core area III: The nine specific diseases covered by the project—epidemiology, etiology, screening, diagnosis, treatment, complications, usual patient problems and nursing interventions, rehabilitation problems and potentials—are thoroughly investigated. The nine sites discussed are cancers of the lung, colon, breast, head and neck, prostate, female genital, and stomach and leukemia and lymphoma. Three weeks.

Core area IV: The process and practicalities of screening, detection, and diagnosis and the importance of pathology are explored and observed. One week.

Core area V: Psychosocial care is handled via lecture, discussion, observation, and practicum. The following topics are covered: primary nursing, nurse-patient relationships, nurse–health professional relationships, I–Thou concept, body image, sexual adjustment, maturational adjustment, gerontology, crisis intervention, group therapy, family counseling, the pain experience, the death experience, grief, the hospice concept, and leisure time. Four weeks.

Core area VI: The team approach, the concept and practicality of continuity of care, and the importance and realities of rehabilitation are explored via lecture, discussion, and observation. One and one-half weeks.

Core area VII: The advanced concepts of the four treatment modalities are explored, and extensive direct patient care is provided. Three weeks.

Core area IX: This is a course, "Experiential Training in Human Relationship," Social Work 755, given at the University of Hawaii. It consists primarily of experiential training in communication and interviewing skills. Four weeks.

Core area X: Each nurse explores various community resources for cancer patients. Four weeks.

Core area XI: Each nurse works and studies directly with referring physicians. Four weeks.

Part Five

Educational Aspects
of Oncology Nursing

Chapter 20

The Detection of Cancer

Patricia Sato

Every day someone is told he or she has a dreaded disease—cancer. The same questions go through each person's mind: Why me? Why now? Why wasn't there some warning? There are usually no answers. Even when there are, the answers are of no benefit to the person to look for warning signals retrospectively. It does not have to be this way, though. There can be some answers or solutions that benefit people. The way to reduce the number of deaths due to cancer is through prevention, and if cancer cannot be prevented, through early detection.

Screening and detection go hand in hand. In order for cancer to be detected, there must be well-established screening tests. These tests cannot be used unless the public is educated that early diagnosis and treatment are necessary and that these two factors are positively related to higher rates of cure from cancer. The ideal situation is to prevent as much cancer as possible; for this ideal to be achieved, the public must be well informed about the factors that seem to increase the chances of getting cancer. This chapter will present these topics and will explore the obstacles to early detection.

SCREENING AND DETECTION

Screening tests can be easily used on large numbers of people without high cost and have a high degree of success in detecting early cancer. For screening tests to be successful, they must meet the following criteria:

1   The test should be available to large numbers of people.
2   The test should be inexpensive.
3   It must be easily reproducible.
4   It must be of proven value.
5   The results must be quickly obtainable.
6   The test must be technically simple.
7   It must be applicable to large numbers of people.
8   It must appeal to people. A test that makes one uncomfortable for long
    periods of time will be avoided by people.

To screen everyone would be very expensive, would be time-consuming, and
might actually defeat the purpose of the screening test, since many people would
be tested who did not have cancer and therefore too many negative results would
be obtained. Screening should be done on that part of the population that has a
high probability of getting cancer.

Identification of High-Risk Groups[1]

High-risk categories for the major cancer sites have been established by the
American Cancer Society by determining the rates of cancer occurrence in each
population group. It is recommended that persons in high-risk groups have
routine screening tests to detect early cancerous or precancerous lesions. These
people can be identified by age, sex, race, occupation, family history, habits, and
physical examination. All of these factors should be considered in recommend-
ing frequency of screening to the patient. Also considered should be convenience to the patient.

   Breast Cancer   This disease occurs mainly in women over the age of 35,
with whites having a greater risk than blacks in the United States. Risks are
greater for those women who have never borne a child and for those who had the
child after age 25. Risk increases with age and is higher for those whose mothers
or sisters had breast cancer. Women who experienced early menarche or late
menopause are also at greater risk, and cancer in one breast increases the risk of
development in the other breast.

   Colorectal Cancer   Since colon cancer occurs more frequently in countries
that are urbanized or highly developed, studies of dietary influence are being
done. Special attention is being paid to those foods that are highly processed and
therefore travel more slowly through the intestine, because there is a concomitant increase in amount of time for exposure of the intestinal tract to carcinogens.
The risk may run as high as 50 percent for those whose close relatives have
familial polyposis and for those who have had ulcerative colitis for more than ten
years.

   Gastric Cancer   The risk for gastric cancer is about three times greater if
one's close relatives have had the disease. While there is some association of

gastric cancer with blood group A, no definite link has yet been found. It is associated with gastric ulcers but rarely, if ever, with duodenal ulcers. Dietary influence may also be important, since the incidence of this type of cancer is higher in those who have a high intake of smoked fish or meats, pickled vegetables, or dried, salted fish. The risk is high for native-born Japanese and decreases for their offspring who live in the United States. Gastric cancer rates are declining in the United States.

Lung Cancer Smoking is stated to cause 80 percent of all lung cancer. Obviously, not all lung cancer victims smoke. Nor do all smokers get lung cancer. The statistics do show, however, that a higher percentage of smokers succumb to lung cancer than do nonsmokers. Smoking is also implicated in cancer of the esophagus and of the bladder. The risk of lung cancer increases if the patient has had a close relative with lung cancer. In men, the risk is greatest for one between the ages of 60 and 69 who has smoked two or more packs of cigarettes a day for 20 years or more and who started smoking before the age of 15. This man's risk of development of lung cancer is 15 to 20 times greater than that of a man who never smoked. For women, the lung cancer risk is greatest for one who is between the ages of 55 and 64, who has smoked up to one or more packs of cigarettes per day for at least 20 years, and who began smoking before the age of 20. This woman would have five times as great the risk of developing lung cancer as would a woman who never smoked.

Oral Cancer The habits of cigarette smoking, tobacco chewing, ingestion of alcohol, poor oral hygiene, and lack of dental care all increase the risk of oral cancer. Lip cancer occurs more frequently in those who have had excessive exposure to sunlight. Blacks, other dark-skinned people, and Orientals have less risk of developing oral cancer than do whites.

Ovarian Cancer This cancer is seldom seen in women under the age of 35 and peaks in occurrence in women between the ages of 65 and 69. The risk rises if close relatives have had cancer of this site.

Prostatic Cancer This cancer is rare in men under the age of 50. It is greater in those whose close relatives have had the disease. It is uncommon in Indians and Mexicans; although some sources state that the rate is low in Orientals and Filipinos, other sources disagree. The latter sources state that the risk for these two cultural groups rises in proportion to increasing age. (The latter statistics include occult carcinoma of the prostate as well as overt states of the disease.)

Skin Cancer The risk for skin cancer is highest for those with outdoor occupations, such as farming, sailing, and fishing. It is also high in those who work with coal, tar, pitch, or creosote. Some families tend to be prone to skin cancer. Fair-skinned people are more susceptible to skin cancer than darker skinned people are, and excessive suntanning can lead to this condition.

Cervical Cancer   This type of cancer occurs most often in the 45- to 69-year age group. Some of the social factors associated with this type of cancer are low-income background, history of sexual intercourse with many different partners, and early onset of sexual activity. Poor care during and following pregnancy and no regular checkups or pap smears are also associated with this type of cancer.

Endometrial Cancer   The risk for endometrial cancer is highest for those in the age group of 50 to 64. Although there is an increased risk for those who have had a late menopause, present knowledge indicates that a family history of the disease does not seem significant. An increased risk for this type of cancer is seen in the obese, the diabetic, and the hypertensive woman.

Other Cancers   Occupational risks occur for some types of cancer. For example, fibers and dust associated with asbestos, glass fiber products, and sawdust increase the risk of cancer. Chemical fumes from manufacturing processes and arsenic compounds used in paints and sprays also contribute to an increased risk factor, as do inks and dyes. Women and young girls whose mothers took diethylstilbestrol during their pregnancies, especially during the first trimester, have a much increased chance of developing vaginal cancer. Those who previously received radiation in any form for treatment of a disease, whether benign or malignant, have an increased chance of developing cancer in the irradiated or an adjacent site many years later.

Once these groups are identified, it is necessary to screen the people for potentially cancerous growth. At present, the best screening procedures are specific rather than general. The sites most commonly and easily screened are the lung, colon, rectum, breast, mouth, and uterus. Fortunately, these are also the sites in which cancer develops most frequently in the United States. Only one cancer that commonly occurs is not included in this list: prostatic cancer. This is not because of the difficulty in examining the prostate, but because few men go each year for this examination. There have been no screening programs organized thus far which focus on this problem.

Attempt at a General Screening Test

A general screening test would be one that could easily detect the presence of cancer in the body but would not necessarily indicate the site of cancer occurrence. So far, however, such a test has not been developed and refined well enough to meet all the criteria for a screening test. One promising test is the carcinoembryonic antigen (CEA) test, which measures the amount of tumor antigen in the serum (see Figure 20-1). At first it was hoped that this test could be used to detect cancer in the asymptomatic person, but it was discovered that too many variables could influence the outcome of the test. The CEA test has been found to be more useful in determining the prognosis of the patient who has already been diagnosed as having cancer. Another important effect of the CEA

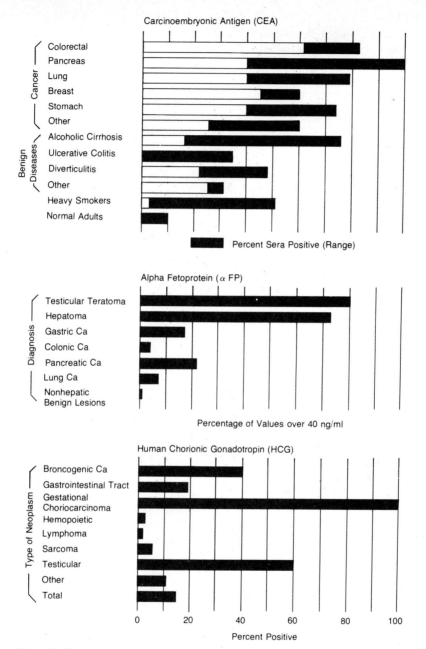

Figure 20-1 An ideal cancer screening test would be one that ran a combination of immunologic, hormonal, and other chemical tests for tumor markers on a single blood sample. Three serum markers with potential diagnostic value, CEA (*top*), alphafetoprotein (*center*), and HCG, have been detected in sera of patients with a variety of tumors. Although the results are promising, these markers are not yet specific enough for screening purposes. *(N. I. Berlin, "Research Strategy in Cancer: Screening, Diagnosis, Prognosis," Hospital Practice, January 1975, p. 89.)*

test has been to prove that substances can be detected in the blood of the cancer patient which are not found in the blood of those who do not have cancer. Other studies are under way to detect tumor-specific antigens in the blood, in an effort to detect cancer in the asymptomatic person, but as yet no tests are well enough developed for use in a routine screening examination.

Specific Screening Tests

Screening for Breast Cancer Since there had been no decrease in the occurrence of breast cancer prior to 1971, the American Cancer Society (ACS) launched a breast cancer screening program that year. The purpose of this program was to determine whether screening of asymptomatic women would lead to earlier detection and therefore better rates of survival from breast cancer. The program was a success and led to the funding of 29 breast cancer demonstration project centers by the American Cancer Society and the National Cancer Institute. At these centers, women are screened by interview, physical examination of the breasts, mammography, and thermography. Women are also taught how to do breast self-examinations. The rate of cancer detection is about 6 cancers per 1000 women. The best rates of survival from breast cancer are seen in women whose disease is localized at the time of primary treatment; and 77 percent of these women have had no metastasis to the axillary nodes at the time of diagnosis and treatment.[1]

With the establishment of breast cancer demonstration projects, more data on the history of each patient are being collected. It is hoped these data will yield more knowledge about the factors surrounding the development of the disease. The popularity of these centers is evidenced by the number of women waiting for appointments.

While thermography and mammography are worthwhile techniques, they are less easily attainable and more expensive than the most simple of all screening techniques—the breast self-examination. The ACS publishes a very good pamphlet on this topic and will distribute a film or provide a speaker to groups upon request. There is no substitute for knowing the physical condition of one's own breasts and for being alert to the changes that occur. Should a suspicious lump occur, a physician can be consulted promptly for early diagnosis and treatment.

Screening for Colon and Rectal Cancer The number of people expected to develop cancer of the colon or rectum is definitely increasing. The ACS feels that three out of four of those who develop this type of cancer could be saved from mutilating surgery or death by early diagnosis and treatment. One important screening device is the examining finger. Another is the proctosigmoidoscopic examination. While the first procedure *may* be uncomfortable, the second usually is. Both may be embarrassing to the patient. These tests should be done by the physicians as a part of the regular physical examination in those over the age of 40.

The value of the occult blood stool test in the screening for cancer of the colon and rectum should not be underestimated. Cancer of the intestine or rectum frequently causes loss of blood; occasionally a great deal will be lost, and the first symptom presented to the physician or nurse may be anemia. This test, therefore, can detect cancers that have remained asymptomatic. If the test is positive for occult blood, further diagnostic tests should be done. Because of the possibility of a false positive due to blood from previously ingested meat, the patient should be placed on a meat-free diet for 3 days prior to the test.

Screening for Cancer of the Lung   The only screening test for cancer of the lung currently available is the chest x-ray. There is some question about whether the annual chest x-ray has any value in the detection of lung cancers. A study is currently being done at the Mayo Clinic with this in mind. Male patients over the age of 45 who smoke a pack of cigarettes a day and who are expected to live for over 5 years are examined by sputum cytology exams and chest x-rays. Those who have no sign of cancer are then randomized into one of two groups. The first group receives annual chest x-rays, while the second group is studied by chest x-rays and sputum cytology every 4 months. While the study is still too new to bring about any definite conclusions, the study should show the effectiveness and reliability of the annual chest x-ray in detecting lung cancer.

Screening for Prostatic Cancer   A simple screening test that can be done by a physician examining for cancer of the prostate is digital palpation of the gland. This examination should be done annually, especially in men over the age of 60.

The Value of the Screening Examination

The value of screening exams can be determined by the number of people who are symptom-free at the time cancer is detected. This is usually the stage at which cancer is confined to the organ of origin. Treatment at such a time would be curative.

The most successful screening test is the pap smear. This test is about 95 percent accurate in the diagnosis of cancer of the cervix. It is very simple and inexpensive. The major drawback to this test is that it can be uncomfortable or embarrassing. The ACS recommends that every woman 20 years of age or older have an annual pap smear. Pap smear screening programs are being done with increasing frequency. A Hawaii law requires all hospitals to offer a pap smear to all women 18 years of age or older when they are admitted to the hospital.

The success of the pap smear, or of any screening test, has been due in large part to public education as to the value of these tests in the early diagnosis of cancer. Because the incidence of cancer of the cervix is particularly high in low-income groups, many educational programs have been designed to reach these women. These programs are continuing despite the fact that they have not been as successful for the low-income group as for the higher-income groups. Other programs are geared to young women who begin having sexual activity early. The proportion of women who begin engaging in sexual activity early is definitely increasing, and it is known that cancer of the cervix is more frequent in such women.

Women in the 50- to 64-year age group need to be educated about endometrial cancer and its occurrence in this age group. A pap smear is of no value in diagnosing endometrial cancer. While women in this age group need pap smears to detect cervical cancer, they also need annual pelvic exams. One new technique is to wash the endometrial cavity and then do cytology studies on the washing. Some physicians do not currently use this technique unless clinical findings indicate possible pathology. Endometrial cancer is less prevalent than cervical cancer and so is overlooked by many people seeking to provide educational programs about cancer. It is hoped that emphasis on the annual pap smear will send many women to their physicians, who will examine them pelvically as well as give a pap smear, especially for the 50 to 64 age group.

After any screening test, if the results are still in doubt, more diagnostic studies should be done. Numerous tests are available. Table 20-1 shows some of the more common tests done to rule out cancer in a specific organ site.

Once screening is done, the diagnosis can usually be made. There is always the possibility of a false positive or a false negative. Therefore more definitive testing may be needed. Confidence in the value of the screening test is important, but it must be remembered that the screening test is not a precise tool. There are other more specific and refined diagnostic tests available. The screening test is merely a simplified method to test a large number of people who are considered to have a high risk of developing cancer.

Detection

Knowing that cancer is present in an organ is not the end of detection. It is important to detect how extensive the cancer is within that organ and whether metastasis to any other organ has occurred. A plan of treatment can then be determined and followed. Curative treatment is always desired, but if it cannot be achieved, detection of the extent of disease will give a more informed estimate of the prognosis or expected outcome of the disease and/or its treatment.

OBSTACLES TO SCREENING AND DETECTION OF CANCER

One of the biggest obstacles in the prevention or detection of cancer has been the public's fear of the disease. Studies done in 1939 showed that the public had a very definite fear of cancer. More recent studies show that instead of blindly fearing cancer, the public now has a more realistic approach and is taking steps to combat the disease. One of the advances made in the area of public education is the emphasis placed on the seven safeguards against cancer rather than only on the seven warning signals of cancer (see Figure 20-2). This emphasis creates a more positive attitude toward cancer detection and treatment than was previously seen. Rather than using "scare" techniques to motivate people to better health practices, those who have assumed the task of public education for cancer

Table 20-1 Summary of Cancer Detection Approaches

Site	Common warning signals	Screening tests available	Diagnostic tests available
Breast	Lump or thickening in the breast	Annual checkup, monthly breast self-exam, mammography, thermography	Aspiration of fluid from breast masses, breast biopsy, chest x-ray, skeletal survey
Colon and rectum	Change in bowel habits, rectal bleeding	Annual checkup, proctosigmoidoscopy (especially over the age of 40), occult blood stool exam, digital exam	Colonoscopy with biopsy, barium enema
Lung	Persistent cough, lingering respiratory ailment	Annual checkup, chest x-rays, sputum cytology studies	X-rays: fluoroscopy, tomography, bronchography, angiography, bronchoscopy; bronchial washings; sputum cytology studies after bronchoscopy; scalene node biopsy; mediastinoscopy; lung scans
Stomach	Indigestion, meat intolerance	Annual checkup, occult blood stool test	Gastric analysis, UGI series, exfoliative studies, endoscopy
Prostate	Urinary difficulty	Annual checkup including digital exam	Needle or open biopsy, serum acid phosphatase, bone scan
Uterus	Unusual bleeding or discharge	Annual checkup including pelvic exam and pap smear, exfoliative studies	Schiller test, tissue biopsy, fractional D & C, cone biopsy, lymphangiography, colposcopy
Kidney and bladder	Urinary difficulty, urinary bleeding	Annual checkup with urinalysis, occasionally exfoliative studies	IVP; retrograde pyelography, nephrotomography, selective renal arteriography, venacavography
Oral (including pharynx)	Sore that does not heal, dysphagia	Annual checkup by physician or dentist	Examination of oral cavity to include nasopharynx, oropharynx, and laryngopharynx; x-rays to include plain films, tomograms, barium swallow, contrast studies of larynx and chest; biopsy of all suspicious lesions
Skin	Sore that does not heal, change in wart or mole	Annual checkup	Excisional or incisional biopsy

prevention are relying more and more on the motivation of most people to remain healthy. Thus, information is presented in a rational manner and is designed to stress the need for more adequate preventative and early diagnostic and therapeutic intervention.

CANCER'S 7 WARNING SIGNALS	THE 7 SAFEGUARDS URGED BY ACS
Change in bowel or bladder habits	**Lung:** Reduction and ultimate elimination of cigarette smoking.
A sore that does not heal	**Colon-Rectum:** Proctoscopic exam as routine in annual checkup for those over 40.
Unusual bleeding or discharge	**Breast:** Self-examination as monthly female practice.
Thickening or lump in breast or elsewhere	**Uterus:** Pap test for all adult and high-risk women.
Indigestion or difficulty in swallowing	**Skin:** Avoidance of excessive sun.
Obivous change in wart or mole	**Oral:** Wider practice of early detection measures.
Nagging cough or hoarseness	**Basic:** Regular physical examination for all adults.
If YOU have a warning signal, see your doctor!	

Figure 20-2 The seven warning signals of cancer as proposed by the American Cancer Society; the newer approach is the seven safeguards against cancer. *(Courtesy American Cancer Society.)*

PREVENTION OF CANCER

The only phase of anticancer efforts more important than screening, detection, and treatment of cancer is prevention. In cancer prevention, techniques based on current knowledge of etiologic factors are applied so that malignant changes do not occur. A study done in 1966 by the American Cancer Society determined why people did not get annual physical examinations that would include some cancer screening tests. The answers of the "nongoers" indicated that they viewed those who got annual physicals as hypochondriacs. This view is irrational, for an annual physical examination can indicate caution on the part of those who are examined regularly. The nongoers seem to have a fear of the unknown, and instead of resolving this fear by obtaining information about their physical condition from a physician, they feel that health problems will resolve themselves spontaneously if they ignore them. Unfortunately, this is not true. More positive public education about cancer is needed to help these people overcome these fears.

In an evaluation of public education efforts regarding cancer, Clifton R. Read lists the following basic concepts of public education:

1 High-fear themes in cancer control are counterproductive.
2 Persons who have had cancer and have been cured are effective in countering the intense, deep-seated fear of the disease.

3 People tend to go to physicians to find out that they do not have cancer, not that they do; thus it is very important for women to know that a breast lump may be many things, and probably is, rather than cancer.

4 Program success will be in relation to the convenience of the action urged and to the immediate availability of the medical procedure advocated.

5 Knowledge and information about cancer are desirable, but they do not necessarily lead to proper or prompt action.

6 The time and expense consumed in "scientifically" pretesting materials can inhibit evaluation. Yet health educators know the value of checking the TV storyboards with network gate-keepers, of reviewing a proposed film for the primary grades before production with teachers and students, of finding out just how women in a lower socioeconomic group actually respond to the text and art in a leaflet while the leaflet is in the planning stage.

7 Potentially, the most creative force in health education is the physician. If we could increase his energy and influence in our cause, more could be accomplished.

8 Face to face education is more effective than a leaflet or the media, although there seems to be a good deal of evidence that television can be nearly as potent as one's neighbor talking over a back fence.

9 Reaching the elderly and disadvantaged (the lower socioeconomic groups who tend to have more cancer) is particularly difficult and requires the use of ideas that complement rather than assault their conviction. It is important that the personnel, staff or volunteers, be acceptable to the target group because of color, native language, and empathy; to me, empathy seems to be more important.

10 A careful stocktaking of health beliefs and habits is an essential preliminary to launching an educational campaign. All ways of communications should be used, including the media, meetings, and person to person approaches. Those who are trained in communications as advertising copy writers, journalists, TV program directors, etc., can be extremely helpful. One nation's program and materials must be adapted with great care for use in another country.

11 Planning for evaluation should begin when an educational project is conceived, the long and short-range measurable objectives must be defined, resources examined, and the machinery for step by step evaluation set up so that there can be periodic evaluation throughout the project, leading to a steady upgrading of the educational process.[2]*

Certain other safeguards to prevent cancer can be taken in addition to those proposed by the American Cancer Society. Prolonged exposure to radiation is known to increase the incidence of cancer, so the amount of radiation a person receives should be reduced to a minimum. Certain chemicals in food are known to be carcinogenic and should be avoided as much as possible. Drugs that contain carcinogenic chemicals should be used only if prescribed by a physician. The value of the drug should be weighed against the risk involved in taking it.

*From Clifton R. Read, "Evaluation of Public Education," in R. L. Clark, R. W. Cumley, J. E. McCay, and M. M. Copeland (eds.), *Oncology 1970,* vol. v. Copyright © 1971 by Year Book Medical Publishers, Inc., Chicago. Used by permission.

Precautions to protect workers from industrial carcinogens should be taken. Persons with diseases that increase the risk of cancer should be examined frequently for early signs and symptoms of cancer.

The ACS, through its public education program, is trying to educate every American about the hazards of cigarette smoking. Lung cancer and its link to cigarette smoking has probably been publicized more than other types of cancer and their possible causes. Surveys done in 1969 showed a dramatic decline in the number of cigarette smokers in the United States. Although no studies on the number of cigarette smokers have been published since 1971, it is felt that there has been a slight increase in the number of smokers since then. Because more women are smoking now than 30 years ago, the rate of lung cancer occurrence in women has been increasing steadily. Soon there will be as many women smokers as men smokers. Because of these trends, the ACS has been waging an all-out battle against smoking. As people become more aware of the facts about smoking and the risks they take in doing so, it is hoped that they will cease this harmful practice. The ACS is backing any legislation that will restrict smoking in public places. This type of legislation will help nonsmokers whose health may also be endangered by the smoke. The ACS also offers free antismoking clinics.

SUMMARY

The ideal situation would be to prevent all cancer. Since the precise cause(s) of cancer is not known, and since more than one etiologic factor is implicated, absolute prevention of cancer seems impossible given current levels of knowledge. Therefore, it is essential to educate the public as to the value of screening examinations as a means of detecting cancer in its early stages. Screening examinations are a method to assess a large number of people for the possibility of cancer. The story does not end there, however. Once cancer is suspected, the individual undergoes more refined examinations to confirm the diagnosis and/or to detect the extent of disease. Early detection is essential in all types of cancer.

Nurses talk to many other people about cancer. They talk to their patients and families and to their own families and friends. In these conversations, the nurse should remember to talk of the successful cancer treatments. In doing so, the nurse can help dispel the cancer phobia felt by the majority of Americans. Thus, education of the public can be accomplished by individual health professionals realizing the impact they can have on the early detection and treatment of cancer in themselves, their patients, their families, or their friends.

REFERENCES

1 '76 Cancer Facts and Figures, New York, American Cancer Society, 1975.
2 Clifton Read in L. R. Clark, R. W. Cumley, J. E. McKay, and M. M. Copeland (eds.), Oncology Yearbook, 1970, vol. V, Yearbook Medical Publishers, Chicago, 1971.

BIBLIOGRAPHY

Ackerman, L. V., and J. A. del Regato, *Cancer,* St. Louis, C. V. Mosby, 1970.

Berlin, N. I., "Research strategy in cancer: Screening, diagnosis, and prognosis," *Hospital Practice,* January 1975, pp. 83–91.

Bouchard, R., *Nursing Care of the Cancer Patient,* St. Louis, C. V. Mosby, 1967.

Donovan, M. I., and Pierce, S. O., *Cancer Care Nursing,* Appleton-Century-Crofts, New York, 1976.

Behnke, H. D., *Guidelines for Comprehensive Nursing Care in Cancer,* New York, Springer Publishing Co., 1973.

Clark, R. L.; Cumley, R. W.; McKay, J. E.; and Copeland, M. M., *Oncology Yearbook, 1970,* vol. III. Yearbook Medical Publishers, Chicago, 1971.

Rubin, P. (ed.), *Clinical Oncology for Medical Students and Physicians,* New York, American Cancer Society, 1970.

Chapter 21

Cancer Quackery: What You Need to Know

Pamela K. Burkhalter

Cancer quackery has evolved into a multimillion dollar annual business in the United States. Cancer patients and their families are subject to financial, medical, and emotional victimization when they seek out or are approached by promotors of unproven cancer treatment or prevention measures. Varying levels of anxiety, fear, anger, or depression tend to make the newly diagnosed cancer patient highly vulnerable to the "miracle cure" offered by the person who calls himself or herself "Doctor." Cancer patients are victimized by the emotionally based but deceptively logical arguments presented by nonmedical purveyors of various forms of unproven treatments.

Although public education programs concerning nonlegitimate cancer treatments and their impact on patients and families are desperately needed, an equally great need exists in the education of health professionals. Nurses, physicians, psychologists, clergy, and other care givers must understand their role in preventing disruption of the effective care cancer patients need and deserve. With understanding of the nature and impact of unproven approaches to cancer treatment, the nurse will be in a better position to clarify misconceptions, facilitate decision making, and provide support for cancer patients who may be searching for that quick, easily accessible, and "guaranteed" cure offered by the cancer quack.

CURRENT CANCER QUACKERY METHODS

Cancer quackery, meaning unproven methods of cancer management, can be defined as the intentional misrepresentation and/or deliberate misapplication of diagnostic or treatment measures which impedes or delays the patient's entry into legitimate, constructive forms of cancer treatment. The most tragic aspect of the entire cancer quackery business is *delay*. The cancer patient may be persuaded by the enticing arguments of instant cure and fail to seek out valid forms of care. When this happens, the "critical interval" comprising early screening and detection of cancer passes without being put to optimal use by the patient. Unfortunately, with passage of time many of the victims of cancer quackery pay the ultimate price for the delay.

Of the multitude of quackery methods currently available via "underground" sales networks, four major categories stand out as the most popular.

Drugs and Chemical Preparations

Throughout human history, herbs, potions, and various combinations of chemical agents have been used and advocated for the treatment of disease. Among the currently used preparations are Krebiozen, Hoxey "chemotherapy," and Laetrile.

Krebiozen (Carcalon)   Since the early 1950s, Krebiozen has been promoted as a cure for cancer. Theoretically this clear liquid substance is manufactured from a horse blood extract. When injected into the cancer patient, it supposedly stimulates the body's inherent anticancer substances, which then slow or arrest growth of the cancer. Although this form of quackery is still promoted in certain foreign countries, it has *never* been found to have any anticancer activity in humans. In-depth research, by the National Cancer Institute, of over 500 case reports supplied by the drug's promoters revealed no substantiated evidence of its efficacy in the treatment of cancer. In addition, long-term scientifically controlled animal research has failed to demonstrate any anticancer effectiveness of Krebiozen.

At various times, Krebiozen has been analyzed as containing mineral oil—at $9.50 per ampule; at other times, mineral oil, a minute amount of amyl alcohol, and creatine—at $9.50 per ampule.

Hoxey "Chemotherapy"   The "secret formula" for the internal Hoxey chemotherapy preparation contains varying quantities of potassium iodide; buckthorn and prickly ash barks; licorice; cascara; alfalfa; and roots of burdock, berberis, stillingia, and poke. Included in the overall Hoxey treatment is an external preparation in paste or liquid form, the latter composed of about 96 percent water. In conjunction with use of the Hoxey chemotherapy, cancer patients may receive prescriptions for calcium tablets, "kidney" tablets, and vitamin C. The diet must exclude sugar, salt, pork, pickles, tomatoes, and bleached flour products. Hoxey chemotherapy preparations continue to be sold and prescribed by quacks in places such as Tijuana, Mexico.

Hoxey chemotherapy has repeatedly been demonstrated to be ineffective in the treatment of cancer. It has no scientifically supported anticancer treatment potential. Case reports collected by the method's advocates contained cure claims made by people who had never had cancer, patients cured of cancer prior to use of the Hoxey method, and cancer patients who received the Hoxey chemotherapy and subsequently died while still using the method.

Laetrile (Amygdalin)   By far the most widely known and promoted unproven drug treatment for cancer is treatment with Laetrile (also known as cyto H-3, Wobe Mugo, and B-17). It has been available for more than 50 years but has received the majority of its attention during the past 20 to 25 years. Derived from apricot and peach kernels, apple seeds, and other fruit pits, Laetrile theoretically acts to halt tumor cell metabolic activities while leaving all surrounding tissue undisturbed. The active ingredient is hydrogen cyanide. The preparation comes in tablet or parenteral form, with the oral form being 40 times more toxic than the injectable route in terms of hydrogen cyanide content.

Repeated, extensive, and vigorously controlled laboratory research into the action of Laetrile on cancer, by such facilities as Memoral Sloan Kettering Cancer Center, National Cancer Institute, Arthur D. Little, Inc., and the Catholic Medical Center, has clearly and conclusively revealed its lack of effectiveness. It does not cure cancer. However, in spite of the overwhelming scientific evidence, proponents of Laetrile claim that it not only can prevent cancer, but also can inhibit metastasis, limit tumor growth, and "control" cancer. These false claims, with their appeal to the emotions, have led to the continuing and burgeoning interest in this form of cancer quackery.

Unfortunately, Laetrile has become somewhat of a political issue. Proponents claim that "Big Government" is preventing the "little guy" from exercising freedom of choice in what can be used for treatment of cancer. Arguments such as these fail to take into account the simple fact that Laetrile has *never* been proven effective as an anticancer agent! To foist this preparation on the public, especially on the cancer patient, as even a possible cure would be to raise false hopes, lure patients away from effective legitimate treatments, and victimize thousands of children who are unable to make a sound choice between quackery and genuine treatment. To prevent such tragedy, Laetrile will continue to be labeled an unproven method of cancer treatment.

One of the main arguments presented by advocates of Laetrile to explain its present illegal status is that doctors, nurses, pharmacists, and hospitals (to name a few) have a financial investment in ensuring that cancer patients remain ill. This highly charged, irrational argument seems to be in conflict with the supposedly altruistic motivations of Laetrile's supporters, who have created excessively lucrative business enterprises devoted to the manufacture and sale of this product. While Laetrile tablets cost about 2 to 3 cents each to produce, they currently cost cancer patients anywhere from $1.25 to $2 or more per tablet. Needless to say, these costs are not covered by third-party health insurance payments. Thus, it appears that it is the quack who convinces the fearful cancer patient to use Laetrile and forego effective treatment who makes a "financial killing."

Krebiozen, Hoxey chemotherapy, and Laetrile are the three most widely used unproven chemical treatments for cancer. Numerous other compounds have and continue to be advocated by the cancer quack. Examples of these "drugs" include male human urine extracts, mistletoe extracts (Iscador), anticancer goat serum, and extract of bamboo grass (Bamfolin). Each of these remedies is completely ineffective in the treatment of cancer and has not been demonstrated as an effective cancer therapy.

Nutritional and Dietary Approaches

Nutrition has always played a large role in health care. Few would argue this point. However, advocates of cancer quackery claim that dietary approaches alone can prevent and cure cancer. Cancer patients have been urged to renounce effective treatment in favor of bizarre and potentially harmful diet regimens (Figure 21-1). The sequence of events may consist of (1) the patient or a concerned relative goes to a health food store, (2) the operator or salesperson, on finding out the situation, directs the person to a particular book or pamphlet containing recipes to cure cancer, (3) the person purchases the recipe ingredients, and (4) the person may be persuaded to also purchase a superblender to

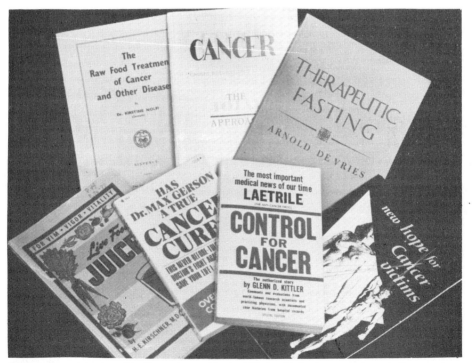

Figure 21-1 A variety of books and pamphlets sold in health food stores advocate the use of unproven methods of cancer management.

ensure proper consistency of the mixture. Many health food stores, conventions, and bookstores have either knowingly or unknowingly taken up the banner of cancer quackery with these tactics. The anxious and fearful cancer patient becomes easy prey to such unscrupulous operators. It must be pointed out, however, that health foods per se have many beneficial effects if used with discretion. It is the presentation of diets and health food recipes as cures for cancer and the encouragement to avoid or abandon legitimate treatment that clearly is equivalent to quackery in its most harmful sense.

Among the phenomenally large number of unproven dietary methods are the raw food treatment and the fasting treatment. In the former, the patient can eat only a raw food diet. In the later, the patient relinquishes all food intake. Water may be ingested during the fast. The consequences of such activity for the nutritionally depleted cancer patient can be devastating. Although Laetrile is considered a chemical preparation, many of its supporters have sought to have it relabeled a vitamin—''a natural food substance.'' Under this label, Laetrile is known as vitamin B_{17} or Aprikern. By promoting these products as nutritional supplements, manufacturers attempted to circumvent the ban on Laetrile. However, the Food and Drug Administration instigated the removal of these products from health food store shelves when it was found that each product contained a potentially lethal amount of cyanide.

Other nutritional approaches list such things as artificially induced fevers; purging of the body with coffee, buttermilk, or yogurt enemas; undereating, taking of vitamin supplements, and fasting-purging schedules. Raw juice and grape diets also are promoted in books and pamphlets sold in many health food stores.

The adverse impact of such methods on the cancer patient can be profound. An already weakened patient is exhausted by the high-colonic enemas, bizarre food intake, lack of protein, and exercise schedules advocated in these methods. It must be emphasized here that no matter how unusual and weird these methods sound, *they are being used* by desperate and fearful cancer patients. Nurses should make themselves aware of what is currently available in their communities. They should visit health food stores. They should browse through the bookshelves and find out what the cancer patient may be exposed to when he or she visits a health food establishment.

Occult or Psychic Techniques

Some forms of cancer quackery are surrounded by a veil of mysticism or religious faith. In some cases, patients attend seances and receive ''miracle'' injections costing as much as $50 or more. The aspect of mystery and the attractiveness of secret ingredients or rituals act as lures to many cancer patients who desperately want to believe in the curative potential of the method.

The most prominent form of psychic cancer quackery is ''psychic surgery,'' based in the Philippines and promoted by the Espiritista Church. Many so-called healers have established businesses devoted exclusively to the performance of ''surgery'' without benefit of anesthesia, aseptic technique, or incisions. Patients present their problem to the healer, undergo surgery, and leave believing that their tumor, gallstone, or whatever has been removed. The technique used is sleight of hand. A patient's abdomen, leg, chest, or other body part is kneaded and manipulated while the operator oozes betel juice or animal blood, concealed in cotton balls in the palm of the hand, onto the skin. After a period of time (determined by the complexity of the surgery), the operator briefly shows a blob of animal fat or small animal organ to the patient and quickly disposes of the material. The skin is then cleansed, and the patient is assured that the cancerous growth has been obliterated.

Some of these psychic healers have established travel agencies with hotel and transportation packages to accommodate patients and families. Cost for a series of treatments, plus expenses, can range from $1000 to $3000 dollars or more. In addition, the "doctor" is paid via donations from grateful patients. The healers call themselves "doctor" but have no formal medical training. In most cases, these people have less than a grade school education.

Study of the psychic surgery method has repeatedly revealed that it is nothing more than a fraud, a con game. Human tissue is not removed by the manipulations and rituals performed by the psychic surgeon. As with most forms of quackery, the patient *wants, needs,* and *must believe* in the ultimate success offered by the quack. With that mind set, the patient willingly submits to the operator, fully believing that the cure is forthcoming. Unfortunately, the transitory psychological relief and feeling of well-being that patients with organic disease may experience following such experiences is just that—transitory. The psychic surgeon did not perform surgery: no tissue was removed, no incisions were made. The cancer remains.

Mechanical Devices

Although waning as a major form of cancer quackery, ozone generators, vibrating machines, orgone accumulators, and innumerable other mechanical devices are still used by cancer patients. In an age in which the public is constantly exposed to the wonders of electrocardiography, radiotherapy, and blood dialysis, the purveyors of worthless devices have little difficulty in convincing the cancer patient to purchase a machine or its services. As a consequence, the person with a bowel cancer, for example, who may benefit optimally by early surgical intervention, may use such a device to treat the cancer. He or she sits in front of it daily, as prescribed, fully expecting that the machine's emanations will cure the cancer. With passage of time, the patient not only still has the disease, but also may have metastasis. Money, faith, and, most of all, precious time are lost. Cost of devices can range from $300 to $2500 each if purchased; the devices can often be rented.

This summary of cancer quackery methods is representative of the most commonly used and promoted approaches offered illegally in the United States* and legally in certain foreign countries. In addition to treatment methods, techniques are available to diagnose cancer and other diseases. For many patients, this kind of quackery represents the only diagnostic work-up the patient

*Several states have legalized the use of Laetrile. However, it remains illegal to transport it across state boundaries.

undergoes. If the quack diagnoses cancer, exact, guaranteed cure is then offered. The patient is told and believes that he or she has cancer, while never having a biopsy, blood chemistry studies, or radiology work-up. Among the more common of these diagnostic methods are the handwriting test, blood smear test, hemacytology index (HCL), and malignancy index. Needless to say, none of these so-called diagnostic methods has been proven effective in diagnosing cancer.

CHARACTERISTICS OF CANCER QUACKS

The cancer patient often is unable to distinguish between the quack and the reputable, well-trained physician for a number of reasons. The promoter of the unproven method *appears* legitimate in many ways. The quack may have a well-appointed office, business cards, a receptionist, and a nurse. How, then, can the patient, the family, and health professionals determine if a practitioner is a quack? The following characteristics can serve as a useful measuring stick, and their initials spell *profits* (see Figure 21-2).

Promotion

The quack or his or her supporters often will promote the product or method at rallies, conventions, and seminars aimed at attracting the lay public. Treatment results, theories, and case reports are published in journals or popular magazines

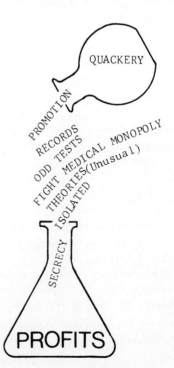

Figure 21-2 Cancer quackery means *profits for the cancer quack.*

lacking scientific standards. In these periodicals and newspapers, the testimonials and exaggerated theories are sensationalized to appeal to the searching cancer patient or person who fears that he or she has cancer. In addition, the quack may recruit entertainers, politicians, or other well-known people to "spread the word." The very prominence of such people tends to lend a sense of legitimacy to the method. Unfortunately, these advocates seldom have the knowledge or scientific background to clearly evaluate the method they become associated with. Organizations that promote and support cancer quackery include The International Association of Cancer Victims and Friends, the National Health Federation, and the Committee for Freedom of Choice in Cancer Therapy.

Records That Are Unreliable

Case histories of patients "cured" by the unproven method are characterized by lack of biopsy evidence, laboratory data, follow-up data, and other forms of scientific proof to substantiate the claims made. Testimonials written in an emotional tone are offered as examples of cure. Records tend to cover short periods of time and may include patients who have died as well as people who did not have cancer. Legitimate cancer treatment measures are in terms of months and years of remission or absence of tumor growth. Some of the case reports consist of patients who continued to use reputable effective cancer treatments while at the same time using an unproven method. When the patient's condition improves, however, the quackery did it, not the legitimate treatment. In reporting such cases, the quack fails to mention the legitimate therapy and its role in the patient's improved status.

Odd Tests and Credentials

The cancer quack often requires the patient to undergo bizarre and unusual diagnostic tests to confirm the patient's or quack's suspicions. In some cases, a genuine non-cancer-related complaint is "upgraded" to a serious malignant condition for which the practitioner has a treatment. The credentials of many quacks are nonexistent; other quacks simply put "Doctor" in front of their names. Still others have degrees such as N.D. (Doctor of Naturopathy), Ph.N. (Philosopher of Naturopathy),* D.A.B.B.-A. (Diplomate of American Board of Bio-Analysts), Ms.D. (Doctor of Metaphysics), or D.N.T., L.P.T., Ph.G., Ph.T., or T.G. (the meaning of the latter five is unknown). A certain number of quacks, however, have legitimate credentials obtained from respected institutions.

Fights against "Medical Monopoly"

Quacks and their supporters repeatedly and vociferously renounce the medical profession and government agencies as perpetrators of a conspiracy against

---

*According to the American Naturopathic Association, naturopathy is "a therapeutic system embracing a complete physianthropy employing Nature's agencies, forces, processes, and products, except major surgery." C. W. Tabor, *Tabor's Cyclopedia Medical Dictionary,* 10th ed., F. A. Davis, Philadelphia, 1965, p. N-4.

them. According to the quacks, all health professionals and care institutions who resist using unproven treatments on cancer patients are unfeeling, uncaring, and motivated solely by financial gain in treatment of patients who have cancer. The conspiracy argument insists that Big Government, is withholding unproven methods to protect the "cancer care racket."

Unfortunately, the advocates of quackery fail to state that their methods can undergo the same testing and evaluation sequence as can any other proposed treatment for cancer. Should the method be proven effective in the treatment of cancer, it would be approved and used.

Isolation

Persons using illegal treatment methods and products in the care of cancer patients are isolated from established, reputable scientific facilities and treatment institutions. At the same time, practitioners of cancer quackery refuse to seek consultation from reputable medical facilities and physicians. To do so, according to the quacks, would be to expose patients to lies and the ineffective rigors of "cutting," "burning," "poison," and "mutilation" found with legitimate cancer treatment. By using such highly charged and false terms to describe surgery, radiotherapy, and chemotherapy, quacks play on the fears patients may have about the unknown. Thus, by refusing consultation, quacks maintain an isolated position in relation to the genuine medical community.

Theories That Are Unusual

In order to create an aura of scientific validity around the unproven method, the quack may devise a new theory of cancer causation. The theory corresponds logically to the unproven method currently being pushed. As a consequence, a very neat, self-perpetuating, closed system is created. Diagrams, formulas, and discussions of the theory, using complex terminology, are presented to the cancer patient as evidence of the efficacy of the entire "package." Because cancer patients, their families, and their friends seldom question such "sophisticated evidence," it serves the quack's purpose well.

Often the quack will cite historical figures who fought to have their ideas and theories accepted as examples of the trials and tribulations the quack must continually face in the never-ending battle to bring his or her method to the patient.

Another characteristic of the theories propounded by the quack is their wide applicability. Any time a theory or corresponding treatment method is found to be applicable to a wide variety of unrelated conditions and illnesses, the patient should question what is being offered. When a juice mixture, for example, can cure anything from halitosis to cancer to acne, one should become suspicious!

Secrecy

The ingredients, active compounds, or specifics of the rituals performed by the cancer quack usually are clouded by secrecy. Many potions and "drugs" used by quacks are not made available for testing. It has been necessary to initiate legal action to obtain certain products for testing purposes.

The cancer quack, then, *can* be identified with attention to the described characteristics. Patients need to be prepared for the smooth sales pitches used by the promoters of unproven methods. Public education is crucial.

MOTIVATIONS FOR USING UNPROVEN METHODS

With all the evidence against quackery, the logical question becomes, Why would an intelligent person go to a quack? It must be remembered that patients who turn to quackery are like anyone else. Some are professionals, while others are blue- or white-collar workers. In other words, the person who goes to a quack may be no different from the nurse who gives care in terms of values, beliefs, and upbringing.

When a diagnosis of cancer has been made or when a person feels that symptoms imply such a diagnosis, the person's motivations to seek out or accept the services of a quack may include one or more of the following.

Fears of Cancer

A diagnosis of cancer arouses intense fear in most people. It often is associated with death, pain, incapacity, and deterioration. There may be a very real fear that after going through all the treatment procedures, the cancer may still be present. A fear of the unknown and with a belief in some of the myths of cancer may act as prods to the patient to seek out a quack.

These fears are all real to the patient. Cancer *is* a devastating disease for many afflicted with it; it cannot always be cured; some of the treatments used are stressful and taxing to the mind and body. Nurses must recognize this fear, attend to it, acknowledge it, and deal with it. By allowing the patient to express these fears, the nurse provides understanding and support as well as an opportunity to assist the patient in mobilizing resources.

Impatience with Progress

Cancer treatment usually is a long process. It can involve an extensive diagnostic work-up, radiation therapy, surgery, chemotherapy, or a combination of these modalities plus others. These treatments are time-consuming. As such, they may foster a sense of restlessness in the patient who expects rapid improvement or immediate cure. The cancer quack, however, offers a quick, rapidly "effective" treatment usually occurring within days. This is most appealing to the restless cancer patient who is not making rapid strides toward recovery.

Need for Control

People are accustomed to exercising varying degrees of control over their daily lives. As a patient, the person loses control over many aspects of life, from mealtime to ambulation time to sleep time. He or she usually has access to family contact during limited hours and may not be allowed to see his or her children or a beloved pet. How often are rounds made during which the patient's bed is surrounded by strangers and the "case" is discussed *over* the patient? How consistently are the patient's needs and goals taken into account in planning treatment? These aspects of control over one's life may be overlooked or ignored completely in the rush to treat cancer. The quack, in contrast, offers the patient an alternative to loss of control. The quack often discusses the treatment in an in-depth manner and makes the patient a partner in the treatment process.

By acknowledging the cancer patient's need to *be* in control of his or her life and treatment and by increasing the patient's control where possible, one can reduce the number of patients who seek out the quack for such an opportunity and consideration.

Frustration with Treatment

Some cancer patients become frustrated with impersonal care received from physicians, nurses, or care institutions. They want and need to have a meaningful relationship with the physician or nurse as they face cancer and its treatment requirements. When this need is unmet by the "busy" physician or nurse, frustration may result which spurs the patient to find someone or something to meet the need. One alternative is the quack, who allows time to listen and commiserate with the patient's problem.

Need for Hope

Some cancer patients feel as if they are "in a dark hole, looking out." When the disease fails to respond to treatment and physical deterioration occurs, the patient may begin to lose hope. Perhaps a human being's central life-sustaining force, hope becomes the cancer patient's primary need. He or she needs hope for remission, if cure is not feasible, for pain control, for maintenance of dignity, for wholeness in body and spirit, and for understanding. When this hope wanes, the patient may turn to the quack, who represents not only hope but cure—a miracle of life. Some cancer patients, upon learning of a terminal prognosis, turn to the quack as the last hope for active treatment.

This need for hope cannot be denied. It must be fostered and nurtured by the physician, nurse, and other care givers with each instance of patient contact. Unrealistic hope should, of course, be avoided. When quantity of life cannot be provided, *quality* of life can be assured by sensitive, caring health professionals.

Lack of Information about Methods

Many cancer patients are simply uninformed when it comes to cancer treatment methods. A well-advertised and promoted unproven method may sound as legitimate as reputable treatment approaches. The patient may feel somewhat insecure because of lack of understanding of the complexities of cancer treatment. Health professionals who fail to simplify explanations and who convey a condescending attitude toward the patient when questions are asked reinforce the patient's feelings of insecurity and may stimulate anger and resentment.

Although some health professionals do provide clear and straightforward explanations of cancer and its treatment, others do not. If patients are to be partners in the treatment and care process, they need to be informed of what the expectations are and what treatment consists of. It is absolutely necessary to plan for time during which the patient unhurriedly is encouraged to formulate questions and receive information.

Suspicion of Care System

Some cancer patients have had unsatisfactory past experiences with the health care system. As a result of these experiences, they have suspicions about the care to be received as a cancer patient. The quack may be an appealing alternative. In addition, the quack may also acquire the appeal of the "underdog": the person being persecuted by the medical establishment.

Patients who circumvent the care system because of past unsatisfactory experiences are difficult to identify until they are encountered after the quackery has failed them. At this time, the patient needs understanding and unbiased explanations of what treatment will consist of. The underdog image of the quack needs to be dispelled and correct information provided in a supportive manner.

NURSING IMPLICATIONS OF CANCER QUACKERY

Provide Information

In order to prevent cancer patients from being victimized by cancer quackery, nurses must know what forms unproven methods take. In part, that has been the purpose of this chapter. With a solid grasp of this information, the nurse will be able to explain to the patient the dangers inherent in delaying and abandoning legitimate treatment in favor of quackery. At the same time, the nurse can present the facts about the method to the patient. As this information is imparted, it is essential that the nurse attend to the nonverbal cues presented by the patient. The nurse needs to focus on the emotional messages conveyed by the patient, the amount of hope that is invested in the unproven method, and the impact it may have on the patient. In the end, however, information alone may not be enough to dissuade the patient who is searching for a miracle. This fact is often difficult to come to terms with. Obviously, there are no quick and easy answers to this dilemma.

Communicate Findings

When one learns that some of the cancer patients one cares for have been approached by promoters of cancer quackery, it is important that one gather as many of the details surrounding the method and the person offering it as possible. This information should then be communicated to such agencies as the local medical association, American Cancer Society, health department, and/or consumer protection office. These agencies often are interested in collecting detailed information on the prevalence of unproven methods in a community as one step in planning legislative efforts and designing public education programs.

Be Nonjudgmental

Cancer patients who have used unproven methods in an unsuccessful attempt to cure the disease often are admitted to a hospital in the latter stages of the illness. They have bypassed the critical interval and may have paid the ultimate price. These patients frequently have feelings of guilt, shame, and loss. When it becomes clear that they have made an error in judgment, feelings of shame are aroused. Their losses are numerous: time, money, health, and possibly life itself. For these patients, the nurse must make every effort to allow the patient to ventilate his or her feelings, especially the frustration and self-blame that can occur. Effort should be made to assist the patient in resolving feelings and at the same time foster attention to the present care the person will receive. Dwelling on the past will not help the patient or the family. Ignoring what has happened is equally inappropriate. A caring, nonjudgmental attitude by the nurse can help the patient and the family regain a sense of hope.

Educate Others

Health care providers from all educational levels need to know what cancer quackery is, who the quacks are, and why patients would seek out such services. In order for this information to be conveyed, in-service and community education programs need to be carried out. The nurse can be instrumental in recognizing the need for this education and in stimulating the development of programs for his or her place of employment or in the community has a whole.

By correcting misconceptions about cancer and providing factual information on the what, who and why of cancer quackery, care givers will be in a better position to prevent its spread and harm to patients.

Support Legislation

Although cancer quackery is regulated at the federal level of government, only 10 states have enacted anticancer laws to control intrastate sale, distribution, and use of unproven methods. These states are California, Colorado, Hawaii, Illinois, Kentucky, Maryland, Nevada, North Dakota, Ohio, and Pennsylvania. Getting such a law passed in the state legislature requires a commitment, a commitment to work hard, and, often for a long time to see that legislation is enacted. Nurses, as primary care providers for cancer patients, can be instrumental in stimulating community interest in controlling cancer quackery. Within the professional association they can form subcommittees devoted to fostering legislation. They can lobby for proposed antiquackery legislation. Nurses can play a tremendous role in securing protection for cancer patients and their families. In this patient advocate role, the nurse truly can have a positive impact on the care received by the cancer patient.

Be There

What does the quack provide the patient that makes him or her so appealing? He provides caring, compassion, dignity, understanding, and time to really be with the patient in a time of great fear. By providing these very services, the nurse can reduce the quack's appeal. *Being there* requires a commitment to stay with the patient when the going gets rough; when he or she expresses fear, anger, resentment, or depression. It means listening actively with full attention to what the patient is saying verbally and nonverbally. It also means knowing personal limitations and making referrals when the feelings expressed are overwhelming to the nurse. Work and time pressures need not necessarily interfere with such interaction. *Quality* of time spent with a patient is infinitely more valuable than quantity alone.

SUMMARY COMMENT

Cancer quackery is devastating. It victimizes cancer patients at a highly vulnerable period in their lives. Nurses can reduce the impact of cancer quackery by becoming committed to decreasing its easy availability. When supporters of unproven methods contact patients or family members, the nurse can discuss the method with the family and patient. If they feel free to talk with the nurse, physician, or other care giver about what they have found, a giant step will have been taken in reducing the attractiveness of quackery.

At bottom, however, nurses must realize that only when the cancer patient's needs are fully met by the legitimate health care system will he or she no longer *need* the cancer quack. Each time the patient's psychological, emotional, and intellectual needs are identified and met, the influence of cancer quackery weakens.

BIBLIOGRAPHY

American Cancer Society Index of Pertinent File Material on Unproven Methods of Cancer Management, 1975, American Cancer Society, New York, 1975.

Brody, Jane E. "Four Cancer Centers Find No Proof of Therapy Value in Illegal Drug," *New York Times,* July 21, 1975.

Brown, Helene. "Cancer Quackery: What Can You Do about It?" *Nursing 75,* **5:**24–26, May 1975.

Brown, Mrs. Robert L. "Do-It-Yourself Guide: Diagnosis, Treatment, and Cure of Cancer or Ducks Aren't the Only Ones that Quack!!!" *Proceedings of the American Cancer Society's National Conference on Human Values and Cancer,* American Cancer Society, New York, 1973.

Burkhalter, Pamela K. "Cancer Quackery," *American Journal of Nursing,* 451–453, March 1977.

"Cancer Victims Go 'Underground' to Mexico," *Medical World News,* 34–43, December 1, 1967.

Committee on Unorthodox Cancer Therapies. "Report of the Committee on Unorthodox Therapies for Cancer, May 1975," American Society of Clinical Oncology, Inc., New Smyrna Beach, Fla., 1975.

"Court Bars Shipment of Laetrile," *FDA Consumer,* News Highlights, May 1975.

"Crackdown on Quackery," *Life,* **55:**72B–83, November 1, 1963.

Culliton, Barbara J. "Sloan-Kettering: The Trials on an Apricot Pit—1973," *Arizona Medicine,* **32:**724–726, September 1975.

Duffy, Paul H. "Cancer Quackery," *Arizona Medicine,* **32:**724–726, September 1975.

"Extra-Dispensary Perceptions," *Time,* 86–87, March 17, 1975.

Eyerly, Robert C. "Laetrile: Focus on the Facts," *American Cancer Society,* New York, 1975, pp. 1–5.

Facts on Quacks: What you should know about health quackery, American Medical Association, New York, 1971.

Feldmann, Edward G. "Harmless, But Ineffective Remedies," *Journal of Pharmaecutical Sciences,* **64:**10, October 1975.

Fishbein, Morris. "History of Cancer Quackery," *Perspectives in Biology and Medicine,* **8:**139–166, 1965.

Goldman, Robert P. "The Fantastic Krebiozen Story," *Saturday Evening Post,* 15–19, January 4, 1964.

Health Quackery: Cancer, American Medical Association, New York, 1970.

Hodges, Frederick B. "The Laetrile Hoax," *California Medicine,* **118:**78, June 1975.

Holland, James F. "The Krebiozen Story," *JAMA,* **200:**125–130, April 17, 1967.

Isler, Charlotte. "The Fatal Choice: Cancer Quackery," *RN,* **37:**55–59, September 1974.

"Laetrile," *FDA Consumer Memo,* November 1974.

Loyd, F. Glen and Irwin, Theodore. "How Quackery Thrives on the Occult," *Today's Health, 21*–23, 87–88, November 1970.

Morris, Neil. "Potential for Tragedy in Public Overplay of Cancer 'Cures,'" *CMA Journal,* **113:**465, 470, September 6, 1975.

Nolan, William A. "A Doctor in Search of a Miracle," "*Honolulu Star-Bulletin, five-part series, August 4*–8, 1975.

Ward, Donovan F. "The Four Horsemen of Quackery: Fear, Gullibility, Deceit, and Deadlines," *Today's Health,* **10:**76–77, January 1965.

"Why Go to a Quack?" *Time,* **64:**40, August 16, 1954.

Young, Mort: "Laetrile," *San Francisco Examiner,* five-part series, November 10–14, 1975.

References Advocating Unproven Cancer Treatment Methods

Airola, Paavo. *Cancer Causes, Prevention and Treatment: The Total Approach,* Health Plus, Publishers: Phoenix, 1972.

DeVries, Arnold. *Therapeutic Fasting,* Chandler, Los Angeles, 1963.

Haught, S. J. *Has Dr. Max Gerson a True Cancer Cure?,* London Press, North Hollywood, 1962.

Kelley, William D.: *New Hope for Cancer Victims,* The Kelley Research Foundation, Grapevine, 1974.

Kirschner, H. E. *Live Food Juices,* H. E. Kirschner Publications, Monrovia, Calif., 1972.

Kittler, Glenn D. *Laetrile: Control for Cancer,* Warner Books, New York, 1963.

Nolfi, Kirstine: *The Raw Food Treatment of Cancer and Other Diseases,* The Vegetarian Society, Manchester, England, 1973.

Chapter 22

Community Resources for the Cancer Patient

Melvin S. Y. Whang

Who provides services for the patient with cancer? How can one find out what is available in one's life setting? To whom may one turn for assistance? What are the economics of the disease? These are questions that the patient and family are confronted with when the initial diagnosis of cancer has been made and the treatment is being planned.

The extent to which the patient and family will require sources of assistance additional to those provided in treatment is dependent on the nature and extent of the cancer and the type of care required, whether in the hospital, in the home, or both. The patient may be entirely incapacitated, requiring hospital or skilled nursing care; partially incapacitated, maintaining some function, and living at home; needing little assistance, life essentially changed very little, and able to work; or requiring no additional help.

Cancer is catastrophic in both its emotional and its financial impact. It is the chief killer of children, a major cause of death in the aged, and a less frequent but devastating illness in younger and middle-aged adults. The following example illustrates the disaster a family may face when cancer strikes:

Mrs. R. W., a 32-year old housewife, was treated for cancer over a period of several years. She had undergone a kidney transplant that was rejected. After hospitalization and treatment in an East Coast hospital, she spent 9 months at a prestigious

Midwest clinic and 6 months in a medical school hospital in Chicago where she died of cancer. The local unit of the American Cancer Society was contacted by the husband regarding financial assistance for the costs incurred by his wife's illness, which amounted to $25,000. Unable to meet this financial burden, he sought legal advice and was given two alternatives: one, file for bankruptcy, or two, have his debtors garnishee his wages as an employee of the state of Illinois.

In 1974, approximately $104.2 billion was the estimate of our national health bill, an increase of 10.6 percent over 1973. An estimated $3 billion was spent on medical treatment and other nonpersonal services for cancer in 1972. The enormous cost is mainly attributed to hospitalization. In 1962 cost for direct patient care per day was $36, as compared with $92+ today. If indirect costs (loss of income, etc.) were included our national bill would be an estimated $15 billion for cancer alone.[1]

In 1977 an estimated 10 million persons will be under medical care for cancer. Cancer affects two out of three American families, and in this decade alone, approximately 6.5 million new cases of cancer and 3.5 million cancer-caused deaths will occur. As estimated by the National Center for Health Statistics, 1,457,527 deaths from cancer occurred from 1973 to 1976, and an additional 385,000 cancer patients, or 1055 per day, will die in 1977. For every six deaths in the United States, one will be due to cancer.[2]

The enormous size of the figures indicates the magnitude of the task of providing the variety of resources, financial and otherwise, which the cancer patient and family may require. In thinking of the resources available to the cancer patient and family, one considers first the private physician, the local hospital and its clinics, and the nurse. By knowing where and how to obtain these services, it is possible for one to maintain the care and rehabilitation of the patient. If health care is needed, it is the individual's and/or the family's primary responsibility to decide that the individual needs a physician, and it is the physician's responsibility to decide that the individual needs hospitalization.

Resources may be in any form from temporary financial assistance to spiritual assistance. When possible, the patient pays for any services rendered. If this is not the case, he or she can be helped by the American Cancer Society, public assistance payments, the church, etc., each alone or in combination.

COMMUNITY RESOURCES FOR CANCER

The types of resources available for the cancer patient and family will vary according to local customs; community size; existence of voluntary health agencies; effectiveness of the local health department; and its relationship to county, state, and federal agencies. Most states have placed the responsibility for aiding cancer patients and families, on the local community. It is usually through the local community that the individual makes person-to-person contact with the public health nurse, the minister, the medical social worker, and other members of the health care team. Resources are most effective when they are established in the community itself. Ideally, elements of the community participate in a coordinated, comprehensive, and economical plan to care for the cancer patient.

Health professionals need to know exactly who can provide transportation, home care, and financial assistance services. Combined efforts can and should, if at all possible, be jointly administered and financed by the patient, family, voluntary agency, etc. Such joint utilization of resources, especially in smaller communities, will provide more and better services for each dollar spent. Needs often exceed available resources, and it is vital that duplication be avoided.

The following are various resources provided by tax-supported or private institutions and fee-for-service or nonprofit organizations. They may not offer services and programs specifically tailored to the cancer patient or his or her family. However, if a combination of agencies working together can meet the needs of the cancer patient, joint services can be made available after eligibility is determined. Rules, regulations, policies, and guidelines may vary from state to state, and one should check them to ascertain the availability of specific services and the eligibility requirements for recipients of the services.

Public Health Nursing

The public health nursing branch of the state department of health provides public health nursing services, including home and office visits, for health counseling, health education, supportive guidance and procedures, referral services when necessary, and nursing care of the sick in the home setting by means of demonstration of care and/or supervision of care given by the family.

Services are available at no charge and are based on health needs. Home care is provided on a temporary basis that is contingent upon the particular type of care required. Depending on the state or county, services may include skilled nursing care.

Vocational Rehabilitation Division, State Health Department

The division of vocational rehabilitation can provide vocational and rehabilitation services in the areas of medical, psychological, social, and vocational evaluation. In addition, the division can provide the following services: counseling and guidance, physical and psychological restoration (including medical care), hospitalization, surgery and artificial appliances, vocational training, maintenance and transportation, tools, equipment, supplies for employment and establishment of small businesses, and job placement and follow-up.

The vocational rehabilitation division does not have programs and/or services outlined specifically for cancer patients. Should the patient meet the intake policy and eligibility requirements, assistance can be offered. The patient must be physically or mentally disabled to qualify.

American Mental Health Association (AMHA) Mental Health Division, Department of Health

The AMHA, a voluntary health agency, has the primary function of educating both the medical and the lay community while providing information and referral services. The mental health division of the state department of health offers clinical consultation for assessment of emotional and mental disorders, inpatient and outpatient psychiatric treatment, and rehabilitation of ex-hospital patients.

Mental health facilities are utilized as a resource for the cancer patient only if other counseling and guidance services are not available within a given community. These agencies do not have programs and/or services geared specifically to the needs of cancer patients. Anyone in need of psychiatric diagnostic, treatment, and consultation service is eligible, provided the patient and/or family income does not allow for private care.

Government Financial and Medical Assistance: Public Welfare Division

Financial assistance is available from state public welfare departments to help meet temporary or long-term requirements, including medical care payments. Disability and unemployment benefits vary according to local regulations, as do child support and assistance to the blind. The Food Stamp Program for welfare and nonwelfare families helps them increase their food-purchasing power. The means of administering the Food Stamp Program, however, do vary in different states. Eligibil ty for financial assistance, medical care, payments and Food Stamps is determined by the family's income and resources in relation to need, in accordance with standards established both by the federal and local governments.

At present, information about the wide variety of local governmental services available is best obtained directly from the staff of the public agencies represented in the community, from hospital social work personnel, or from the American Cancer Society, as will be described. Discussed below are some of the most important government programs whose administration is generally not subject to local governmental regulation and whose provisions cover a very large number of patients with cancer.

U.S. Veterans Administration

Veterans, their dependents, and their beneficiaries are eligible to receive medical and dental services, hospitalization and ancillary medical services including outpatient visits, rehabilitation, and education and counseling services. Disability compensation and pension, death compensation and pension, and dependency and indemnity compensation are available, as is reimbursement for transportation, funeral, and burial expenses for deceased veterans. Mentioned are only those sources that might pertain to the cancer patient and family.

Medicare/Medicaid

Anyone age 65 or older and anyone under 65 who is disabled qualify for Medicare, which is financed by the federal government under the Social Security Administration and has two parts. Part A of the Social Security Act provides hospital insurance, which includes inpatient hospital care and services of an extended care/skilled nursing facility or care in the patient's own private home by a home health agency.

Part B provides for medical insurance at a cost of $7.20 per month (July 1976) and is optional. It pays for doctor's bills, outpatient hospital services, medical supplies and services, and home health services. Prosthetic devices and durable medical equipment are also covered. If a person has been disabled for at least 2 years, he or she is eligible for Supplemental Security Income in addition to Medicare.

Medicaid is supported jointly by the federal and state governments, and anyone qualifying for welfare or old age assistance is eligible. Medicaid covers doctor's and some hospital services including extended care/skilled nursing facilities, depending on the state and the policies of the department of social services that administers the program.[3]

Health Planning and Resources Development Act of 1974

The national Health Planning and Resources Development Act is a 3-year program that was authorized by President Ford on January 4, 1975. It involves a $1 billion program of health planning and resources development. Its enactment adds two new titles to the public Health Services Act. The first (Title XV) is to establish new programs for health planning and resources development, and the second (Title XVI) replaces the Hill-Burton program, revising the construction and modernization of the health care facilities programs and allocating additional funds for the development of health resources. Among the 10 guidelines for health resources proposed by the National Council of Health, Education and Welfare, the following appear to be of direct value as community resources for cancer patients:

1 To train and increase the use of physician assistants, particularly nurse clinicians
2 To develop a multi-institutional relationship enabling support services to be shared
3 To promote specific programs for improving the quality of health care services
4 To promote specific methods for the prevention of diseases, including nutritional and environmental factors relevant to health and health care prevention services
5 To develop public education programs promoting improvement in personal health care and better use of health services[4]

Among the guidelines for planning methods and technology is the establishment of a national center for all health planning information. The center will collate and provide information regarding all existing health services and resources, planning of new resources development, and methods of application and procedure.

There are other sources to assist the cancer patient. The Visiting Nurse Association can provide services in the home on the request of the attending physician. These services may include part-time nursing and physical therapy, injections and other prescribed treatment, and education of both patient and family in self-care and rehabilitation. The association is nonprofit, and fees are minimal; adjustments can be made for either partial payment or no fee for those who cannot afford to pay. In many communities, the public health nurse may function as the Visiting Nurse.

Convalescent homes are available for the patient who is not quite ready to assume his or her normal life-style but needs little or no nursing care. Skilled nursing facilities or long-term custodial care may include both bed and ambulatory patients.

TREATMENT

Cancer, with its variety of primary and metastatic sites, makes up a bewildering array of different diseases, each treated by specific techniques that were developed for the particular type of cancer and which may include a combination of the various modalities of therapy. Since the establishment of the first radium institutes, when the cost of radium was beyond the reach of individual institutions, many facilities treating cancer have become available for treating cancer. In many states throughout the nation, varying institutions are equipped to treat specific types of cancers. There are 15 federally supported comprehensive cancer centers that are equipped and able to treat an array of cancers, utilizing up-to-date equipment, procedures, and techniques.

Some of these specialized or comprehensive institutions offer their services at no cost or at low cost. Some are nonprofit institutions supported by the public through donations, while others are supported by public and/or government funds. Examples of these institutions would be the Memorial Hospital for Cancer and Allied Diseases in New York and the M. D. Anderson Institute and Hospital in Houston.

There are county or state hospitals for the medically indigent as well as private cancer clinics and hospitals that operate on a partial payment basis. Service organizations such as the Lions Club, the Shriners, and community Parent-Teacher Associations often underwrite costs of medical supplies for special groups, such as children, the aged, or the blind.

AMERICAN CANCER SOCIETY, INC.

The American Cancer Society is a nonprofit, voluntary organization of several million volunteers fighting cancer through a threefold program of research, education, and patient service and rehabilitation. Its national headquarters is located in New York City, and there are 58 chartered divisions and 2792 local units throughout the United States and its territories—American Samoa, Guam, and Puerto Rico.[5]

It is at the local level that the personnel and resources of the American Cancer Society are rendered to the community through various programs and services that help meet the needs of the particular locale. The society's service program includes rehabilitation services through organized rehabilitation teams; information and counseling services; loan closet equipment, such as wheelchairs, blenders, and hospital beds; dressings and other gift items for the patient during convalescence; and transportation to and from medical facilities for treatment.

The resources available from the American Cancer Society will vary according to local policies and may include homemaker services, such as patient sitting and patient visiting; home health care services; rehabilitation services; social work assistance; help with employment problems; help with medications; and blood donor programs. An example of the rehabilitation services offered by the society is presented in Figure 22-1.

The objective of the rehabilitation programs is to assist new laryngectomy, mastectomy, and ostomy patients. These rehabilitation programs offer the patient psychological and physiological assistance and seek to improve the quality of life of the survivors. The American Cancer Society has trained and utilized thousands of volunteers who have successfully adjusted to their own encounters with cancer and who are willing and eager to help others.

The program is a team effort of the society and the medical community, as it relieves the latter from spending valuable time in an activity that is not medically oriented but nonetheless is a very important aspect of the maintenance and care of the cancer patient. Whether the head of a household, single, married, child, or parent, the patient or potential patient is a functioning human being who hopes to remain in a functioning condition as long as possible at a minimum cost to all concerned—the individual, the family, and the society. The overall objective is to increase the individual's length of life and to help the person be as active as possible.

American Cancer Society Community Resources

An increasingly vital aspect of the ACS professional education program is formation of nursing education committees. By incorporating volunteer nurses from the various areas of nursing, e.g., staff nurse, public health nurse, clinic or office nurse, nursing home personnel, L.P.N., etc., these committees can generate ideas for nursing education programs and develop and implement them. If a community does not have an active and working nursing education committee and would like to see one established, the local unit of the American Cancer Society can be contacted. If there is one interested nurse, he or she can instigate such an action.

A wide range of rehabilitation facilities, both public and private, are available to the cancer patient: the health department vocational rehabilitation divisions, the American Cancer Society, the Veterans Administration, etc., have established programs in rehabilitation. With funds from the federal government, pilot projects in rehabilitation have been developed throughout these special and comprehensive centers, one of which is described in Chapter 10 of this text.

Laryngectomy Rehabilitation Program (International Association of Laryngectomies)

The International Association of Laryngectomies (IAL) has been sponsored nationally by the American Cancer Society since 1952. On the local level most of the IAL clubs are sponsored by the local units of the Cancer Society. The

Discovering that you or a loved one has cancer can be a frightening experience. Call someone who understands!

We are here to help you and your family. Many of us have been through the same experiences and can share your concerns and refer you to people and services in the community who can best help you. Some of the services listed here are available to all cancer patients. Contact your local unit office of the American Cancer Society's Hawaii Division.

SOME THINGS WE DO TO HELP CANCER PATIENTS

COUNSELING The American Cancer Society provides experienced counseling for cancer patients and their families.

REFERRALS The Society knows the available community resources and works closely with existing local health and welfare agencies. If a patient has a special need, the society knows where assistance can be obtained.

TRANSPOR-TATION In cases of need, transportation to treatment centers and clinics will be provided to the patient by volunteer drivers. Provision for service by taxi or bus may be provided to the medically indigent patient if volunteer service is not available. Transportation may be provided from neighbor islands to Honolulu for special diagnostic tests and treatment if such service is not available on that island.

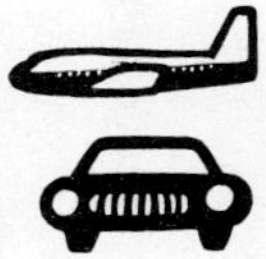

LOAN AND GIFT SERVICES Loan items range from small appliances such as blenders to larger equipment, including wheelchairs, beds and bedside tables. Gift and comfort items cover a wide variety of articles depending upon the patient's needs.

SURGICAL DRESSINGS Various sizes of surgical dressings and tapes are available.

HOMEMAKER SERVICES Assistance can be given in arranging for homemaker services for patients in need.

HOUSING With special permission of the physician and the American Cancer Society Unit in whose area the patient resides, arrangements for temporary housing may be made when required.

REHABILITATION SERVICES PROVIDED

The increasing demand for rehabilitation services reflects the growing rate of survival of cancer patients, brought about by earlier diagnosis and improved treatment. These services are provided by cancer patients who themselves have recovered from similar surgery and are willing to visit and counsel others.

LARYNGECTOMY Most patients who have had their voice boxes (Larynxes) removed learn to speak again using esophageal speech or a mechanical aid called an electrolarynx. Laryngectomees and their families receive information and counseling. Gift items (shower guards, bibs, etc.) are available. Also, rehabilitated Laryngectomees are available to visit patients in the hospital before and after surgery upon request of the physician.

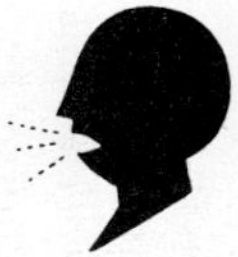

On Oahu, Laryngectomees have formed a Lost Chord Club for the purpose of receiving encouragement and giving understanding and assistance to new Laryngectomees and their families during the adjustment period following surgery.

MASTECTOMY The Reach to Recovery Program is a rehabilitation program for women who have had breast surgery. It is designed to help them meet their physical, psychological and cosmetic needs. With the aid of a volunteer visitor (a woman who has had a mastectomy) the patient can see first hand that she too will be able to successfully adjust to her surgery. The volunteer will provide her with a kit containing temporary prosthesis and exercise instructions.

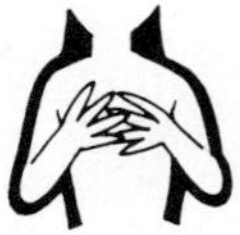

OSTOMY The American Cancer Society has rehabilitative programs for the ostomate, one whose diseased or injured intestine has been removed and there is an opening in the abdominal wall. Ostomates who have successfully adjusted to this surgery have been trained and are available to visit patients upon the physician's request.

Figure 22-1   Some services provided by the American Cancer Society. *(Courtesy American Cancer Society, Hawaii Division, Inc.)*

purpose of the IAL is to promote and assist in the rehabilitation of the laryngectomy patient. The group sponsors training in esophageal speech and assists the
patient to return to his or her former employment or to obtain training and
employment in a new area suited to the individual.

Mastectomy Rehabilitation Program (Reach to Recovery)

The Reach to Recovery program (R-R) of the American Cancer Society was
established to assist women who have undergone breast cancer surgery. The
program is designed to help with physical, psychological, and cosmetic needs.
The program involves a corps of qualified and trained mastectomy volunteers
who visit the pre- or postoperative patient. The volunteer visitor is able to
support the patient and to give visible evidence that she can recover and adjust to
breast surgery. Helpful hints, care, and exercises are taught the new mastectomy
patient.

Ostomy Rehabilitation Program (United Ostomy Association)

The American Cancer Society's Ostomy Rehabilitation Program includes all
ostomy patients, including colostomy, ileostomy, and urinary bypass patients,
whose psychological and physiological needs are similar. Like the mastectomy
program, the "ostomees" have a corps of qualified and trained volunteers who
have undergone and adjusted to similar surgery. They visit and assist new ostomy patients. Some of the local units work hand in hand with the United
Ostomy Association, and assistance can be sought from either group depending
on the local situation.[6]

Patient Transportation

The American Cancer Society has also established guidelines to assist a community in need of a patient transportation corps. Should this resource be needed
in an area, write or call the nearest local office of the American Cancer Society
and a staff member and/or volunteer will be able to assist in setting up such a
system.

   With advanced technology, life expectancy has increased over the decade.
The increased knowledge obtained through research, the development of better
techniques in the treatment of the disease, and the demand for rehabilitative
services are all reflected in the increasingly better survival rates of those diagnosed as having cancer. Should any community need one or all of the above
mentioned services, contact the local ACS and/or those affiliated agencies.

Nursing Education Committee

As was mentioned earlier, a working cancer nursing education committee can be
an asset to the nursing and health care community. Members of such a committee are in a position to generate and develop ideas for nursing programs that seek
to inform and assist nurses in the care, treatment, and rehabilitation of the cancer
patient. The committee should be composed of at least 5 members representing

the various disciplines in nursing. Meetings can be scheduled according to the current needs and trends of the community, but it is suggested that at least three meetings be scheduled per year.

Ancillary Resources

The clergy have always played a major role in the support and comfort of the cancer patient and have been increasingly recognized as part of the health care team. They are able to give added assistance to the patient who has been treated for cancer, ensuring that he or she receives comprehensive rehabilitative care.

More recently, the concept of "self-help" groups comprised of persons with advanced cancers and their families has been developed. Since these individuals are experiencing similar problems, the group meeting provides an opportunity to air feelings and maintain an atmosphere of hope. This approach has also proved very effective for the families of children with cancer. The ACS, the Leukemia Society, and in some communities the Candlelighters can identify these groups.

BLOOD PROGRAMS

American Cancer Society

The American Cancer Society is encouraging its divisions throughout the nation to develop volunteer blood donor programs (VBDP). A national work-study group has been organized, and a meeting was held in May of 1976. As a result of the meeting, two major problems were identified as follows:

1   The increased need for blood components as a result of chemotherapy and radiation therapy treatments
2   The lack of public awareness of the blood needs of the cancer patient

The purpose of the VBDP is to recruit and maintain a list of qualified volunteer blood donors who can be called upon to ensure the availability of blood supply to meet the ever increasing needs of the cancer patient at minimal cost to the patient. Fees for a unit of blood fall into three categories:

1   Cost of the blood
2   Cost to process the blood
3   Cost of cross matching the blood

With such a volunteer program, there would be no cost for the blood, and most insurance plans cover the cost of processing. One ACS division is presently working on a "Blood Reserve Account" with its local Blood Bank. One blood donation would be equivalent to one ACS blood credit and would cover the cost of the blood replacement fee. With two additional blood credits, the processing fee would be covered.

American Red Cross

The blood program of the American Red Cross helps to supply the nation with over 5 million units of blood and blood components annually. Blood is obtained strictly on a voluntary basis. The cost to the patient in need of such treatment is not for the blood itself but for the process required to recruit the necessary donors, to collect and process the blood, and to distribute it. Most health insurance policies cover blood-processing fees.

The program is community-oriented. Should a family require a large quantity of blood, as in the case of leukemia patients, what is necessary can be obtained without a replacement charge if relatives and friends in the community volunteer as blood donors, thereby assuring the constant supply of blood to the community.[7]

Nationwide Blood Services and Facilities

Blood services throughout the United States fall into two major categories: blood banking and the pharmaceutical industry. The present discussion is confined to the blood banking sector. Table 22-1 illustrates the number and types of blood banks and transfusion services available:

Table 22-1   Blood Banks and Transfusion Services

Type	Number	Percentage
Dependent hospitals	4158	84
Collecting hospitals	687	14
Collecting and supplying hospitals	118	2
Total nonmilitary hospitals	4963	100
Military hospitals	161	3
Community blood banks	154	3
Commercial blood banks	63	1
Red Cross regional blood centers	59	1
Total blood banks and transfusion services	5400	

The majority of blood banks and transfusion services are operated on a voluntary, nonprofit basis, as illustrated in Table 22-2.

HOSPICE

New to the United States is the concept of the "hospice," which is a nonprofit corporation supported through funds received from various foundations. One has been established in New Haven, Connecticut, modeled after the original hospice in England. Services are offered to terminally ill patients. The hospice complements the efforts of the medical and health care team within the area. Its

**Table 22-2 Transfusion Service
Support Systems**

Agency	Total	Percentage
Voluntary	2786	52
Government	1892	35
Proprietary	663	12
American Red Cross	59	1
Total	5400	100

Source: Summary Report: NHLI's Blood Resources Studies,
DHEW Pub. No. (NIH) 73-416, Washington, D.C., Government
Printing Office, 1972, pp. 16 and 18.

purpose is to care for persons suffering with chronic degenerative disease and to
help them live out their remaining lives with dignity. Services are offered to those
patients who by physician estimate have less than 3 months to live.

Comprehensive care and support, including medical, nursing, social,
psychological, and spiritual care, is given to the patient. The facility itself is a
"homelike" and natural setting unlike most hospitals. The atmosphere is designed to promote a community feeling, with the patients and their families
interacting with staff and volunteers. The objective here is to prevent isolation.
Those patients confined to bed are able to be moved about so that they may
continue to participate in the functions of the hospice. The facility is so designed
that the presence of staff is sensed at all times. Symptoms that must be managed
by medical care are given priority; they include physical pain, anorexia, mood
and alertness, nausea and vomiting, and respiratory distress. The overall purpose of the hospice is to foster well-being among patients and their families and to
help the patient live as natural and comfortable a life as possible until death.[8]

FAMILY SERVICE ASSOCIATION OF AMERICA

The Family Service Association of America is a counseling agency whose
primary objective is to strengthen family life and to assist families and individuals
to cope with and overcome their problems. For the cancer patient and/or his or
her family, counseling services would concern themselves with problems resulting from physical and psychological illnesses.

The agency's services are available to anyone. It does not provide financial
assistance, but for those who are able to pay for services rendered, the agency
has a sliding fee scale based on annual income and family size. Regardless of the
economic position of the family or individual, services are not withheld because
of lack of funds. Persons seeking help should call their local Family Service
Association for an appointment and if on public assistance, can use this for
payment. Referrals from other agencies or interested individuals can be similarly
handled. In cases of emergency, applicants can be interviewed without previous
appointments.

FRIENDS IN SEARCH OF HELP (FISH)

The Friends in Search of Help (FISH) is a nonprofit good-neighbor program of volunteers to help anyone who needs help of any kind. FISH is an international organization. Each community group decides what services to offer. Some of the types of services offered in one community include the following:

- Transportation in emergencies, for shut-ins, for the handicapped, and for others
- Babysitting if the need is unexpected
- Housework for the suddenly ill
- Needs caused by tragedies or disasters
- Provision or preparation of meals
- Reading to the blind and being a companion to the elderly
- Referrals to community agencies for more specialized professional help when needed[9]

Local churches and religious groups; fraternal, social, and patriotic organizations; and the Salvation Army are all able to provide the cancer patient and the family with volunteer and financial assistance for homemaker service, counseling, and medical and surgical clinics in cooperation with other agencies. Home health services provided by other members of the health care team are increasingly being made available and include the help of physical, occupational, and inhalation therapists. Some of these therapists are in private practice, but the majority are employed by local hospitals and clinics.

INFORMATION AND REFERRAL SERVICE ASSOCIATION

The Information and Referral Service Association provides immediate telephone response to help persons experiencing crisis. Referral is made to agencies for those persons with emergency health and/or related social problems. The service is also an up-to-date source of information about health, social welfare, and related agencies and supplies this information to individuals or agency workers upon request.

Other sources of counseling and referral service include the family clergyperson (see Chapter 15, ''Spiritual Ministries with Cancer Patients''). In some larger metropolitan areas, there is a welfare information service that publishes directories and employs social workers to answer questions and direct people to appropriate resources.

EASTER SEAL ASSOCIATION OF AMERICA

Unlike most private or public agencies, which offer their services to specific groups, the Easter Seal Association will assist any crippled or handicapped person needing rehabilitation. The association offers direct services in physical, speech, and occupational therapy; education; recreation; and audiological services. It also assists, within budget limitation, with special orthopedic appliances and transportation.

For death and burial assistance, government departments of social service or welfare have programs that vary from state to state. For those qualified, the Veterans Administration and Social Security Administration will provide help for funerals and burial. In most large cities, funeral and memorial societies now exist which will be able to work out an economical plan to assist a family facing the crisis of death.

SUMMARY

This chapter has attempted to present an overview of the many potential sources of support that can be called upon to meet the multitude of needs of the cancer patient and family. No two communities are alike, and, as such, each agency or department that is able to render some form of service to the patient will undoubtedly vary according to local policies and funds available.

With the assistance and interest of the federal government, there soon may be an established center of resource information. Until that becomes a reality, however, it is necessary for health professionals who are concerned for the cancer patient—for the quality of care and follow-up rehabilitative procedures—to know what resources are available in each community. By working in cooperation with local agencies, organizations, and departments, it will be possible to ensure the ultimate assistance and care of the cancer patient and family in understanding and coping with the disease. In this way, the patient and family may be helped with the sometimes disastrous financial and emotional burdens of the disease while the patient is restored to as near a normal and productive life as possible.

REFERENCES

1 Thomas H. Ainsworth, Jr.: "The Cost of Cancer," *Proceedings of the American Cancer Society's National Conference on Human Values and Cancer*. (New York: American Cancer Society, 1973), p. 74.
2 *Cancer Facts and Figures*. (New York: American Cancer Society, 1977), pp. 3–4, 29.
3 *Medicare Handbook*. (Washington: U.S. Government Printing Office, DHEW Pub. No. [SSA] 74-10050, 1974), p. 40.
4 Health Planning and Resources Development Act of 1974. (Washington: U.S. Government Printing Office, DHEW Pub. No. [HRA] 75-14015, 1975), pp. 1, 16, 18.
5 *Administration and Information Manual*. (New York: American Cancer Society, 1972), pp. 1, 2.
6 Ibid.
7 Donald R. Avoy: *Blood: The River of Life*. (American Red Cross, 1976), pp. 67–68.
8 Edward F. Dobihal, Jr.: "Hospice: Caring for Life," *Hospital Cancer Coordinator Newsletter*, **IX** (1974), pp. 1–2.
9 *FISH Organization* (FISH of Honolulu, 1976).

BIBLIOGRAPHY

Administration and Information Manual. New York: American Cancer Society, 1972.

Ainsworth, Thomas H., Jr.: "The Cost of Cancer," *Proceedings of the American Cancer Society's National Conference on Human Values and Cancer*. (New York: American Cancer Society, 1973.)

Avoy, Donald R.: *Blood: The River of Life*. (American Red Cross, 1976.)

Cancer Facts and Figures. (New York: American Cancer Society, 1975.)

Dobihal, Edward F., Jr.: "Hospice: Caring for Life," *Hospital Cancer Coordinator Newsletter,* **IX,** 1974.

FISH Organization. (Honolulu: FISH, 1976.)

Health Planning and Resources Development Act of 1974. (Washington: U.S. Government Printing Office, DHEW Pub. No. [HRA] 75-14015, 1975.)

Medicare Handbook. (Washington: U.S. Government Printing Office, DHEW Pub. No. [SSA] 74-10050, 1974).

Summary Report: NHLI's Blood Resource Studies. (Washington: U. S. Government Printing Office, DHEW Pub. No. [NIH] 73-416, 1972.)

Chapter 23

Continuing Education in Oncology Nursing: One Community's Experience

Sharon S. Ogi

BACKGROUND

Oncology is another world for *cancer*. *Cancer* . . . what does it mean? What does it mean to you? What does it mean to those who have the diagnosis of cancer? What does it mean to their families?

In 1971, the U.S. Congress established the National Cancer Institute (NCI)'s Cancer Control Program (CCP) with its goal as developing and implementing a coordinated national effort toward reducing the nation's cancer incidence, morbidity, and mortality. The program's objective is to ensure that existing knowledge about cancer is disseminated and applied as rapidly and as effectively as possible to benefit the people. To accomplish this, the CCP provides for (1) education of health professionals and the public; (2) demonstrations of currently available preventive, diagnostic, and therapeutic measures to the medical community; and (3) improvements in cancer rehabilitation methods. These efforts are designed to ultimately promote the prevention of cancer, to increase the number of cures, to decrease the far-reaching effects of the disease, and to improve the quality of life for cancer patients.

The National Cancer Program (NCP) looks toward providing better care for the patients with cancer and, in this light, recognizes the serious need for well-educated personnel to provide the specialized care the cancer patient requires. Federal funding has provided 15 oncology nursing education contracts through cancer centers, medical centers, and community hospitals across the nation.

THE COMMUNITY ONCOLOGY NURSING PROJECT (CONP)

As nurses, we come into daily contact with cancer—with a cancer patient or a patient's family. As humans we encounter cancer—in a neighbor, a friend, or a loved one. As nurses we must deal with patient's, family's, and other health professionals' reactions to diagnosis, prognosis, and treatment. As humans, we must deal with our own feelings and attitudes towards cancer. Working with the cancer patient is often frightening, frustrating, and painful, and yet oncology nursing can be one of the most challenging and rewarding aspects of nursing.

Although numerous cancer centers and medical centers across the nation specializing in cancer care exist today, the majority of patients with cancer are cared for in community hospitals. In recognition of this situation, the National Cancer Institute provided funding for the development and implementation of easily accessible continuing education programs in nursing based in community hospitals. These continuing education programs relate to the nursing service needs of cancer patients in the community setting, to ongoing continuing education activities, and to available consultation services and resources in the field of cancer.

One such continuing nursing education program is the Community Oncology Nursing Project (CONP).* The CONP is based on the belief that the education of community nurses in oncology and oncology nursing will lead to the ultimate goal of quality care for the cancer patient and his or her family.

The CONP has several objectives that are designed to upgrade and expand the knowledge, attitudes, and practices of community nurses in relation to cancer and cancer nursing. The objectives are as follows:

1   To meet the stated needs of the community nurses in relation to oncology and oncology nursing
2   To provide core education offerings—theory and clinical application—in oncology and oncology nursing
3   To provide ongoing education in specialty areas or aspects related to oncology
4   To act as a resource consultation center for community nurses, agencies, professionals, etc.
5   To participate actively in other NCI and community activities

*Community Oncology Nursing Project, Contract No. NIH-NCI-N01-CN-45153, National Cancer Institute—Division of Cancer Control and Rehabilitation, The Queen's Medical Center, Honolulu, Hawaii.

THE BEGINNING OF THE CONP

Basic Beliefs

The CONP's philosophy serves as the foundation for all programs offered under this contract and is stated in terms of basic beliefs of the project. The nurse is considered to be a worthy individual, and his or her education is worthwhile. Nursing education is seen as a way of learning the more abstract, theoretical concepts and relating them to the more practical, clinical applications in the delivery of care. The responsibility for self-learning and for helping others to learn is seen as the best motivation to learning.

A continuing education program for nurses is designed to meet the learning needs as identified by a community of nurses. Within such a program, clinical experiences with the pathophysiological and psychological aspects of cancer care are essential, and the nurse is viewed as being accountable and responsible for the acquisition of these learning experiences. The utilization of the nursing process in delivery of care fosters independent thinking, accountability, and responsibility. Therefore, a worthwhile theory of learning in continuing education programs for nurses is one consisting of practical involvement leading to application—an active learning process. As learning is an active process, the role of the teacher is that of a facilitator, a catalyst, a resource person, and a didactic communicator.

The CONP is based on the belief that the nursing care of the cancer patient will be improved through the knowledge and expertise gained via a continuing education program.

Educational Model

An educational model was designed, in harmony with the basic beliefs of the CONP (see Figure 23-1). The ultimate outcome of the model, or project, is not to produce a specialist in oncology, but rather to prepare a nurse to be a resource person to peers as they deal with the cancer patient and family and/or to be a more proficient general practitioner in oncology.

In the model, the preliminary plan was initially outlined. The first completed tasks were to obtain administrative and technical proposal approval. The next item of work was that of analyzing major community facilities with the purpose of gaining insight as to the settings from which the nurse trainees would come and providing an opportunity for facility participation in the planning process. Through site visits and interviews at the facilities, the following areas were examined:

1 The number of beds in the facility
2 The number and type of nursing units in which the majority of cancer patients were accommodated
3 The bed capacity of the unit
4 The R.N.'s role in the facility
5 The L.P.N.'s role

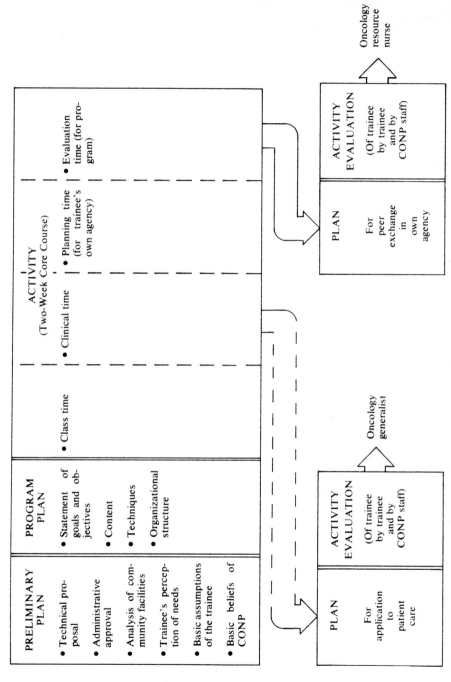

Figure 23-1 Community oncology nursing project educational model.

6   The expected number of trainees to be sent to the CONP's core courses
7   Any special considerations

The results of this analysis indicated that the majority of cancer patients were scattered throughout the units of the facilities, e.g., on medical, surgical, or specialty units such as urology, orthopedics, neurology, etc. The majority of the R.N.s were in leadership roles on a nursing team, while the L.P.N.s delivered direct patient care as team members.

A second analysis centered on the prospective nurse trainee's perceived needs in oncology nursing. Questionnaires (see Appendix), circulated to R.N.s and L.P.N.s in the major community facilities, sought to determine their perceived educational needs in relation to oncology nursing as well as their preferred method of learning. Questionnaire results indicated that R.N.s identified their major learning needs in the following areas: (1) helping families cope with the diagnosis of cancer, (2) helping patients cope with the diagnosis of cancer, (3) pathophysiology of cancer, (4) surgical management, and (5) immunotherapy. The L.P.N.s identified (1) surgical management; (2) screening, detection, and prevention; (3) helping families cope with the diagnosis of cancer; (4) helping patients cope with the diagnosis of cancer; and (5) services available to cancer patients as their major areas of learning need. The preferred methods of learning for both groups were lectures, films, and discussion groups.

Basic assumptions were formulated with respect to the trainees' experiential and educational background, e.g., a course in anatomy and physiology, social and technical skills, past experiences with cancer, and motivation and interest in learning more about oncology nursing. The perceptions of the prospective R.N.s and L.P.N.s with reference to their needs in oncology nursing were also considered, as was the capacity of the prospective trainees to meet the goals and general objectives of the course.

From this preliminary plan, the program plan evolved. The goals and general objectives were identified and the core content and specific objectives delineated.

The next phase of the educational model was the activity phase, in which the trainee entered the actual education period. This period was divided into class time, clinical time, planning time, and evaluation time. Upon completion of the activity phase, the nurse could be designated as an oncology resource nurse and/or an oncology generalist, i.e., a direct care giver.

Time Line

A modified version of the Performance and Evaluation Review Technique (PERT) was utilized to develop a time line. A list of all critical events for the 3 years of the contract was developed and plotted on a time line. This chart served as a guideline for the project staff as to the activity level and deadlines within the project at a specific time.

PROGRAMS

Various kinds of educational program offerings were designed, based on both the basic beliefs and the educational model of the project. A variety of teaching aids and methodologies were utilized throughout the program offerings and included 35mm slides, 16mm films, filmstrips, cassette tapes, video-tapes, overhead transparencies, handouts, lecture/discussion, role playing, seminars, etc.

Core Course

Eighty-hour (10 day) intensive courses in oncology and oncology nursing were designated as core courses. These courses include structured classes, clinical application, independent study time, exposure to a community nursing prac-ticum, and individualized counseling with project staff. Role playing, discussion and sharing groups, and the group process were utilized and provided oppor-tunities for increasing one's self-awareness. The faculty for these courses in-cludes the project staff and area experts: nurses, physicians, and other health professionals. The core courses were offered six times each in the first and second years of the project and three times in the third year; they had a limitation as to class size.

The overall goals and general objectives for the core courses are presented in Table 23-1. In addition, each specific class content area throughout the course contained specific behavioral objectives.

In looking at the overall flow of the core course schedule, several major content areas were identified, as listed in Table 23-2. Each core course was modified and improved upon from previous participant evaluations.

A specific core course was designated for nurses who were employed in education or supervision; e.g., in-service instructors; faculties of schools of nursing; head nurses and supervisors in community health agencies, hospitals, and medical centers. The course offered a core content of material, provided opportunities for individualized activities, and enabled the nurses to implement the nursing process as it related to their individual job situations.

Core Workshops

Because of the unique nature of the state of Hawaii and the Pacific Basin, project staff modified the core course content and presented core workshops on each of the major neighboring islands within the state and on Guam. These core work-shops were intensive 24-hour (3-day) courses and included an overview of oncology and oncology nursing. The workshops were primarily didactic in nature, but provided role playing and discussion groups. Emphasis was placed on communication skill development; increased self-awareness; and current advances in research, diagnosis, treatment, and rehabilitation of the patient and family. Each workshop was also modified to meet the needs of the area's nurses as identified by them. The core workshops were offered once a year on each of

Table 23-1 Community Oncology Nursing Projects: Overall Goals and General Objectives

Goal	General objectives
1 To increase the nurses' baseline of knowledge and awareness of their own attitudes and practices in oncology nursing and its related aspects	a The nurse shows an increased awareness of his or her therapeutic communication and interviewing skills. b The nurse knows the epidemiology and pathophysiology of neoplastic disease. c The nurse knows the nursing process. d The nurse utilizes the nursing process in correlating the nursing action for patient problems to the pathophysiology and clinical manifestations of cancer and its treatment modalties. d The nurse shows an increased awareness of his or her attitudes towards cancer, death, and care of the cancer patient/family.
2 To assist nurses in recognizing the impact of cancer on the patient, family, health professional, and community	1 The nurse knows his or her role in the rehabilitation process associated with cancer. b The nurse knows his or her role in the prevention, screening, and detection associated with cancer. c The nurse is aware of the roles, responsibilities, skills, and needs of other health professionals. d The nurse is aware of cancer quackery and its nursing implications.
3 To assist nurses in the dissemination of their knowledge, attitudes, and practices in oncology nursing to peers	

the neighboring islands of the state in years 01 and 02 of the project. The Guam core workshop was offered once in year 02.

The overall goals, general objectives, and content areas for these core workshops were similar to those of the core courses, with minor modifications (see Table 23-3).

Special Seminars

Special seminars in oncology nursing were designed to meet the continuing educational needs of the nurses who had graduated from the core courses or core workshops. Specific seminar content was suggested by project graduates, and the curricula and behavioral objectives were developed by project staff. Each seminar included a faculty of area experts. Seven special seminars were offered

Table 23-2   Community Oncology Nursing Project: Core Course Content Areas

1 Project philosphy and overview	16 Infectious complications and nursing complications
2 Communication and interviewing: theoretical and practical concepts	17 Clinical experience and conference time
3 Epidemiology	18 Independent study time
4 Carcinogenesis	19 Nursing role in prevention, screening, and detection
5 Diagnostic procedures	
6 Pathophysiology of neoplastic disease	20 Organizations for cancer in Hawaii
7 Immune system and immunotherapy	21 Multidisciplinary approach to continuity of care, rehabilitation, and discharge planning: theoretical and practical concepts
8 Clinical manifestations and nursing implications of specific malignant neoplasms	
	22 Community nursing practicum
9 Pain theory and management	23 Terminal care of the patient and family dealing with cancer
10 Cancer quackery	
11 Nursing process	24 Site visitation of community facilities working for cancer
12 Psychosocial aspects	
13 Family theory and counseling	25 Individual counseling and planning
14 Physicians' outlooks	
15 Treatment modalities and nursing implications: surgery, radiotherapy, and chemotherapy	

in year 02 and 10 in year 03 in Honolulu as well as on each of the neighboring islands. Seminar content areas included titles such as

1 "The Group Process"
2 "Talking with Patients—Practical Application"
3 "Nursing Approaches to Denial"
4 "Leukemia"
5 "Genitourinary Cancers in Males"
6 "Cancer Research: Carcinogenesis and Therapies"
7 "Leukemia/Lymphoma"
8 "Oncology Nursing as a Specialty"
9 "Fourth Treatment Modality: Immunotherapy"

Table 23-3   Community Oncology Nursing Project: Core Workshop Content Areas

1 Project philosophy and overview	8 Epidemiology, clinical manifestations, and nursing implications of specific malignant neoplasms
2 Pathophysiology of neoplastic diseases	
3 Modalities of treatment and nursing implications: surgery, radiotherapy, chemotherapy, and immunotherapy	
	9 Nursing role in prevention, screening, and detection
4 Communication and interviewing: theoretical and practical concepts	10 Multidisciplinary approach to continuity of care, rehabilitation, and discharge planning
5 Nursing process and planning conference	11 Terminal care of the patient and family dealing with cancer
6 Family theory and counseling	
7 Psychological implications	12 New developments in cancer care
	13 Individual counseling

Table 23-4   Community Oncology Nursing Project: Post–Core Course Expectations

Anecdotal records	1	The purposes for the completion of the anecdotal record form by the trainee at specified intervals after completion of the core course are a To demonstrate the trainee's utilization of the nursing process in a patient/family situation in his or her own setting b To ensure the trainee's continued usage of knowledge and practices learned in the core course c To monitor the trainee's awareness of his or her own attitudes over a period of 6 months d To monitor the trainee's dissemination of knowledge, attitudes, and practices gained in the core course
or		
Individual project	1	The purposes for the development and implementation (as appropriate) of an individual project by the trainee are a To demonstrate the trainee's utilization of ideas and knowledge gained in the core course in his or her own work situation and to meet his or her own agency needs b To ensure the trainee's integration of knowledge and practices learned in the core course into the clinical setting c To monitor the trainee's dissemination of knowledge, attitudes, and practices gained in the core course d To enhance the quality of care delivered to the patient with cancer
	2	The project is to be any research, report, in-service, teaching-tool, or any other project chosen by the trainee to be presented and/or implemented in his or her own work situation. A synopsis of the project shall be written or taped for analysis purposes by the project staff and is due within 6 months of completion of the core course.
Patient care conferences	1	The purposes for the conduct of a patient care conference by the trainee are a To demonstrate the trainee's utilization of nursing process in relation to a specific patient/family situation b To ensure the trainee's integration of knowledge and practices learned in the core course into the clinical setting c To monitor the trainee's dissemination of knowledge, attitudes, and practices gained in the core course d to enhance the quality of care delivered to the patient with cancer
	2	The trainee must hold a patient care conference in his or her clinical setting which is approximately 10–15 minutes in length. Either the conference must be taped and the tape then sent to the project office or the conference must be scheduled so that a project staff member may be present for analysis purposes.
Evening get-togethers	1	The purpose of these evening get-togethers is to allow for peer exchange, sharing, and problem-solving sessions.
	2	Once a month, beginning 1 month after completion of the course, there will be a get-together of all trainees of the core course. Each trainee is required to attend three get-together sessions within the first 6 months after the completion of the core course.
	3	Responsibility for organization of these meetings lies with the trainee group.

Table 23-5   Community Oncology Nursing Project: Core Course: Follow-up Reaction Form for Employed Participants

This form is sent to all employed graduates six-months after completion of the core course and records the following items in relation to his or her employment:

1   The current work load and percentage of time spent in various activity areas
2   The types of cancer patients cared for by the nurse
3   Determines if the nurse now works more in oncology nursing than prior to the course
4   Requests information on changes in the nature of the nurse's work since taking the course
5   Seeks to determine whether the nurse has applied acquired learning, and if not, identifies barriers to such practical application
6   Records instances of recognition from supervisors or peers
7   Asks if the nurse initiated any peer support groups
8   Checklists activities in which the nurse's behavior has changed
9   Provides an opportunity for the nurse to express any other impact the course may have had on herself or on others through him or her
10   Asks if the nurse plans to practice oncology nursing in the future
11   Rates the course in relationship to work and personal expectations
12   Determines level of satisfaction in working with cancer patients
13   Measures the nurse's ability to provide high quality of care to cancer patients

Source: Printed with permission from forms originated by Jane K. Dixon, Ph.D., as part of the Yale University Oncology Nursing Program, Contract No. 1-CN-45138.

(2) level of presentation, (3) instructor competence, and (4) applicability to work situations, etc.

Impact of the Program

Originally, the CONP devised two tools to measure the project graduate's effectiveness upon patient/family outcomes in the community postcourse. It was found that while the tools provided much general information, there were too many uncontrolled variables. Because the obtained results could not be satisfactorily analyzed, use of these forms was discontinued.

The project then adopted three Yale University Oncology Nursing Program* forms that measure the effect of the program on graduates following the course as they function within the community. These forms are entitled Core Course: Follow-up Reaction Form for Employed Participants (Table 23-5), Core Course: Follow-up Reaction Form for Participants Not Currently Employed (Table 23-6), and a Supervisor's Follow-up Reaction Form (Table 23-7).

A one-time evaluation form was sent to all directors of nursing whose employees participated in the project. These data were collected midway through the project and measured the following:

1   The number of nurses expressing interest in attending the project's programs

*Written permission was obtained from the Yale University Oncology Nursing Program. Contract No. 1-CN-45138, Jane K. Dixon, Ph.D., Research Associate.

   2 The number of nurses actually sent to participate
   3 The reaction of the director to nurses in sending nurses to participate in
the program
   4 If the director had reservations in sending nurses to participate, sources
that could be identified
   5 The potential benefit of the program to their agency
   6 Comments to project staff

The majority of comments made by the directors were favorable. The few
directors expressing reservations listed them as being related to financial constraints, staffing problems, and/or staff apathy.

SUMMARY

Continuing nursing education programs provide a means by which nurses can
upgrade and expand their knowledge, attitudes, and practices in nursing. The

**Table 23-6   Community Oncology Nursing Project: Core Course: Follow-up Reac-
tion Form for Participations Not Currently Employed**

This form is sent to all unemployed graduates six months after completion of the core course and
records the following items:
1   The reason for present unemployment
2   If employed at some future time, would the nurse specialize in oncology nursing
3   In seeking a job, the nurse's feeling about seeking a job in oncology nursing
4   The nurse's ability to provide high quality of care to cancer patients
5   The nurse's activities related to oncology nursing—future plans, reading, lectures attended,
    writing, lectures given, professional organization activities, and volunteer work
6   Any other way in which course had an impact on self or on others through him or her

Source: Printed with permission from forms originated by Jane K. Dixon, Ph.D., as part of the Yale University Oncology Nursing
Program, Contract No. 1-CN-45138.

**Table 23-7   Community Oncology Nursing Project: Supervisor's Follow-up Reac-
tion Form**

This form is sent to the employed graduate's immediate supervisor and records the following items:
1   The extent to which the nurse's participation in the program is valuable to the agency
2   The nature of the nurse's work—changed or not
3   The percentage of time the nurse cares for cancer patients
4   Any perceived barriers to nurse's ability to apply what has been learned
5   Checklist of activities related to oncology nursing designed to measure if the nurse has changed
     as a result of the program
6   Comfortableness of the nurse in caring for cancer patients
7   If satisfaction of the nurse in caring for cancer patients is apparent
8   Quality of care delivered by the nurse
9   Recommendation of program to other nurses
10   Messages to project staff

Source: Printed with permission from forms originated by Jane K. Dixon, Ph.D., as part of the Yale University Oncology Nursing
Program, Contract No. 1-CN-45138.

advances that occur daily in the cancer field, in both research and management, challenge the nurse to participate in such programs in order to be knowledgeable and capable of delivering updated, quality care to cancer patients and their families.

This chapter has described the Community Oncology Nursing Project, a continuing education project in oncology and oncology nursing. This project responded to the needs present in a community of nurses and utilized area experts involved in cancer research and management to meet those needs. The benefits to the nursing community were many and included the following:

1 The opportunity to tailor a program for the nurses' specific needs
2 Exposure to the most current trends in cancer research and management
3 Clinically oriented cancer experiences
4 The opportunity for personal as well as professional growth
5 Opportunities for interested and motivated nurses to meet and to share ideas and feelings
6 The opportunity for involvement in community cancer activities
7 The enhancement of competence in nursing care for cancer patients and families

Nurses owe it to themselves, to their patients and their families, and to the profession to provide the highest level of care possible and hence must be responsible and motivated to continue their own education.

COMMUNITY ONCOLOGY NURSING PROJECT   **Appendix 1**
Honolulu, Hawaii

Questionnaire — Nurses

1. Please check the following items as they apply to you:
   a. R.N._____ L.P.N._____
   b. Where do you work:

1. Medical unit	5. Skilled nursing facility
2. Surgical unit	6. Community setting
3. Medical/surgical unit	7. Clinic
4. Specialty unit (please specify)	8. Physician's office

   c. Educational background

1. R.N. = Diploma	2. L.P.N.

2. If you work in a hospital, what is the bed capacity of your unit? What is the average number of cancer patients on your unit per day?
3. If you work in the community setting, what is the average number of cancer patients/families on your caseload?
4. How would you describe your attitude (feelings) in dealing with cancer patients/ families?
5. Have you ever attended any conferences, workshops, or seminars focused on cancer nursing within the last few years? Yes _____ No _____

6. In column 1, list in order of priority (1 to 5), the topics you feel confident about.

	Column 1	Column 2
A. Prevention, screening, and detection methods.....	_____	_____
B. Pathological process of cancer	_____	_____

C. Understanding current treatment modalities for
cancer and nurse's role:

	Column 1	Column 2
1. Surgery	_____	_____
2. Chemotherapy	_____	_____
3. Radiation therapy.....................	_____	_____
4. Immunotherapy	_____	_____
D. Helping patients cope with the diagnosis of cancer..	_____	_____
E. Helping families cope with the diagnosis of cancer..	_____	_____
F. Services available to cancer patients	_____	_____

G. Nursing care of patients with specific problems:

	Column 1	Column 2
1. Mastectomy...........................	_____	_____
2. Colostomy	_____	_____
3. Laryngectomy	_____	_____
4. Others (specify)	_____	_____
H. Patient/family teaching	_____	_____
I Nurse's role in rehabilitation	_____	_____
J. Supportive care of the dying patient	_____	_____
K. Cancer quackery	_____	_____
L. Others (specify)	_____	_____

7. In column 2, list in order of priority (1 to 5), the topics you feel you need more education in. (Refer to list in #6.)

8. If given time off from work, would you be interested in attending a course plus follow-up conferences and seminars in oncology nursing? Yes _____ No _____

9. What method of learning would interest you most (list in order of priority if more than one):
   a. Films
   b. Lectures
   c. Demonstrations
   d. Clinical application
   e. Role playing
   f. Seminars (discussion groups)
   g. Others (specify)

10. After attending a course in oncology nursing, would you be:
   a. Able to teach your peers about cancer nursing without any restrictions?
      Yes _____   No _____   If no, list restrictions
   b. Willing to teach your peers to help others to know about cancer nursing?
      Yes _____   No _____

Name (optional)

Index